Joint Models for Longitudinal and Time-to-Event Data

With Applications in R

Chapman & Hall/CRC Biostatistics Series

Editor-in-Chief

Shein-Chung Chow, Ph.D.
Professor
Department of Biostatistics and Bioinformatics
Duke University School of Medicine
Durham, North Carolina

Series Editors

Byron Jones
Biometrical Fellow
Statistical Methodology
Integrated Information Sciences
Novartis Pharma AG
Basel, Switzerland

Jen-pei Liu
Professor
Division of Biometry
Department of Agronomy
National Taiwan University
Taipei, Taiwan

Karl E. Peace
Georgia Cancer Coalition
Distinguished Cancer Scholar
Senior Research Scientist and
Professor of Biostatistics
Jiann-Ping Hsu College of Public Health
Georgia Southern University
Statesboro, Georgia

Bruce W. Turnbull
Professor
School of Operations Research
and Industrial Engineering
Cornell University
Ithaca, New York

Chapman & Hall/CRC Biostatistics Series

Chapman & Hall/CRC Biostatistics Series

Joint Models for Longitudinal and Time-to-Event Data

With Applications in R

Dimitris Rizopoulos

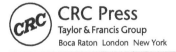

CRC Press
Taylor & Francis Group
Boca Raton London New York

CRC Press is an imprint of the
Taylor & Francis Group, an **informa** business
A CHAPMAN & HALL BOOK

Chapman & Hall/CRC Press
Taylor & Francis Group
6000 Broken Sound Parkway NW, Suite 300
Boca Raton, FL 33487-2742

First issued in paperback 2022

Version Date: 20120525

ISBN 13: 978-1-03-247756-5 (pbk)
ISBN 13: 978-1-4398-7286-4 (hbk)

DOI: 10.1201/b12208

Library of Congress Cataloging-in-Publication Data

Rizopoulos, Dimitris.
    Joint models for longitudinal and time-to-event data : with applications in R / Dimitris Rizopoulos.
        p. cm. -- (Chapman & Hall/CRC biostatistics series ; 6)
    Includes bibliographical references and index.
    ISBN 978-1-4398-7286-4 (hardback)
    1. Numerical analysis--Data processing. 2. R (Computer program language) I. Title.

QA279.R59 2012
518--dc23   2012014570

Visit the Taylor & Francis Web site at
http://www.taylorandfrancis.com

and the CRC Press Web site at
http://www.crcpress.com

To Roula and my parents

To the memory of my grandmother

Preface

Joint models for longitudinal and time-to-event data have become a valuable tool in the analysis of follow-up data. These models are applicable mainly in two settings: First, when the focus is on the survival outcome and we wish to account for the effect of an endogenous time-dependent covariate measured with error, and second, when the focus is on the longitudinal outcome and we wish to correct for nonrandom dropout. Due to the capability of joint models to provide valid inferences in settings where simpler statistical tools fail to do so, and their wide range of applications, the last 25 years have seen many advances in the joint modeling field. Even though interest and developments in joint models have been widespread, information about them has been equally scattered in articles, presenting recent advances in the field, and in book chapters in a few texts dedicated either to longitudinal or survival data analysis. However, no single monograph or text dedicated to this type of models seems to be available.

The purpose in writing this book, therefore, is to provide an overview of the theory and application of joint models for longitudinal and survival data. In the literature two main frameworks have been proposed, namely the random effects joint model that uses latent variables to capture the associations between the two outcomes (Tsiatis and Davidian, 2004), and the marginal structural joint models based on G estimators (Robins et al., 1999, 2000). In this book we focus on the former. Both subfields of joint modeling, i.e., handling of endogenous time-varying covariates and nonrandom dropout, are equally covered and presented in real datasets. Motivated by the background and collaborations of the author, these examples come from the medical field and in particular from biomarker research. Nevertheless, joint models of this type can be employed whenever there is interest in the association between a longitudinal and an event time outcome, and therefore have numerous applications in other fields as well. In addition, several extensions are presented, including among others, different types of association structure between the longitudinal and survival outcomes, inclusion of stratification factors, incorporation of lagged effects, the handling of exogenous time-dependent covariates, and competing risks settings. For the longitudinal part, primary focus is given on continuous longitudinal outcomes and the use of linear mixed-effects models.

All the analyses included in the book are implemented in the R software environment for statistical computing and graphics, using the freely available package **JM** written by the author. This package fits a wide range of joint models, including the extensions mentioned above. However, it does not cover all of the types of joint models that have been proposed in the literature, and therefore, some extensions, such as joint models for categorical longitudinal markers and multiple longitudinal markers are introduced in the text, but without any software illustration. The results presented in the text were produced using version 1.0-0 of package **JM** and R 2.15.0. The current version of the package can be obtained from the Comprehensive R Archive Network (`http://cran.r-project.org`). Because of platform dependencies, the analysis results may be expected to vary slightly with different computers or operating systems, and future versions of R and the package. All the code used in the text is available from the supporting Web site

`http://jmr.r-forge.r-project.org`

The author would appreciate being informed of typos, errors and improvements to the contents of this book, and may be contacted via electronic mail at

`d.rizopoulos@erasmusmc.nl`

Prerequisites

The contents in this book assume familiarity with basic concepts of statistical data analysis at the level of an introductory course in statistics, including standard maximum likelihood theory, and a strong background in regression analysis. Some background knowledge of mixed effects models and survival analysis would also be beneficial but is not required. Similarly, with respect to R, the book does not assume any prior knowledge, but basic familiarity with the language would be helpful.

Typographical Conventions

R language objects, commands and output referenced throughout this book are printed in a monospace **typewriter** font. Code that could be interactively entered at the R command line is formatted as:

```
> x <- 5
```

where > denotes the R command-line prompt and everything else is what the user should enter. In addition, R expressions that do not fit in a single line will be appropriately indented like this:

```
> jointModel(lmeFit, coxFit, timeVar = "time",
    method = "weibull-PH-aGH", parameterization = "both")
```

When referring to a function within the main text, it will be formatted in a typewriter font and will have parentheses after the function name, e.g., jointModel(). Similarly, function arguments and value specified for these arguments will also be formatted in a typewriter font, but with no parentheses at the end, e.g., method = "weibull-PH-aGH".

To save space, some of the R output has been edited. Omission of complete lines is indicated by

. . .

but some blank lines have been removed without indication.

Acknowledgements

Many pieces of the work presented in this monograph are based on joint research with Geert Verbeke and Geert Molenberghs, with whom it has been my great pleasure to collaborate. I would also like to thank Emmanuel Lesaffre for useful discussions on joint modeling topics, and for creating a stimulating work environment. Special thanks also goes to all users of **JM** whose input has greatly benefitted the development of the package.

With regard to this book in particular, I would like to thank the anonymous reviewers for valuable feedback on earlier versions of the manuscript, and John Kimmel at Chapman and Hall/CRC for his help and support during the whole production process. This monograph was written using a combination of Friedrich Leisch's Sweave package, the LaTeX document preparation system, and, of course, R.

Dimitris Rizopoulos
Rotterdam, April 2012

Contents

xiii

Chapter 1

Introduction

1.1 Goals

In follow-up studies different types of outcomes are typically collected for each sample unit, which may include several longitudinally measured responses, and the time until an event of particular interest occurs. The research questions of interest in such studies often require the separate analysis of the recorded outcomes, but in many occasions interest may also lie in studying their association structure. A frequently encountered example of the latter case can be found in biomarker research, where many clinical studies are designed to identify biomarkers with strong prognostic capabilities for event time outcomes. Standard examples include among others, human immunodeficiency virus (HIV) research in which interest lies in the association between CD4 cell counts or viral load and the time to Acquired immune deficiency syndrom (AIDS), liver cirrhosis studies which investigate the association between serum bilirubin and the time to death, and prostate cancer studies in which interest lies in the association between prostate-specific antigen (PSA) levels and the time to the development of prostate cancer. An important inherent characteristic of these medical conditions is their dynamic nature. That is, the rate of progression is not only different from patient to patient but also dynamically changes in time for the same patient. Thus, the true potential of a biomarker in describing disease progression and its association with survival can only be revealed when repeated evaluations of the marker are considered in the analysis.

1

To address research questions involving the association structure between repeated measures and event times, a class of statistical models has been developed known as joint models for longitudinal and time-to-event data. Currently, the study of these models constitutes an active area of statistics research that has received a lot of attention in the recent years. In particular, after the early work on joint modeling approaches with application in AIDS research by Self and Pawitan (1992) and DeGruttola and Tu (1994), and the seminal papers by Faucett and Thomas (1996) and Wulfsohn and Tsiatis (1997) who introduced what could nowadays be called the standard joint model, there has been an explosion of developments in this field. Numerous papers have appeared proposing several extensions of the standard joint model including, among others, the flexible modeling of longitudinal trajectories, the incorporation of latent classes to account for population heterogeneity, the consideration of multiple longitudinal markers, modeling multiple failure times, and the calculation of dynamic predictions and accuracy measures.

The primary goal of this book is to offer a comprehensive introduction to this joint modeling framework. In particular, we will focus on the type of research questions joint models attempt to answer and the circumstances under which these models are appropriate to answer these questions. We will explain which are the key assumptions behind them, and how they can be optimally utilized to extract relevant information from the data. An additional aim of this book is to promote the use of these models in everyday statistical practice. To this end, (almost) all the theoretical material covered in the text is illustrated in real data examples using package **JM** (Rizopoulos, 2012b, 2010) developed for the R software environment for statistical computing and graphics (R Development Core Team, 2012).

1.2   Motivating Studies

1.2.1   *Primary Biliary Cirrhosis Data*

Primary biliary cirrhosis (PBC) is a chronic, fatal, but rare liver disease characterized by inflammatory destruction of the small bile ducts within the liver, which eventually leads to cirrhosis of the liver. The dataset we consider here comes from a study conducted by the Mayo Clinic from 1974 to 1984 (Murtaugh et al., 1994) that includes 312 patients, 158 randomized to D-penicillamine and 154 to placebo. The outcome of primary interest was patient survival and whether this could be prolonged by D-penicillamine. In addition, we have information on baseline covariates (e.g., age at baseline, gender, etc.), and follow-up measurements for several biomarkers. These included, among others, serum bilirubin, the presence of spiders (blood vessel malformations in the skin) and hepatomegaly (enlarged liver). Here we will focus on the serum bilirubin level which is considered a strong indicator of

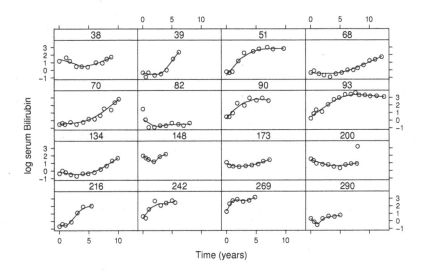

FIGURE 1.1: Smooth longitudinal profiles of 16 subjects from the PBC dataset. The solid line represents the fit of the loess smoother.

disease progression, and, in particular, we are interested in the association of this marker with survival. The original clinical protocol for these patients specified visits at six months, one year, and annually thereafter. However, due to death and censoring, patients made on average 6.2 visits (st.dev. 3.8 visits), resulting in a total of 1945 observations of serum bilirubin. By the end of the study 140 patients had died, 29 received a transplant, and 143 were still alive. Figure 1.1 shows smoothed longitudinal profiles of the log serum bilirubn for a sample of patients, from which it can be seen that many of these profiles are nonlinear in time.

1.2.2   AIDS Data

In the AIDS dataset we consider 467 patients with advanced human immun-odeficiency virus infection during antiretroviral treatment who had failed or were intolerant to zidovudine therapy. The main aim of this study was to compare the efficacy and safety of two alternative antiretroviral drugs, namely didanosine (ddI) and zalcitabine (ddC), in the time-to-death. Patients were randomly assigned to receive either ddI or ddC, and CD4 cell counts were recorded at study entry, where randomization took place, as well as at 2, 6, 12, and 18 months thereafter. More details regarding the design of this study can be found in Abrams et al. (1994).

By the end of the study 188 patients had died, resulting in about 59.7% censoring, and out of the 2335 planned measurements, 1405 were actually

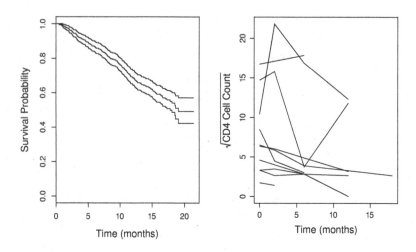

FIGURE 1.2: Left panel: Kaplan-Meier estimate of the survival function for the time-to-death in the AIDS dataset. The dashed lines correspond to 95% pointwise confidence intervals. Right panel: Longitudinal trajectories for square root CD4 cell counts for six randomly selected subjects in the AIDS dataset.

recorded, leading to 39.8% of missing responses. Figure 1.2 presents the Kaplan-Meier estimate of the survival function for the time to death as well as longitudinal trajectories of the square root of the CD4 cell count for a random sample of ten patients (for more details on the Kaplan-Meier estimator the reader is referred to Section 3.2). For our illustrations we focus on one of the secondary aims of this study, which was to study the association structure between the CD4 count and the risk for death for these advanced HIV-infected patients. In particular, the CD4 cells are a type of white blood cells made in the spleen, lymph nodes, and thymus gland and are part of the infection-fighting system. The CD4 count measures the number of CD4 cells in a sample of blood and constitutes an important marker of the strength of the immune system. Therefore, a decrease in the CD4 cell count over time is indicative of a worsening of the condition of the immune system of the patient, and thus to higher susceptibility to infection.

1.2.3 Liver Cirrhosis Data

The Liver Cirrhosis dataset includes 488 patients with histologically verified liver cirrhosis, with 237 patients randomized to a treatment with prednisone and the remaining receiving a placebo. Liver cirrhosis is a generic term that

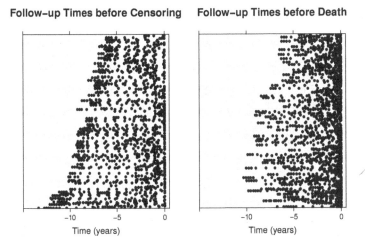

FIGURE 1.3: Distribution of follow-up times before censoring (left panel) and death (right panel) for the Liver Cirrhosis data.

includes all forms of chronic diffuse liver disease characterized by extensive loss of liver cells and extensive disorganization of the hepatic lobular architecture. The study took place from 1962 to 1974 in Copenhagen, and its main purpose was to evaluate whether prednisone prolongs survival for patients with cirrhosis (Andersen et al., 1993). By the end of follow-up, 150 (63.3%) prednisone-treated, and 142 (56.6%) placebo-treated patients died.

Patients were scheduled to return at 3, 6, and 12 months, and yearly thereafter, and provide records for several clinical and biochemical variables. The clinical variables included information on alcohol consumption, nutritional status, bleeding and degree of ascites, whereas the most important biochemical variables are albumin, bilirubin, alkaline phosphatase and prothrombin. Even though patients were supposed to provide measurements on the aforementioned predetermined visit times, the actual follow-up times varied considerably around the scheduled visits. Moreover, as can be seen from Figure 1.3, patients who died had more visits taking place shortly prior to death.

For our illustrations we will concentrate on the association between the prothrombin index and the risk for death. This index is a measurement based on a blood test of coagulation factors II, VII, and X produced by the liver. Figure 1.4 depicts the subject-specific longitudinal trajectories per treatment group. In addition, we are interested in investigating the capability of the prothrombin index in discriminating between subjects who died within a medically relevant time interval after their last assessment and subjects who lived longer than that. For example, for a future patient from the same population, we would like to inform the treating physicians about her survival probability which is calculated based on her baseline covariates and her available

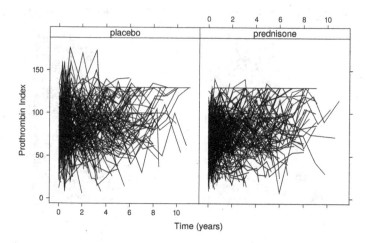

FIGURE 1.4: Subject-specific longitudinal trajectories of the prothrombin index for the Liver Cirrhosis data per treatment group.

prothrombin measurements, and assist them in further deciding upon their actions.

1.2.4   Aortic Valve Data

The Aortic Valve dataset includes 289 patients with aortic valve stenosis (AS) who underwent allograft aortic root replacement (RR) or subcoronary implantation (SI) procedures at Erasmus University Medical Center between 1992 and 2005 (Takkenberg et al., 2002, 2006). Aortic stenosis occurs when the opening of the aortic valve located between the left ventricle of the heart and the aorta is narrowed, and is one of the most common valvular heart diseases. All patients in this dataset have been followed up prospectively by annual telephone interviews and through visits to their cardiologist. Echocardiographic follow-ups at Erasmus MC were obtained at six months postoperative, one year postoperative, and thereafter, biennially by means of serial standardized echocardiography. By the end of the study, 61 (21.1%) patients had died and 78 (27%) had a re-operation.

Here we are interested in the association between the aortic jet velocity (aortic gradient) and the risk for death or re-operation. Due to the fact that the aortic gradient levels exhibit right skewed shapes of distribution, we typically work with their square root transform. Figure 1.5 shows the scatterplots of the subject-specific intercepts and slopes, from a simple linear regression for the square root of the aortic gradient, ordered according to the event time. We observe much greater variability in the subject-specific intercepts than in the slopes, and for the latter we see that the variability decreases for later

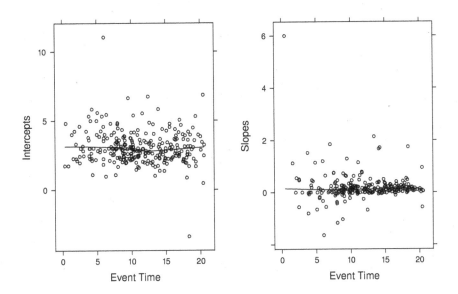

FIGURE 1.5: Subject-specific intercepts and slopes per type of operation for the evolution of the square root of the aortic gradient in time for the Aortic Valve Dataset. Solid lines denote the fit of the loess smoother.

event times. This is partially explained by the fact that as time progresses more aortic gradient measurements are recorded for each patient, which in turn results in a more accurate estimate of the slope.

1.2.5 Other Applications

The previous sections have focused on datasets from human studies focusing on the association between longitudinal biomarker measurements and patient survival. Nevertheless, the interrelationships between longitudinal responses and event times are of interest in many other disciplines as well. Below we give three such examples from areas other than biomarker research.

Ex1: In gregarious animal studies longitudinal measurements of the sociodynamics of the herd may be associated with the time to relocation to an other area.

Ex2: In sociology and educational testing, but also in some epidemiological studies, it is often of interest to relate the performance of respondents to questionnaires to event time outcomes. For example, dementia research questionnaires are used to measure the status of a patient's mood, and her memory and communication capabilities. Since dementia is progressive, patients are given these questionnaires at frequent intervals and interest lies in the relation between the evolution of the performance of a patient in these psychometric tests and the clinical onset of the disease.

Ex3: In civil engineering it is often of interest to study the time until a building is no longer useable. To achieve this, several indicators of structural integrity are recorded at regular time intervals, with the aim to evaluate if these indicators are strong predictors for the risk of failure of the structure in question.

1.3 Inferential Objectives in Longitudinal Studies

It is evident from the previous section that in longitudinal studies typically a wealth of information is recorded for each patient, and interest often lies in complex associations between these different pieces of information. Before discussing in more detail possible interrelationships that could be of interest in a longitudinal setting, we will first make a distinction between two types of outcomes recorded in these studies. First, we will call *explicit* outcomes the outcomes that are explicitly specified in the study protocol to be recorded during follow-up. For example, in the PBC study these include the survival information on the patients, and the longitudinal measurements on biomarkers. The second type of outcomes, which we call *implicit* outcomes, are the outcomes that are not of direct interest but nonetheless may complicate the analysis of the explicit ones. A characteristic example is missing data. In particular, even though according to the protocol patients are typically required to appear at the study center(s) at prespecified occasions to provide information, this is rarely done in practice. Patients often miss some of their visits or they may completely drop out from the study for a variety of reasons. For instance, as we saw in the AIDS dataset, out of the 2335 planned measurements, 1405 were actually recorded, leading to 39.8% of missing responses. Another example of an implicit outcome, closely related to the missing data, is the visiting process, which is defined as the mechanism (stochastic or deterministic) that generates the time points at which longitudinal measurements are collected (Lipsitz et al., 2002). Random visit times are more often encountered in observational studies where the time points at which the longitudinal measurements are taken are not fixed by design but rather determined by the physician or even the patients themselves. Nonetheless, random visit times may even occur in randomized studies that have been pre-specified by the protocol visit times. For example, for the PBC dataset and during the first two years of follow-up, measurements of serum bilirubin were taken at baseline, half, one, and two years, with little variability, whereas, in later years the variability in the visit times increased considerably. In the following we present a categorization of the possible research questions we could formulate in a longitudinal study (Rizopoulos and Lesaffre, 2012).

1.3.1 Effect of Covariates on a Single Outcome

The most common type of research questions in medical studies, in general, is to estimate or test for the effect of a set of covariates in some outcomes of interest. For example, for the AIDS patients we would like to know whether ddI improves the survival rates, or whether there is a difference in the average longitudinal profiles of the CD4 cell counts between males and females. The answer to such questions requires one to postulate a suitable statistical model that relates the covariate(s) to the outcome of interest. Depending on the nature of the outcome several types of statistical models are available. A review of the basic modeling frameworks for longitudinal and event time data is given in Chapters 2 and 3, respectively.

1.3.2 Association between Outcomes

Often it is also of interest to investigate the association structure between outcomes. For instance, in the PBC dataset physicians are interested in measuring how strongly associated the current level of serum bilirubin is with the risk for death. A similar example occurs in asthma studies, where the risk for an asthma attack may be correlated with the levels of air pollution. At first glance, these research questions seem similar in spirit to the ones posed in Section 1.3.1, with the only difference being that the covariate process is now time-dependent. Thus, one could simply proceed by postulating suitable models that relate the two outcomes of interest. For example, we could simply formulate a time-dependent Cox model for the hazard for death and include the longitudinal CD4 cell count measurements as a time-dependent covariate (Andersen and Gill, 1982). Nevertheless, an important feature that we need to carefully consider is the fact that in such models the outcome variables play the role of both the response and the covariate. To proceed in this setting we first need to discern the type of the covariate-outcome process, and in particular whether the covariate-outcome is internal (also known as endogenous) or external (also known as exogenous) to the response-outcome. Formal definitions of endogeneity are given later in Chapter 3. However, a more intuitive manner to distinguish between internal and external covariates is by understanding the nature of a time-dependent covariate process. To put it loosely, internal covariates are generated from the patient herself and therefore require the existence of the patient. Revisiting the previous two examples, we note that the CD4 cell count and the hazard for death are stochastic processes generated by the patient herself, and therefore the CD4 cell count constitutes an internal covariate process. On the other hand, air pollution is an external covariate to asthma attacks, since the patient has no influence on air pollution. When the covariate-outcome is external to the response-outcome, we can use the majority of the standard models mentioned in Section 1.3.1, with relatively small modifications. However, as we will see later, statistical analysis with internal covariates poses several additional difficulties.

1.3.3 Complex Hypothesis Testing

Combinations of the previous two types of research questions are also often of interest. A typical example of this setting constitutes the evaluation of surrogate markers. In particular, for chronic conditions, such as PBC, we could be interested to assess treatment efficacy using the short-term longitudinal serum bilirubin measurements instead of the survival endpoint, which is lengthy to ascertain. Prentice (1989) set three conditions for surrogacy: (I) treatment must have an effect on patient survival; (II) treatment must have an effect on the marker, i.e., serum bilirubin; and (III) the effect of treatment should manifest through the marker, i.e., the risk for death given a specific marker trajectory should be independent of treatment. It is evident that to assess conditions (I) and (II) we need to posit separate models for the survival and longitudinal outcomes each one containing treatment as a predictor. However, to check condition (III) a model for the survival outcome that conditions on both treatment and serum bilirubin is required instead. Given the special characteristics of serum bilirubin as an endogenous time-dependent covariate explained above, joint models provide a flexible modeling framework to determine whether treatment has an effect on survival after accounting for serum bilirubin.

A similar type of analysis is required when we are interested in simultaneously testing for the effect of a baseline covariate in several outcomes. For instance, continuing on the same example mentioned above, serum bilirubin may not be a good biomarker in describing disease progression, and therefore treatment may still have an influence on patient survival, even after conditioning on serum bilirubin. In this situation we could extend our analysis, and include additional biomarkers of disease progression, such as spiders and hepatomegaly. Interest could then be in testing for the effect of treatment in all markers simultaneously or in testing for the association of one specific marker with the risk for death after correcting for the other markers. It is evident that in order to perform such tests we need a modeling approach that can flexibly capture the interrelationships between these outcomes.

1.3.4 Prediction

Statistical models are also often built to provide predictions of patient-related outcomes. In particular, due to current trends in medical practice towards personalized medicine, models that can provide subject-specific predictions of high quality can prove to be quite valuable. In practice, for a specific patient and at a specific time point during follow-up, physicians would like to utilize all available information they have at hand (including both baseline information and accumulated biomarker levels) to produce predictions of medically relevant outcomes, gain a better understanding of the disease dynamics, and ultimately make the most optimal decision at that time. When new information is recorded, physicians would be interested in updating these predictions, and therefore proceed in a time dynamic manner.

When good quality predictions are of interest, it would be useful to combine all available information we have for a patient in order to account for the biological interrelationships between the outcomes. In the PBC dataset for example, it is clear from the definition of the biomarkers that they measure different aspects of liver functioning. Thus, if we were to base predictions on one of those markers and ignore the others, we would discard valuable information. This would unavoidably imply that we would not reach the maximum of the predictive capability that we could have achieved had all biomarkers been simultaneously combined. It is evident, therefore, that a modeling approach that combines all markers in a single model is advantageous because it utilizes all available information. The added value of combining markers for prediction has been empirically illustrated by Fieuws et al. (2008) who noted that predictions of graft failure in a kidney transplant study based on a joint model using all recorded biomarkers of kidney functioning substantially outperformed the separate analysis per marker.

1.3.5 Statistical Analysis with Implicit Outcomes

In all the above types of research questions we have focused on explicit outcomes. However, as mentioned earlier, in longitudinal studies more often than not implicit outcomes are also generated and their appropriate handling is required even though they are not the outcomes of primary interest. In particular, in the presence of implicit outcomes, and before proceeding in the analysis of interest one must carefully consider the nature of the probabilistic mechanism describing the process generating the implicit outcome(s) (missing data and/or visit times) because it can greatly determine how the analysis should be adjusted in order to obtain valid inferences.

1.4 Overview

Chapters 2 and 3 aim at introducing the building blocks of joint models, namely linear mixed-effects models for longitudinal data and relative risk models for survival data. In particular, in Chapter 2 we discuss the complications arising in the analysis of longitudinal responses, and we introduce the linear mixed-effects model as a flexible modeling framework to handle correlated data. We refer to estimation and inference, and then focus on the problem of missing data that is frequently encountered in longitudinal studies. We define the different missing data mechanisms and explain under which circumstances the linear mixed model provides valid inferences.

Chapter 3 starts by explaining the special features of event time data, such as censoring and truncation, and how they complicate the analysis of such data. Next, we introduce relative risk models and in particular the Cox model. As in Chapter 2, we briefly refer to estimation, under partial and full likelihood, and inference. In the final section we focus on time-dependent covariates. More specifically, we provide the definitions of endogenous and exogenous time-dependent covariates, and we discuss under which settings the extended (time-dependent) Cox model provides valid inferences.

Chapter 4 introduces the basics of the joint modeling framework. In particular, continuing from the end of Chapter 3, we motivate joint models first from the survival point of view as a modeling framework to handle endogenous time-dependent covariates. We introduce the standard joint model, discuss the assumptions behind it, and present maximum likelihood estimation. Following, we make the connection with the missing data framework presented in Chapter 2, and additionally motivate joint models as models that can handle nonrandom dropout.

In Chapter 5 we explore several extensions of the standard joint model. Extensions for the survival part include different types of parameterizations between the longitudinal and survival outcomes, stratified relative risk models, handling of multiple failure times, and the consideration of accelerated failure time models. With respect to the longitudinal part we first present joint models with categorical longitudinal markers, and then we extend to multivariate joint models with multiple longitudinal outcomes. Finally, as an alternative to the standard joint model we present the latent class joint model, which assumes that the association between the longitudinal and event time processes is due to the existence of latent heterogeneity in the population.

In Chapter 6 we present several diagnostic tools to assess the assumptions behind joint models based on residuals. We focus on separate types of residuals for the survival and longitudinal parts, respectively, and special attention is given on how these residuals can be affected by the nonrandom dropout induced by the occurrence of events. In addition, we also refer to misspecification of the random-effects distribution and how this affects the derived inferences.

Chapter 7 focuses on prediction and discrimination. More specifically, we illustrate how joint models can be used to estimate survival probabilities for the event time outcome and predictions for the longitudinal outcome, and illustrate how these are dynamically updated as additional information is collected for each subject. Next, we turn our attention to prospective accuracy measures for the longitudinal marker, and assess its capability in distinguishing between subjects who are about to experience the event and subjects who have a much lower risk. In particular, under a general definition of prediction rules, we present suitable definitions of sensitivity and specificity measures, and we determine the longitudinal marker's accuracy using receiver operating characteristic methodology.

Finally, Appendix A provides a brief introduction to the R language such that readers with no or little experience with this software package can obtain the minimal required background knowledge to enable them to apply the joint modeling techniques presented in this text in their own datasets.

Chapter 2

Longitudinal Data Analysis

This chapter introduces the linear mixed-effects model for the analysis of continuous longitudinal responses that constitutes the first building block of joint models for longitudinal and event time data. Special attention is given on the frequently encountered problem of missing data. In particular, we present the different types of mechanisms describing the association structure between the longitudinal responses and the missingness process, and we explain under which circumstances a joint modeling analysis of the two outcomes is required.

2.1 Features of Longitudinal Data

The collection of correlated data is very common in many fields of quantitative research. Following Verbeke and Molenberghs (2000) and Molenberghs and Verbeke (2005), the generic term *correlated data* encompasses several multivariate data structures, such as clustered data, repeated measurements, longitudinal data, and spatially correlated data. Our focus in this chapter is on longitudinal data, which can be broadly defined as the data resulting from the observations of subjects (e.g., human beings, animals, or laboratory samples) that are measured repeatedly over time. Such data are frequently encountered in health sciences in which longitudinal studies play a prominent role in enhancing our understanding of the development and persistence of disease. The distinguishing feature of longitudinal studies is that they permit the direct assessment of changes in the response variable over time, by measuring subjects repeatedly throughout the duration of the study. For example, in a longitudinal study in which patients are (randomly) assigned to take different treatments at the start of the study and are followed up over time, we can investigate both

1. how treatment means differ at specific time points, e.g., at the end of the study (cross-sectional effect), and

2. how treatment means or differences between means of treatments change over time (longitudinal effect).

From the above descriptions, it is evident that in a longitudinal setting we expect repeated measurements taken on the same subject to exhibit positive correlation. This feature implies that standard statistical tools, such as the t-test and simple linear regression that assume independent observations, are not appropriate for longitudinal data analysis.

2.2   Linear Mixed-Effects Models

An intuitive approach for the analysis of longitudinal data is based on the idea that each individual in the population has her own subject-specific mean response profile over time, which has a specific functional form. A graphical representation of this idea is given in Figure 2.1, which shows the longitudinal responses of two hypothetical subjects (points), and their corresponding linear mean trajectories (dashed lines). The average evolution over all the subjects is depicted by the solid line. To formally introduce this representation of longitudinal data, we let y_{ij} denote the response of subject i, $i = 1, \ldots, n$ at time t_{ij}, $j = 1, \ldots, n_i$. Figure 2.1 suggests that a simple linear regression model with an intercept and a linear time effect seems adequate to describe separately the data of each subject. However, different subjects tend to have different intercepts and slopes. Therefore, a plausible model for the observed responses y_{ij} is

$$y_{ij} = \tilde{\beta}_{i0} + \tilde{\beta}_{i1} t_{ij} + \varepsilon_{ij},$$

where the error terms ε_{ij} are assumed to come from a normal distribution with mean zero and variance σ^2. Since subjects are randomly sampled from a population of subjects, it is reasonable to assume that the subject-specific regression coefficients $\tilde{\beta}_{i0}$ and $\tilde{\beta}_{i1}$ also will be randomly sampled from the corresponding population of regression coefficients. It is customary to assume that the distribution of the regression coefficients in the population is a bivariate normal distribution with mean vector $\beta = (\beta_0, \beta_1)^{\top}$ and variance-covariance matrix D. Under this setup, we can reformulate the model as

$$y_{ij} = (\beta_0 + b_{i0}) + (\beta_1 + b_{i1}) t_{ij} + \varepsilon_{ij},$$

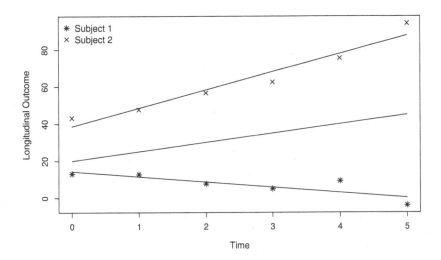

FIGURE 2.1: Intuitive representation of a linear mixed-effects model. The points represent hypothetical longitudinal responses of two subjects in a longitudinal study. The dashed lines represent the subject-specific longitudinal evolutions. The solid line represents the population-averaged evolution.

where $\tilde{\beta}_{i0} = \beta_0 + b_{i0}$, $\tilde{\beta}_{i1} = \beta_1 + b_{i1}$, and the new terms $b_i = (b_{i0}, b_{i1})^\top$ are called *random effects*, having a bivariate normal distribution with mean zero and covariance matrix D. The parameters β_0 and β_1 describe the average longitudinal evolution in the population (i.e., averaged over the subjects) and are called *fixed effects*.

The generalization of the above model, allowing additional predictors and additional regression coefficients to vary randomly, is known as the linear mixed-effects model (Laird and Ware, 1982; Harville, 1977; Verbeke and Molenberghs, 2000), and it is one of the most frequently used models for the analysis of longitudinal responses. The general linear mixed model has the form:

$$
\begin{cases}
y_i &= X_i\beta + Z_i b_i + \varepsilon_i, \\[2mm]
b_i &\sim \mathcal{N}(0, D), \\[2mm]
\varepsilon_i &\sim \mathcal{N}(0, \sigma^2 I_{n_i}),
\end{cases}
\tag{2.1}
$$

where X_i and Z_i are known design matrices, for the fixed-effects regression coefficients β, and the random-effects regression coefficients b_i, respectively, and I_{n_i} denotes the n_i-dimensional identity matrix. The random effects are assumed to be normally distributed with mean zero and variance-covariance matrix D, and are assumed independent of the error terms ε_i, i.e., $\mathrm{cov}(b_i, \varepsilon_i) = 0$. The interpretation of the fixed effects β is exactly the same as in a simple linear regression model, namely, assuming we have p covariates in the design matrix X, the coefficient β_j, $j = 1, \ldots, p$ denotes the change in the average y_i when the corresponding covariate x_j is increased by one unit, while all other predictors are held constant. Similarly, the random effects b_i are interpreted in terms of how a subset of the regression parameters for the ith subject deviates from those in the population.

An advantageous characteristic of mixed models is that it is not only possible to estimate parameters that describe how the mean response changes in the population of interest, but it also is possible to predict how individual response trajectories change over time. This is one of the main reasons for the use of these models in the joint modeling framework for longitudinal and time-to-event data, which will be introduced in Chapter 4. In addition, mixed models can accommodate any degree of imbalance in the data, that is, we do not require the same number of measurements on each subject nor that these measurements be taken at the same set of occasions. Moreover, the random effects account for the correlation between the repeated measurements of each subject in a relative parsimonious way. In particular, the outcomes of the ith subject will be marginally correlated because they share the same random effect b_i. To put it another way, we assume that the longitudinal responses of a subject are independent conditionally on her random effect, i.e.,

$$p(y_i \mid b_i; \theta) = \prod_{j=1}^{n_i} p(y_{ij} \mid b_i; \theta).$$

When the chosen random-effects structure is not sufficient to capture the correlation in the data (especially for models with few random effects), we can extend the linear mixed model defined above and allow for an appropriate, more general, covariance matrix for the subject-specific error components, i.e., $\varepsilon_i \sim \mathcal{N}(0, \Sigma_i)$, with Σ_i depending on i only through its dimensions n_i. In the literature, there have been several proposals of different models for Σ_i that lead to different types of serial correlation functions. Some of the most frequently used are the first order autoregressive, exponential, and Gaussian correlation structures, but standard statistical software for fitting linear mixed models provide many more options (Verbeke and Molenberghs, 2000; Pinheiro and Bates, 2000).

2.2.1   Estimation

The estimation of the parameters of linear mixed-effects models is often based on maximum likelihood (ML) principles. In particular, the marginal density of the observed response data for the ith subject is given by the expression:

$$p(y_i) = \int p(y_i \mid b_i) \, p(b_i) \, db_i.$$

Taking advantage of the fact that the random effects enter linearly in the specification of the conditional mean $E(y_i \mid b_i)$, and that both the conditional distribution of the longitudinal responses given the random effects $\{y_i \mid b_i\}$ and the distribution of the random effects b_i are normal, the above integral has a closed-form solution, and leads to an n_i-dimensional normal distribution with mean $X_i \beta$ and variance-covariance matrix $V_i = Z_i D Z_i^\top + \sigma^2 I_{n_i}$. Therefore, assuming independence across subjects, the log-likelihood of a linear mixed model takes the form

$$
\begin{aligned}
\ell(\theta) &= \sum_{i=1}^{n} \log p(y_i; \theta) \\
&= \sum_{i=1}^{n} \log \int p(y_i \mid b_i; \beta, \sigma^2) \, p(b_i; \theta_b) \, db_i,
\end{aligned}
\tag{2.2}
$$

where θ denotes the full parameter vector decomposed into the subvectors $\theta^\top = (\beta^\top, \sigma^2, \theta_b^\top)$, with $\theta_b = \text{vech}(D)$, and

$$p(y_i; \theta) = (2\pi)^{-n_i/2} |V_i|^{-1/2} \exp\left\{ -\frac{1}{2}(y_i - X_i\beta)^\top V_i^{-1}(y_i - X_i\beta) \right\},$$

with $|A|$ denoting the determinant of the square matrix A.

If we assume that V_i is known, then the maximum likelihood estimator of the fixed-effects vector β, obtained by maximizing (2.2) conditional on the parameters in V_i, has a closed form and corresponds to the generalized least squares estimator:

$$\hat{\beta} = \left(\sum_{i=1}^{n} X_i^\top V_i^{-1} X_i \right)^{-1} \sum_{i=1}^{n} X_i^\top V_i^{-1} y_i.
\tag{2.3}$$

When V_i is not known, but an estimate of this matrix is available, then we can estimate β using expression (2.3), in which V_i is replaced by $\widehat{V}_i$. To obtain an estimate for V_i, we can again employ the maximum likelihood method, and maximize the log-likelihood $\ell(\theta_b, \sigma^2)$ for a given value of β. As it is known from standard asymptotic maximum likelihood theory, and under certain regularity conditions, the maximum likelihood estimate of V_i will be asymptotically unbiased. However, in small samples, the ML estimate of V_i will be biased. This is, in fact, the same phenomenon encountered in simple linear regression, where the maximum likelihood estimate of the error terms variance, defined as:

$$\hat{\sigma}^2 = \frac{\sum_i (y_i - x_i^\top \hat{\beta})^2}{n},$$

is known to be biased. This bias arises because the ML estimate of σ^2 has not taken into account the fact that β is estimated from the data as well. An unbiased estimator is obtained by dividing the residual sum of squares with $n - p$ (the residual degrees of freedom), i.e.,

$$\hat{\sigma}^2 = \frac{\sum_i (y_i - x_i^\top \hat{\beta})^2}{n - p},$$

where p denotes the dimensionality of the covariate vector x_i. To address the same problem of maximum likelihood estimation, but in the more general case of multivariate regression when estimating matrix V_i, the theory of restricted maximum likelihood (REML) estimation has been developed (Harville, 1974). The main idea behind REML estimation is to separate the part of the data used in the estimation of V_i from the part used for the estimation of β. In other words, the fundamental idea in REML estimation of V_i is to eliminate β from the likelihood so that it is defined only in terms of V_i. REML estimation proceeds by maximizing the slightly modified log-likelihood function:

$$\begin{aligned}
\ell(\theta_b, \sigma^2) &= -\frac{n-p}{2} \log(2\pi) + \frac{1}{2} \log \left| \sum_{i=1}^{n} X_i^\top X_i \right| - \frac{1}{2} \log \left| \sum_{i=1}^{n} X_i^\top V_i^{-1} X_i \right| \\
&\quad - \frac{1}{2} \sum_{i=1}^{n} \left\{ \log |V_i| + (y_i - X_i \hat{\beta})^\top V_i^{-1} (y_i - X_i \hat{\beta}) \right\} \\
&\propto -\frac{1}{2} \sum_{i=1}^{n} \log |V_i| - \frac{1}{2} \sum_{i=1}^{n} (y_i - X_i \hat{\beta})^\top V_i^{-1} (y_i - X_i \hat{\beta}) \\
&\quad - \frac{1}{2} \log \left| \sum_{i=1}^{n} X_i^\top V_i^{-1} X_i \right|,
\end{aligned}$$

where $\hat{\beta}$ is given by (2.3). The estimate $\hat{V}_i$ obtained by maximizing this modified log-likelihood corrects for the fact that β also has been estimated. Contrary to the estimator of β, neither the maximum likelihood nor the restricted maximum likelihood estimator for the unique parameters in V_i can be written, in general, in closed form. Hence, in order to obtain $\hat{V}_i$, a numerical optimization routine is required. Two frequently used algorithms are the Expectation-Maximization (Dempster et al., 1977), and Newton-Raphson algorithms (Lange, 2004), whose implementation for linear mixed-effects models can be found in Laird and Ware (1982), and Lindstrom and Bates (1988).

Standard errors for the fixed-effects regression coefficients can be directly obtained by calculating the variance of the generalized least squares estimator

(2.3), i.e.:

$$\text{vâr}(\hat{\beta})$$

$$= \left(\sum_{i=1}^{n} X_i^{\top} \widehat{Q}_i X_i \right)^{-1} \left(\sum_{i=1}^{n} X_i^{\top} \widehat{Q}_i \text{vâr}(y_i) Q_i X_i \right) \left(\sum_{i=1}^{n} X_i^{\top} \widehat{Q}_i X_i \right)^{-1} \quad (2.4)$$

$$= \left(\sum_{i=1}^{n} X_i^{\top} \widehat{Q}_i X_i \right)^{-1}, \quad (2.5)$$

where $\widehat{Q}_i = \widehat{V}_i^{-1}$, and $\widehat{V}_i$ denotes either the REML or ML estimate of the covariance matrix V_i. The simplification from the first to the second line requires that the model is correctly specified and $\text{vâr}(y_i) = \widehat{V}_i$. If we would like to protect inferences for β from a potential misspecification of the covariance structure of the model, we can use instead the so-called sandwich or robust estimator for $\text{vâr}(\hat{\beta})$ (White, 1982). This is obtained by replacing in (2.4) the empirical estimator for the variance of y_i:

$$\text{vâr}(y_i) = \left(y_i - X_i \hat{\beta} \right) \left(y_i - X_i \hat{\beta} \right)^{\top}.$$

Standard errors based on the sandwich estimator will be consistent, as long as the mean structure $X_i \beta$ of the model is correctly specified, but they will be less efficient than standard errors based on (2.5) when V_i is correctly specified. Standard errors for the estimates of the unique parameters in V_i are obtained from the inverse of the corresponding block of the Fisher information matrix, i.e.,

$$\text{vâr}(\hat{\theta}_{b,\sigma}) = \left\{ E \left(- \sum_{i=1}^{n} \frac{\partial^2 \ell_i(\theta)}{\partial \theta_{b,\sigma}^{\top} \partial \theta_{b,\sigma}} \Big|_{\theta_{b,\sigma} = \hat{\theta}_{b,\sigma}} \right) \right\}^{-1}.$$

2.2.2 Implementation in R

R has extensive capabilities for mixed modeling, with several available packages that can fit different types of mixed-effects models. For linear mixed-effects models in particular, the two main packages are **nlme** (Pinheiro et al., 2012; Pinheiro and Bates, 2000) and **lme4** (Bates et al., 2011). The former can be used only for continuous data, but also can fit models with more complex error structures (i.e., correlated and/or heteroscedastic error terms), whereas the latter fits mixed models for both continuous and categorical responses,[1] but it only accounts for the correlation in the repeated measurements of the subjects using the random effects. In this book we will fit linear mixed-effects models using function `lme()` from package **nlme** because package **JM** that will be used later on to fit joint models is based on the output of this function.

---

[1]For more information on mixed models for categorical responses, the reader is referred to Section 5.7.1.

To illustrate the use of `lme()`, we perform a mixed model analysis to describe the evolution in time of the square root CD4 cell count of the patients in the AIDS dataset. This dataset is available in R as the data frame `aids` in package **JM** (Rizopoulos, 2012b) and can be loaded using the command

```
> data(aids, package = "JM")
```

We should note that in order to fit a mixed model using function `lme()` the data need to be arranged in the so-called *long* format, in which the measurements of each patient are stored in multiple lines.[2] The AIDS dataset is already organized in this format; for example, the longitudinal responses for the first two patients are located in the first seven lines:

```
> aids[aids$patient %in% c(1,2), c("patient", "CD4", "obstime")]
  patient        CD4 obstime
1       1 10.677078       0
2       1  8.426150       6
3       1  9.433981      12
4       2  6.324555       0
5       2  8.124038       6
6       2  4.582576      12
7       2  5.000000      18
```

Column `CD4` contains the square root CD4 cell count measurements, and column `obstime` the time points at which the corresponding longitudinal response was recorded. We start our analysis with a simple linear mixed model that assumes a linear average evolution in time and includes a single random effect term for each patient:

$$\begin{cases} y_{ij} = \beta_0 + \beta_1 t_{ij} + b_{i0} + \varepsilon_{ij}, \\ b_{i0} \sim \mathcal{N}(0, \sigma_b^2), \quad \varepsilon_{ij} \sim \mathcal{N}(0, \sigma^2). \end{cases}$$

This model postulates that the square root CD4 cell counts of all patients have exactly the same evolution in time, but the patients differ at baseline, i.e., each patient has her own intercept with some patients starting with a higher CD4 count and some with lower. This special type of linear mixed model is known as the random-intercepts model, and its graphical presentation is provided in the left panel of Figure 2.2. The basic syntax of `lme()` is based on two arguments, named `fixed` and `random`, which are R formulas used to specify the fixed- and random-effects parts of the model (for more information on the basics of R formulas, the reader is referred to Appendix A). For the formula in the `random` argument, the user also should specify the name of the grouping

---

[2] If the dataset is in the *wide* format with the measurements of each patient stored in multiple columns, it can be transformed to the long format using either function `reshape()` from the **stats** package or the functions in the **reshape** package (Wickham, 2007).

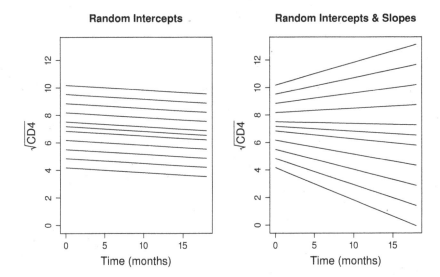

FIGURE 2.2: Graphical representation of the random-intercepts (left panel), and the random-intercepts and random-slopes (right panel) model for the evolution of the square root CD4 cell count in time for the patients in the AIDS dataset. Solid lines represent the average longitudinal evolutions, and dashed lines the subject-specific evolutions.

variable, identifying which repeated measurements belong to the same group (in our example, the groups are the patients). The **data** argument is used to provide the data frame in which all variables are stored. The corresponding call to fit the random-intercepts model is

```
> lmeFit.int <- lme(CD4 ~ obstime, random = ~ 1 | patient,
    data = aids)

> summary(lmeFit.int)

Linear mixed-effects model fit by REML
 Data: aids
       AIC      BIC    logLik
  7176.633 7197.618 -3584.316

Random effects:
 Formula: ~1 | patient
         (Intercept) Residual
StdDev:    4.506494 1.961662
```

```
Fixed effects: CD4 ~ obstime
                Value   Std.Error   DF   t-value   p-value
(Intercept)  7.188663  0.22061320  937  32.58492        0
obstime     -0.148500  0.01218699  937 -12.18513        0
 Correlation:
         (Intr)
obstime -0.194


Standardized Within-Group Residuals:
      Min          Q1          Med          Q3          Max
-3.84004681 -0.44310988 -0.05388055  0.43593364  6.09265321


Number of Observations: 1405
Number of Groups: 467
```

By default, `lme()` performs REML estimation. The `summary()` function returns a detailed output for the fitted model, including the estimates for all the parameters in the model, location measures for the standardized residuals, and information for the data used to fit the model. The estimates for the variance components, i.e., parameters σ_b and σ, are given under the **Random effects** heading, whereas the estimated regression coefficients β, along with the corresponding standard errors, t-values and p-values are provided under the **Fixed effects** heading. As expected, the coefficient for the time effect has a negative sign indicating that on average the square root CD4 cell counts declines in time. The implied marginal covariance structure for the longitudinal responses under the random-intercepts model, having the form

$$V_i = \sigma_b^2 1_{n_i} 1_{n_i}^\top + \sigma^2 I_{n_i},$$

with 1_{n_i} denoting the n_i-dimensional unit vector, assumes constant variance $\sigma_b^2 + \sigma^2$ over time as well as equal positive correlation $\rho = \sigma_b^2/(\sigma_b^2 + \sigma^2)$ between the measurements of any two time points. This covariance matrix is called *compound symmetric*, and the common correlation ρ is often termed the *intra-class correlation coefficient* (Hand and Crowder, 1996). The estimated marginal covariance matrix $\widehat{V}_i$ for a specific patient can be extracted from a fitted linear mixed model using function `getVarCov()`. For our example, we extract the covariance matrix for Patient 12, who is the first patient in the dataset that has all five planned measurements available:

```
> margCov.int <- getVarCov(lmeFit.int, individuals = 12,
      type = "marginal")

> margCov.int
```

```
patient 12
Marginal variance covariance matrix
         1       2       3       4       5
1 24.157 20.308 20.308 20.308 20.308
2 20.308 24.157 20.308 20.308 20.308
3 20.308 20.308 24.157 20.308 20.308
4 20.308 20.308 20.308 24.157 20.308
5 20.308 20.308 20.308 20.308 24.157
   Standard Deviations: 4.9149 4.9149 4.9149 4.9149 4.9149
```

Thus, according to the random-intercepts model, the estimated measurement error variance for each time point equals 24.2, and the estimated covariance between any pair of times is 20.3. The induced correlation matrix from this covariance matrix is calculated by function cov2cor():

```
> cov2cor(margCov.int[[1]])
          1         2         3         4         5
1 1.0000000 0.8407012 0.8407012 0.8407012 0.8407012
2 0.8407012 1.0000000 0.8407012 0.8407012 0.8407012
3 0.8407012 0.8407012 1.0000000 0.8407012 0.8407012
4 0.8407012 0.8407012 0.8407012 1.0000000 0.8407012
5 0.8407012 0.8407012 0.8407012 0.8407012 1.0000000
```

Even though the simplicity of the random-intercepts model is appealing, it poses the unrealistic restriction that the correlation between the repeated measurements remains constant over time. Intuitively, we would expect that measurements that are farther apart in time to be less correlated than measurements taken at subsequent time points. An extension that allows for a more flexible specification of the covariance structure is the random-intercepts and random-slopes model:

$$\begin{cases} y_{ij} = \beta_0 + \beta_1 t_{ij} + b_{i0} + b_{i1} t_{ij} + \varepsilon_{ij}, \\ b_i \sim \mathcal{N}(0, D), \quad \varepsilon_{ij} \sim \mathcal{N}(0, \sigma^2), \end{cases}$$

with $b_i = (b_{i0}, b_{i1})$. This model introduces an additional random effects term, and assumes that the rate of change in the CD4 cell count is different from patient to patient. Its graphical representation is given in the right panel of Figure 2.2. To fit this model with lme(), we specify in the **random** argument a formula that includes the time variable (the intercept is always included by default):

```
> lmeFit.slp <- lme(CD4 ~ obstime, random = ~ obstime | patient,
      data = aids)

> summary(lmeFit.slp)
```

```
Linear mixed-effects model fit by REML
 Data: aids
       AIC      BIC     logLik
  7141.282 7172.76 -3564.641

Random effects:
 Formula: ~obstime | patient
 Structure: General positive-definite, Log-Cholesky parametrization
            StdDev    Corr
(Intercept) 4.5898495 (Intr)
obstime     0.1728724 -0.152
Residual    1.7507933

Fixed effects: CD4 ~ obstime
                Value  Std.Error  DF  t-value p-value
(Intercept)  7.189048 0.22215431 937 32.36061       0
obstime     -0.150059 0.01518147 937 -9.88434       0
 Correlation:
        (Intr)
obstime -0.218

Standardized Within-Group Residuals:
       Min          Q1         Med          Q3         Max
-4.31678303 -0.41425113 -0.05227692  0.41094133  4.37412901

Number of Observations: 1405
Number of Groups: 467
```

Compared to the random-intercepts model, we observe very minor differences in the estimated fixed-effect parameters. For the random effects, we can observe that there is greater variability between patients in the baseline levels of CD4 than in the evolutions of the marker in time. Under the random-intercepts and random-slopes model, the implied marginal covariance function for any pair of responses of the same individual takes form:

$$\mathrm{cov}(y_{ij}, y_{ij'}) = \begin{bmatrix} 1 & t_{ij} \end{bmatrix} D \begin{bmatrix} 1 \\ t_{ij'} \end{bmatrix} + \sigma^2$$

$$= d_{22}t_{ij}t_{ij'} + d_{12}(t_{ij} + t_{ij'}) + d_{11} + \sigma^2, \qquad (2.6)$$

where d_{kl} denotes the klth element of the covariance matrix D. For the same time point $t_{ij} = t_{ij'} = t$, the variance function is $d_{22}t^2 + 2d_{12}t + d_{11} + \sigma^2$, which is quadratic over time with positive curvature d_{22}. Thus, the implied marginal model

$$y_i = X_i\beta + \varepsilon_i^*, \quad \varepsilon_i^* \sim \mathcal{N}(0, Z_i D Z_i^\top + \sigma^2 \mathrm{I}_{n_i}),$$

has heteroscedastic error terms. In the AIDS dataset, the estimated marginal covariance matrix is

```
> margCov.slp <- getVarCov(lmeFit.slp, individuals = 12,
    type = "marginal")

> margCov.slp
patient 12
Marginal variance covariance matrix
         1      2      3      4      5
1 24.132 20.826 20.345 19.624 18.902
2 20.826 23.771 20.463 20.101 19.738
3 20.345 20.463 23.765 21.054 21.408
4 19.624 20.101 21.054 25.550 23.915
5 18.902 19.738 21.408 23.915 29.486
  Standard Deviations: 4.9124 4.8755 4.8749 5.0547 5.4301
```

with corresponding correlation matrix

```
> cov2cor(margCov.slp[[1]])
          1         2         3         4         5
1 1.0000000 0.8695496 0.8495684 0.7903050 0.7086173
2 0.8695496 1.0000000 0.8609732 0.8156361 0.7455380
3 0.8495684 0.8609732 1.0000000 0.8544282 0.8087412
4 0.7903050 0.8156361 0.8544282 1.0000000 0.8712906
5 0.7086173 0.7455380 0.8087412 0.8712906 1.0000000
```

As expected, we observe that the variances increase over time, whereas the correlations decrease. It is evident that the random-intercepts and random-slopes model offers greater flexibility in modeling the marginal covariance matrix, but again it imposes the specific relationship (2.6) that may not always be supported by the data at hand. For instance, the variance function may not be quadratic in time. In order to allow for greater flexibility, and following the same recipe as before, we can include extra random-effect terms and thereby better capture the shapes of the subject-specific longitudinal trajectories. This could be achieved using, for instance, polynomials or regression splines in the specification of the random-effects design matrix Z_i. Nevertheless, we should note that because D needs to be a valid, positive definite, covariance matrix, any random-effects structure will always imply positive marginal correlations.

2.3 Missing Data in Longitudinal Studies

A major challenge for the analysis of longitudinal data is the problem of missing data. Although longitudinal studies are designed to collect data on every subject in the sample at a set of prespecified follow-up times, it is very often

TABLE 2.1: Examples of missing data patterns in a hypothetical longitudinal study with five planned measurements; 'x' denotes an observed measurement and '?' a missing longitudinal response

Subject	Visits				
	1	2	3	4	5
1	x	x	x	x	x
2	x	x	x	?	?
3	?	x	x	x	x
4	?	x	?	x	?

the case that some subjects miss some of their planned measurements for a variety of reasons. Depending on the features of the missing data patterns we can distinguish two types of missingness, namely monotone and non-monotone missingness. Monotone patterns of missingness cover the case of *attrition* or *dropout* when a subject is withdrawn from the study before its intended completion, and *late entry* when a subject does not provide some of her initial response measurements, but appears later on and stays in the study until completion. On the other hand, non-monotone missingness, also known as *intermittent* missingness, is a more general type that covers cases in which, for example, the response of a subject is missing at one follow-up time, she comes back at the next one, but then can be missing again at later time points. An illustrative example of the different missingness data patterns is given in Table 2.1, where Subject 1 is a completer, Subject 2 dropped out at visit four, Subject 3 did not provide the first measurement, and Subject 4 was only present at visits two and four.

The potential for missing data poses several challenges in the design of longitudinal studies and the analysis of data from these studies. The first and most obvious implication is the loss of efficiency, in the sense that changes in the average longitudinal evolutions are less precisely estimated than they would have been when all data were available. This has important consequences in the design of longitudinal studies, because we will need to enroll more individuals to achieve the same levels of power in detecting important effects. The reduction in precision is directly related to the amount of missing data and also is influenced by the chosen method of analysis. In addition, missingness results in unbalanced datasets over time because not all subjects have the same number of measurements at a common set of occasions. This creates complications for methods of analysis that require balanced data, but it does not pose any concern for the linear mixed-effect model introduced earlier. Finally, under certain circumstances and if improperly handled, missing data can introduce bias and thereby lead to misleading inferences. It is this last factor that poses the greatest concern in the analysis of incomplete longitudinal responses. Before discussing in more detail how bias problems may arise, we first need to introduce additional terminology that allow us to place formal conditions on the missing value mechanism and determine how this mechanism may influence subsequent inferences. In general, we assume that each subject i in the study is designed to be measured at occasions $j = 1, \ldots, n_i$, meaning that, for this subject, we expect to collect the vector of measurements $y_i = (y_{i1}, \ldots, y_{in_i})^\top$. To distinguish between the response measurements we actually collected from the ones we have planned to collect, we introduce the missing data indicator defined as:

$$r_{ij} = \begin{cases} 1 & \text{if } y_{ij} \text{ is observed} \\ 0 & \text{otherwise.} \end{cases}$$

Therefore, we obtain a partition of the *complete* response vector y_i into two subvectors, the observed data subvector y_i^o containing those y_{ij} for which $r_{ij} = 1$, and the missing data subvector y_i^m containing the remaining components. The vector $r_i = (r_{i1}, \ldots, r_{in_i})^\top$ and the process generating r_i are referred to as the *missing data process*.

When missingness is restricted to dropout or attrition, the missing data indicator r_i is always of the form $(1, \ldots, 1, 0, \ldots, 0)$, and therefore can be replaced by the scalar variable r_i^d, defined as

$$r_i^d = 1 + \sum_{j=1}^{n_i} r_{ij}.$$

For an incomplete sequence, r_i^d denotes the occasion at which dropout occurs, whereas for a complete sequence, $r_i^d = n_i + 1$. In both cases, r_i^d equals one plus the length of the observed measurement sequence, whether this is complete or incomplete.

2.3.1 Missing Data Mechanisms

The appropriateness of different methods of analysis of incomplete longitudinal data is determined by the *missing data mechanism*. The missing data mechanism can be thought of as the probability model describing the relation between the missing data r_i and response data y_i processes. A taxonomy of missing data mechanisms, first proposed by Rubin (1976), and further developed in Little and Rubin (2002), is based on the conditional density of the missingness process r_i given the complete response vector $y_i = (y_i^o, y_i^m)$:

$$p(r_i \mid y_i^o, y_i^m; \theta_r),$$

where θ_r denotes the corresponding parameter vector. The three types of mechanisms are (Fitzmaurice et al., 2004; Molenberghs and Kenward, 2007):

Missing Completely at Random (MCAR), which postulates that the probability that responses are missing is unrelated to both the specific values that they would have been obtained and the set of observed responses. That is, longitudinal data are MCAR when r_i is independent of both y_i^o and y_i^m,

$$p(r_i \mid y_i^o, y_i^m; \theta_r) = p(r_i; \theta_r). \qquad (2.7)$$

An example of MCAR longitudinal data is encountered in health surveys in which subjects go in and out of the study after providing a pre-determined number of repeated measurements (Fitzmaurice et al., 2004). Since the number and timing of the measurements is determined by design, the probability of obtaining a response is unrelated to the actual measurements. The important characteristic of MCAR is that the observed data y_i^o can be considered as a random sample of the complete data y_i. This, in turn, means that the distribution of the observed data does not differ from the distribution of the complete data. As a result, under MCAR we can obtain valid inferences using any valid statistical procedure for the data at hand, while ignoring the process(es) generating the missing values.

Missing at Random (MAR), assumes that the probability of missingness depends on the set of observed responses, but is unrelated to the outcomes that should have been obtained. That is, longitudinal data are MAR when r_i is conditionally independent of y_i^m given y_i^o,

$$p(r_i \mid y_i^o, y_i^m; \theta_r) = p(r_i \mid y_i^o; \theta_r). \qquad (2.8)$$

An equivalent formulation of MAR is in terms of the predictive distribution of the missing longitudinal responses y_i^m given the observed data y_i^o and r_i. In particular, under MAR this distribution takes the following form:

$$
\begin{aligned}
p(y_i^m \mid y_i^o, r_i; \theta) &= \frac{p(y_i^m, y_i^o, r_i; \theta)}{p(y_i^o, r_i; \theta)} \\[2mm]
&= \frac{p(r_i \mid y_i^o, y_i^m; \theta_r)\, p(y_i^o, y_i^m; \theta_y)}{p(r_i \mid y_i^o; \theta_r)\, p(y_i^o; \theta_y)} \\[2mm]
&= \frac{p(r_i \mid y_i^o; \theta_r)\, p(y_i^o, y_i^m; \theta_y)}{p(r_i \mid y_i^o; \theta_r)\, p(y_i^o; \theta_y)} \\[2mm]
&= \frac{p(y_i^o, y_i^m; \theta_y)}{p(y_i^o; \theta_y)} \\[2mm]
&= p(y_i^m \mid y_i^o; \theta_y),
\end{aligned}
$$

where θ denotes the parameter vector of the joint distribution of the measurements and missingness processes, and θ_y the parameter vector of the measurement model. MAR missingness also is very often called *random missingness* and, in the case of dropout, *random dropout*. A standard example of MAR longitudinal data arises when a study protocol requires patients whose response value exceeds a specific medically relevant threshold to be removed from the study. In this case, missingness is under the control of the investigator and is related to the observed components of y_i only. Due to the fact that the missing data mechanism depends on y_i^o, the distribution of y_i^o does not coincide with the distribution of y_i, and therefore the observed data cannot be considered a random sample from the target population. Only the distribution of each subject's missing values y_i^m, conditioned on her observed values y_i^o, is the same as the distribution of the corresponding observations in the target population. Thus, missing values can be validly predicted using the observed data under a model for the joint distribution $\{y_i^o, y_i^m\}$. The important implication of this feature of MAR is that sample moments are not unbiased estimates of the same moments in the target population. Thus, statistics based on these moments without accounting for MAR, such as scatterplots of the sample average longitudinal evolutions, may prove misleading. On the other hand, under MAR, likelihood-based analyses based on the observed data can provide valid inferences even if we ignore the contribution of r_i, provided that the model for the measurement process y_i is correctly specified. This can be seen from the fact that the likelihood contribution of the complete data (y_i^o, y_i^m, r_i) for the ith subject is factorized as follows:

$$
\begin{aligned}
L_i(\theta) &= \int p(y_i, r_i; \theta) \, dy_i^m \\[2mm]
&= \int p(y_i^o, y_i^m; \theta_y) \, p(r_i \mid y_i^o, y_i^m; \theta_r) \, dy_i^m \\[2mm]
&= \int p(y_i^o, y_i^m; \theta_y) \, p(r_i \mid y_i^o; \theta_r) \, dy_i^m \\[2mm]
&= p(y_i^o; \theta_y) \, p(r_i \mid y_i^o; \theta_r) \\[2mm]
&= L_i(\theta_y) \times L_i(\theta_r).
\end{aligned}
$$

Thus, if θ_y and θ_r are disjoint in the sense that the parameter space of the full vector $\theta = (\theta_y^\top, \theta_r^\top)^\top$ equals to the product of the parameter spaces of θ_y and θ_r, respectively, inference for θ_y can be based on the marginal observed data density $p(y_i^o; \theta_y)$ ignoring the likelihood of the missingness process. This property of likelihood-based inferences under MAR is known as *ignorability*.

Missing Not at Random (MNAR) posits that the probability that longitudinal responses are missing depends on a subset of the responses we would have observed. In particular, the distribution of r_i depends on at least some elements of the subvector y_i^m, even if we condition on y_i^o, i.e.,

$$p(r_i \mid y_i^m; \theta_r) \quad \text{or} \quad p(r_i \mid y_i^o, y_i^m; \theta_r). \tag{2.9}$$

Similarly to MAR, MNAR missingness also is often called *nonrandom missingness*, and in the case of dropout *nonrandom dropout*. An example of MNAR longitudinal data arises in pain studies in which patients may ask for rescue medication when their pain levels exceed the threshold they can tolerate. When patients drop out from the study and ask for rescue medication, we typically do not have a record of their outcome. As was also the case in MAR, under MNAR the observed data do not constitute a random sample from the target population. However, contrary to MAR, the predictive distribution of y_i^m conditional on y_i^o is not the same as in the target population, but rather depends on both y_i^o and on $p(r_i \mid y_i)$. Thus, the model assumed for the missingness process is crucial and must be included in the analysis.

To illustrate how the different missingness mechanisms may affect inferences based on the observed data alone, we show in Figure 2.3 the fit of the loess scatterplot smoother to a single dataset simulated from a linear mixed-effects model in which data have been deleted under the MAR and MNAR mechanisms. We can clearly observe discrepancies, especially in the MNAR case, between the loess smoother fits (solid lines) and the true average evolution (dashed lines).

A final remark regarding the above definitions of the missing data mechanisms is that we have implicitly assumed that the probability of missingness may depend on covariates. This raises a subtle but important point. For example, if missingness is related to a covariate but not to y_i (i.e., MCAR), and in our analysis of the measurement process we do not condition on this covariate, then MCAR can no longer be considered valid.

2.3.2 Missing Not at Random Model Families

From the descriptions provided in the previous section, it is evident that the most difficult type of missing data mechanism to handle is the MNAR mechanism. When longitudinal data are MNAR, we can only obtain valid inferences from an analysis that is based on the joint distribution of the measurement and missing processes. In the literature, three main model families have been proposed for this joint distribution: *selection models, pattern mixture models*, and *shared-parameter models* (Little, 1995; Molenberghs and Kenward, 2007).

The selection model factorization is based on

$$p(y_i^o, y_i^m, r_i; \theta) = p(y_i^o, y_i^m; \theta_y) \, p(r_i \mid y_i^o, y_i^m; \theta_r),$$

where the first factor is the marginal density for the measurement process and

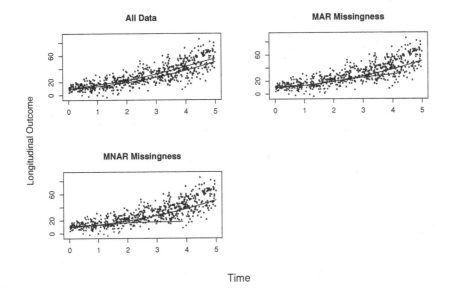

FIGURE 2.3: Graphical illustration of the effect of the MAR and MNAR missing data mechanisms. Solid lines denote the fit of the loess smoother to the observed data. Dashed lines denote the true average longitudinal evolution under which the data have been simulated.

the second one is the density of the missingness process conditional on the longitudinal outcomes. The name of this modeling framework comes from the econometric literature (Heckman, 1976) and is based on the fact that term $p(r_i \mid y_i^o, y_i^m; \theta_r)$ can be seen as the probabilistic mechanism describing each subject's self-selection to either continue or drop out from the study. Selection models for the analysis of longitudinal data with nonrandom (i.e., MNAR) dropout have been mainly brought into focus after the seminal work of Diggle and Kenward (1994).

Pattern mixture models (Little, 1993, 1994) are based on the opposite factorization of the joint distribution, i.e.,

$$p(y_i^o, y_i^m, r_i; \theta) = p(y_i^o, y_i^m \mid r_i; \theta_y)\, p(r_i; \theta_r),$$

where now we have a conditional model for the measurement process given the missingness process, and a marginal model for the missingness process. As the name also implies, pattern mixture models allow for a different measurement model for each pattern of missing values. Therefore, the marginal distribution of the measurements process is a mixture with weights the probability of each missingness pattern.

Shared-parameter models (Wu and Carroll, 1988; Wu and Bailey, 1988, 1989; Follmann and Wu, 1995; Hogan and Laird, 1997, 1998) introduce random effects to capture the association between the measurement and missingness process, i.e.,

$$p(y_i^o, y_i^m, r_i; \theta) = \int p(y_i^o, y_i^m \mid b_i; \theta_y)\, p(r_i \mid b_i; \theta_r)\, p(b_i; \theta_b)\, db_i.$$

Thus, given the random effects, the two processes are assumed independent. The idea behind this modeling framework is that there is an underlying latent process, described by the random effects, that drives both directly observed processes.

A comprehensive presentation of the features and idiosyncrasies of the selection and pattern mixture modeling frameworks for the analysis of incomplete longitudinal data is given in Verbeke and Molenberghs (2000), Molenberghs and Verbeke (2005), and Molenberghs and Kenward (2007). Shared parameter models are the focus of this monograph and will be covered in greater detail in the following chapters.

2.4   Further Reading

In this chapter, we introduced the basics of linear mixed-effects models that will be used later as one of the building blocks for joint models for longitudinal and survival data. For a more comprehensive overview of mixed models, and longitudinal data analysis in general, the interested reader is referred to the excellent texts available in the literature. In particular, mixed-effects models for continuous data are covered in Verbeke and Molenberghs (2000) and Pinheiro and Bates (2000). The first text provides a complete treatment of the linear mixed model, with a good portion of the book focusing on the handling of missing data in longitudinal studies, while the second text presents the software implementation of linear and nonlinear mixed models in S and R using package **nlme**. The related class of hierarchical and multilevel models is covered in Gelman and Hill (2007) and Snijders and Bosker (1999), with a detailed presentation of the relevant theory of variance component estimation given by Searle et al. (1992) and Rao (1997). Mixed models for both continuous and categorical data are treated in Demidenko (2004), McCulloch et al. (2008), and Jiang (2010). Molenberghs and Verbeke (2005) focus on models for the analysis of discrete longitudinal data, including both mixed-effects and marginal models. A more general overview of the different modeling frameworks for the analysis of longitudinal data, for both continuous and categorical, is provided by Diggle et al. (2002), Fitzmaurice et al. (2004), and Hedeker and Gibbons (2006). Skrondal and Rabe-Hesketh (2004) discuss the more general class of latent variable models that has as a special case the mixed-effects model.

Chapter 3

Analysis of Event Time Data

This chapter introduces basic concepts for the analysis of survival data and the class of relative risk models that constitute the second building block of joint models for longitudinal and event time data. Special attention is given to the handling of time-dependent covariates. In particular, we present the two types of time-varying covariates (i.e., endogenous and exogenous), and explain when a joint model for the covariate process and the risk for an event is required to provide valid inferences.

3.1 Features of Event Time Data

The primary aim of many studies is to analyze the time until a prespecified event of interest occurs. In these settings, the response variable is the time until that event, which is often called *failure time*, *survival time*, or *event time*. Survival analysis is most heavily used in clinical and epidemiologic studies, in which the event may be death, the appearance of a tumor, the development of some disease, recurrence of a disease, conception, or cessation of smoking. However, event times also are frequently encountered in other disciplines. For example, in sociology we could be interested in the duration of a first marriage, in marketing the length of subscription to a newspaper or a magazine, and in industry the time a component of machine operates without any failures. In the past, the study of survival data has focused on estimating the probability of survival, and simple group comparisons of the survival distributions of experimental subjects under different conditions. In recent years, focus has mainly turned to the statistical modeling of survival data. The advantages of regression models used in survival analysis are numerous. Multiple independent prognostic factors can be analyzed simultaneously, treatment differences can be assessed while adjusting for heterogeneity and imbalances in baseline characteristics, and predictions can become better calibrated.

When it comes to the statistical analysis of failure times, the first feature that must be taken into account is the shape of their distribution. In particular, due to the fact that event times must be positive, they very often have skewed shapes of distribution. Thus, statistical methods that rely on normality are not directly applicable, and, if used for survival data, may produce invalid results. This problem, however, can be easily overcome in many occasions by working with a suitable transformation of the event times, such as the logarithm or the square root. The most important characteristic that distinguishes the analysis of survival times from other areas in statistics is censoring. The defining feature of censored data is that the event time of interest is not fully observed on all subjects under study. The implications are twofold. First, standard statistical tools, such as the sample average and standard deviation, the *t*-test, and linear regression cannot be used because they assume that we have complete information, and therefore produce biased estimates of the distribution of event times and related quantities. Second, inferences can be more sensitive to a misspecification of the distribution of survival times compared to complete data. The analysis of censored data depends on the nature of the censoring mechanism that describes how censoring occurs. A first classification of censoring mechanisms is with regard to the relative positioning on the time axis of the censoring and true event times. In particular, we have the following categorization:

Right censoring: For a subset of the subjects under study, the event of interest is only known to occur after a certain time point. For example, a subject may reach the end of the study without yet having experienced the event of interest (fixed Type I censoring), or the study may be terminated after a prespecified number of events has been recorded and, thus, not all subjects had an event when the study was closed (fixed Type II censoring) or a subject may move away from the study area and thus not be available to continue (random censoring). In all these examples for some of the subjects under study it is known that their event times took place after the last time point they had been observed.

Left censoring: For a subset of the subjects under study, the event of interest is only known to occur before a certain time point. A typical example of left censoring is the age at which first grade children are able to spell their name. Some children are able to do so before the first grade, but when exactly is not precisely known.

Interval censoring: For a subset of the subjects under study, the event of interest is only known to occur between two certain time points. Interval censoring typically occurs in studies in which interest lies in the time to onset of a disease. For example, HIV-infected patients are periodically tested for the onset of AIDS. When a patient is found positive, then what is actually known is that this patient developed the disease at some point in between the pre-last and last visits.

Interval censoring is the most general type of censoring because it in fact includes both right and left censoring when the upper or lower limits of the interval that contains the true failure time are infinity or zero, respectively.

A second classification of censoring mechanisms has to do with whether or not the probability of a subject being censored depends on the failure process. More specifically, we have,

Informative censoring: When a subject withdraws from the study for reasons directly related to the expected failure time, for example, because of a worsening of her prognosis. To put it more formally, a censoring mechanism is informative if at any time t, the failure rates that apply to the subject still in the study are different from those that apply to subjects who have dropped out of the study. In a sense, informative censoring is similar in spirit to the MNAR missing data mechanism in longitudinal studies introduced in Section 2.3.1.

Noninformative censoring: When a subject withdraws from the study for reasons not related to her prognosis, but it can depend on covariates. Making the same analogy with longitudinal studies, noninformative censoring corresponds to a MCAR missing data mechanism.

Depending on the type of censoring mechanism, different inferential procedures should be followed. With respect to the first categorization, the majority of the literature has focused on methods that can handle right censored data because these are the most frequently encountered. With respect to the second categorization, and when the censoring mechanism is informative, unfortunately, very few things can be done. Similarly to the MNAR missing data mechanism in longitudinal studies, the problem is that the observed data do not contain enough information to model the censoring mechanism. Therefore, unless external information is provided, the possibilities for a meaningful analysis in these cases are rather limited. Due to these complications, the majority of the literature has focused on methods for noninformatively censored data. In this book we also will only consider noninformative right censoring.

3.2 Basic Functions in Survival Analysis

Let T^* denote the random variable of failure times under study. The function that is primarily used to describe the distribution of T^* is the survival function.

If the event is death, it expresses the probability that death occurs after t, that is the probability of surviving time t. Assuming that T^* is continuous, the survival function is defined as

$$S(t) = \Pr(T^* > t) = \int_t^\infty p(s)\, ds,$$

where $p(\cdot)$ denotes the corresponding probability density function. The survival function must be nonincreasing as t increases, with $S(t = 0)$ always equal to one. Another function that plays a prominent role in survival analysis is the hazard function. This describes the instantaneous risk for an event in the time interval $[t, t + dt)$ provided survival up to t, and is defined as

$$h(t) = \lim_{dt \to 0} \frac{\Pr(t \leq T^* < t + dt \mid T^* \geq t)}{dt}, \quad t > 0.$$

Due to its definition, $h(\cdot)$ is also called the instantaneous risk function or simply risk function. The survival also can be expressed in terms of the risk function as

$$S(t) = \exp\{-\mathcal{H}(t)\} = \exp\left\{-\int_0^t h(s)\, ds\right\}, \tag{3.1}$$

where $\mathcal{H}(\cdot)$ is known as the cumulative risk (or cumulative hazard) function that describes the accumulated risk up until time t. Function $\mathcal{H}(t)$ also can be interpreted as the expected number of events to be observed by time t.

When we are interested in estimating these two functions or any other characteristic of the event times distribution, from a random sample at hand, censoring must be taken into account. In particular, we let T_i denote the observed event time for subject i, defined as the minimum of the true event time and the censoring time C_i. We also introduce the event indicator $\delta_i = I(T_i^* \leq C_i)$ that takes the value 1 if the observed event time corresponds to a true event time and 0 otherwise, where $I(\cdot)$ denotes the indicator function. In general, in survival analysis, we are interested in estimating characteristics of the distribution of T_i^* using only the available information, i.e., using $\{T_i, \delta_i\}$. We first discuss the estimation of the survival function. The most well-known estimator has been proposed by Kaplan and Meier (1958). This is a nonparametric estimator that does not make any assumptions for the underlying distribution of the failure times. To introduce this estimator, let $t_1, \ldots, t_k$ denote the unique event times in the sample at hand. Using the law of total probability, the probability of surviving any time point t can be written as the product of the conditional probabilities:

$$\Pr(T^* > t) = \Pr(T^* > t \mid T^* > t - 1) \times \Pr(T^* > t - 1 \mid T^* > t - 2) \times \ldots$$

To estimate survival probabilities at each unique event time, we utilize the above expansion, and in the calculation of the conditional probabilities, we account for censoring by suitably adjusting the number of subjects at risk (i.e., the subjects who have not experienced the event and are not censored), which leads to the estimator:

$$\hat{S}_{KM}(t) = \prod_{i:t_i \leq t} \frac{r_i - d_i}{r_i}, \tag{3.2}$$

where r_i denotes the number of subjects still at risk at the unique event t_i, and d_i is the number of events at t_i. The variance of $\hat{S}_{KM}(t)$ can be calculated using Greenwood's formula (Greenwood, 1926; Kalbfleisch and Prentice, 2002, Section 1.4), and using asymptotic normality for $\hat{S}_{KM}(t)$, a confidence interval for $\mathcal{S}(t)$ can be derived. However, a better approach is to derive an asymmetric confidence interval for $\mathcal{S}(t)$ based on a symmetric interval for $\log \mathcal{H}(t)$. This ensures that the confidence limits for $\mathcal{S}(t)$ will not cross the boundaries of the interval $[0, 1]$. The variance of $\log \hat{\mathcal{H}}_{KM}(t)$ is derived using similar arguments as in Greenwood's formula for $\hat{S}_{KM}(t)$, and equals

$$\hat{\mathrm{var}}\{\log \hat{\mathcal{H}}_{KM}(t)\} = \frac{\sum_{i:t_i \leq t} d_i/\{r_i(r_i - d_i)\}}{\left[\sum_{i:t_i \leq t} \log\{(r_i - d_i)/r_i\}\right]^2}.$$

In the above derivation of the asymmetric confidence interval for $\mathcal{S}(t)$, we used the Kaplan-Meier estimate of the cumulative hazard function $\hat{\mathcal{H}}_{KM}(t)$. Utilizing relation (3.1), this is in fact given by $\hat{\mathcal{H}}_{KM}(t) = -\log \hat{S}_{KM}(t)$. Another similar nonparametric estimator for the cumulative hazard function, for which a wealth of asymptotic theory has been developed, is the Nelson-Aalen estimator (Altschuler, 1970; Nelson, 1972; Aalen, 1976; Fleming and Harrington, 1991),

$$\hat{\mathcal{H}}_{NA}(t) = \sum_{i:t_i \leq t} \frac{d_i}{r_i},$$

where d_i and r_i have the same interpretation as for the Kaplan-Meier estimator. Based on the Nelson-Aalen estimator and using again relation (3.1), we can derive the following estimator for the survival function,

$$\hat{S}_B(t) = \exp\{-\hat{\mathcal{H}}_{NA}(t)\} = \prod_{i:t_i \leq t} \exp(-d_i/r_i), \tag{3.3}$$

which has been suggested by Breslow (1972). To derive a confidence interval for $\mathcal{S}(t)$ based on the Breslow estimator, we again estimate the variance of $\log \hat{\mathcal{H}}_{NA}(t)$ using a formula similar to Greenwood's formula for $\log \hat{\mathcal{H}}_{KM}(t)$. The two estimators of the survival function are asymptotically equivalent. However, in finite samples $\hat{S}_B(t) \geq \hat{S}_{KM}(t)$, and most notably, if the largest observed event time T_i corresponds to a true event time, then $\hat{S}_{KM}(T_i) = 0$, whereas $\hat{S}_B(T_i) > 0$. In general, the Breslow estimator has uniformly lower variance than the Kaplan-Meier, but it is biased upward, especially when $\hat{S}(t)$ is close to zero. When comparing mean square error these aspects trade off (Fleming and Harrington, 1984). An illustration of the Kaplan-Meier and Nelson-Aalen estimators for the survival and cumulative hazard functions, respectively, for the PBC dataset is given in Figure 3.1.

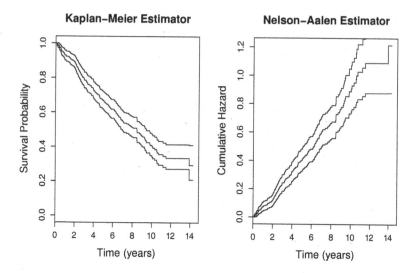

FIGURE 3.1: Left panel: Kaplan-Meier estimate (with associated 95% confidence interval) of the survival function for the PBC dataset. Right panel: Nelson-Aalen estimate (with associated 95% confidence interval) of the cumulative hazard function for the PBC dataset.

3.2.1   Likelihood Construction for Censored Data

When the survival function $\mathcal{S}(t)$ is assumed to be of a specific parametric form, estimation of the parameters of interest is often based on the maximum likelihood method. In particular, let $\{T_i, \delta_i\}$, $i = 1, \ldots, n$, denote the survival information in a random sample from a distribution function $\mathcal{P}$, parameterized by θ, with probability density function $p(t; \theta)$. In the construction of the likelihood function we need to account for censoring. More specifically, a subject i for whom an event is observed at time T_i contributes $p(T_i; \theta)$ to the likelihood, whereas for a subject i who is censored at time T_i, all we know is that she survived up to that point, i.e., $T_i^* > T_i = C_i$, and therefore this subject contributes $\mathcal{S}_i(T_i; \theta)$ to the likelihood. Thus, combining the information from the censored and uncensored observations, we obtain the log-likelihood function:

$$\ell(\theta) = \sum_{i=1}^{n} \delta_i \log p(T_i; \theta) + (1 - \delta_i) \log \mathcal{S}_i(T_i; \theta). \qquad (3.4)$$

Using the relations $h(t) = p(t)/\mathcal{S}(t)$ and $\mathcal{S}(t) = \exp\{-\mathcal{H}(t)\}$, the log-likelihood can be also rewritten in terms of the hazard function as,

$$\ell(\theta) = \sum_{i=1}^{n} \delta_i \log h_i(T_i; \theta) - \int_0^{T_i} h_i(s; \theta)\, ds. \qquad (3.5)$$

From this equivalent formulation it is clear that all subjects contribute an amount to the log-likelihood equal to the negative of the cumulative hazard function evaluated at their corresponding observed event time T_i. Subjects who experienced the event additionally contribute an amount equal to the log hazard function evaluated at $T_i = T_i^*$. Thus, censored observations contribute less information to the statistical inference than uncensored observations. Once the log-likelihood has been formulated, iterative optimization procedures, such as the Newton-Raphson algorithm (Lange, 2004), can be utilized to locate the maximum likelihood estimates $\hat{\theta}$. Inference then proceeds under the classical asymptotic maximum likelihood theory paradigm (Cox and Hinkley, 1974).

3.3   Relative Risk Regression Models

Due to the popularity of the Cox model (Cox, 1972) in modern survival analysis, proportional hazards models (also known as relative risk or relative hazard models) have prevailed. These models assume that covariates have a multiplicative effect on the hazard for an event, and they are formulated as,

$$
\begin{aligned}
h_i(t \mid w_i) &= \lim_{dt \to 0} \Pr(t \le T^* < t + dt \mid T^* \ge t, w_i)/dt \\
&= h_0(t) \exp(\gamma^\top w_i),
\end{aligned}
\tag{3.6}
$$

where $w_i^\top = (w_{i1}, \ldots, w_{ip})$ denotes the vector of covariates that are assumed to be associated with the hazard of each subject, and γ denotes the corresponding vector of regression coefficients. Function $h_0(t)$ is called *baseline hazard* or *baseline risk* function and corresponds to the hazard function of a subject that has $\gamma^\top w_i = 0$. Depending on whether the baseline risk function has a constant scale parameter, $\gamma^\top w_i$ may or may not include an intercept γ_0. Writing model (3.6) in the log scale,

$$
\log h_i(t \mid w_i) = \log h_0(t) + \gamma_1 w_{i1} + \gamma_2 w_{i2} + \ldots + \gamma_p w_{ip},
$$

we observe that the regression coefficient γ_j, for predictor w_j, denotes the change in the log hazard at any fixed time point t if w_j is increased by one unit while all other predictors are held constant. Analogously, $\exp(\gamma_j)$ denotes the ratio of hazards for one unit change in w_{ij} at any time t. In general, the ratio of hazards for a subject i with covariate vector w_i compared to subject k with covariate vector w_k is:

$$
\frac{h_i(t \mid w_i)}{h_k(t \mid w_k)} = \exp\{\gamma^\top(w_i - w_k)\}.
$$

As noted in Section 3.1, one of the implications of censoring is that inferences may be sensitive to misspecification of the distribution of the event times. Under the relative risk model (3.6), the distributional assumptions for T_i^* are hidden in the specification of the baseline hazard function. For example, when T_i^* follows the Weibull distribution, the baseline hazard function takes the form $h_0(t) = \phi\sigma_t t^{\sigma_t - 1}$. In this case estimation of all model parameters, that is the regression coefficients γ and the parameters in the specification of $h_0(t)$, proceeds by maximizing the corresponding log-likelihood function (3.5). However, Cox (1972) showed that estimation of the primary parameters of interest, namely γ, can be alternatively based on the partial log-likelihood function,

$$p\ell(\gamma) = \sum_{i=1}^{n} \delta_i \left[\gamma^\top w_i - \log\left\{ \sum_{T_j \geq T_i} \exp(\gamma^\top w_j) \right\} \right], \qquad (3.7)$$

that does not require specification of $h_0(\cdot)$, that is, without having to specify the distribution of T_i^*. Thus, the relative risk model (3.6) with an unspecified baseline risk function is a semiparametric model that does not make any assumption for the distribution of the event times, but assumes that the covariates act multiplicatively on the hazard rate. Intuitively, the partial likelihood can be considered as a measure of how well the model can order the patients with respect to their survival time. Even though this is not equivalent to a full log-likelihood (3.5), it can be treated as such. In particular, the maximum partial likelihood estimators are found by solving the partial log-likelihood score equations:

$$\frac{\partial p\ell(\gamma)}{\partial \gamma^\top} = \sum_{i=1}^{n} \delta_i \left\{ w_i - \frac{\sum_{T_j \geq T_i} w_j \exp(\gamma^\top w_j)}{\sum_{T_j \geq T_i} \exp(\gamma^\top w_j)} \right\} = 0.$$

The solution $\hat{\gamma}$ is consistent and asymptotically normally distributed with mean γ^0, the true parameter vector, and variance $\left[E\{\mathcal{I}(\gamma^0)\} \right]^{-1}$, the inverse of the expected information matrix corresponding to (3.7). Due to the fact that the expectation requires knowledge of the censoring distribution, standard errors are typically estimated using the observed information $\{\mathcal{I}(\hat{\gamma})\}^{-1}$, where

$$\mathcal{I}(\hat{\gamma}) = -\sum_{i=1}^{n} \frac{\partial^2 p\ell_i(\gamma)}{\partial \gamma^\top \partial \gamma} \Big|_{\gamma = \hat{\gamma}}.$$

For a thorough discussion of the relative efficiency of the maximum partial likelihood estimator with respect to that of a maximum likelihood estimator, in which $h_0(\cdot)$ is specified up to certain unknown parameters, we refer to Kalbfleisch and Prentice (2002, Section 5.9).

3.3.1 *Implementation in R*

The primary R package for the analysis of event time data is the **survival** package (Therneau and Lumley, 2012). To load this package we use the command `library("survival")`. A comprehensive list of other packages in CRAN related to survival analysis is available from the CRAN Task View: Survival

Analysis (Allignol and Latouche, 2012). The function used to fit Cox models is coxph(), which has two main arguments, the formula argument that specifies the relationship between the observed failure times and covariates, and the data argument that specifies the data frame that contains these variables. In the left-hand side of the formula argument, function Surv() is used to specify the available information for the failure times, that is the observed failure times and the type of censoring (i.e., right, left, interval, and counting[1]). The following commands illustrate the use of coxph() to fit a Cox model to the PBC dataset, which is available as the data frame pbc2.id from package **JM**.

```
> data(pbc2.id, package = "JM")

> pbc2.id$status2 <- as.numeric(pbc2.id$status != "alive")

> coxFit <- coxph(Surv(years, status2) ~ drug + age + sex,
    data = pbc2.id)

> summary(coxFit)
Call:
coxph(formula = Surv(years, status2) ~ drug + age + sex, data = pbc2.id)

  n= 312, number of events= 169

                  coef exp(coef) se(coef)      z Pr(>|z|)
drugD-penicil -0.13759   0.87146  0.15597 -0.882  0.37770
age            0.02149   1.02172  0.00772  2.784  0.00537
sexfemale     -0.49330   0.61061  0.20735 -2.379  0.01735

                exp(coef) exp(-coef) lower .95 upper .95
drugD-penicil    0.8715     1.1475    0.6419    1.1831
age              1.0217     0.9787    1.0064    1.0373
sexfemale        0.6106     1.6377    0.4067    0.9168


Concordance= 0.573  (se = 0.024 )
Rsquare= 0.047   (max possible= 0.996 )
Likelihood ratio test= 14.97  on 3 df,   p=0.001844
Wald test            = 16.1  on 3 df,   p=0.001081
Score (logrank) test = 16.3  on 3 df,   p=0.0009836
```

In the first two lines we load and we define the indicator for the composite event, that is, death or transplantation, whichever comes first. The third line fits the Cox model. In function Surv() we specify that variable **years** denotes the observed event times and variable **status2** the event indicator. By default, right censoring is assumed. In the right-hand side of the formula argument

---

[1]Option 'counting' refers to the counting process formulation of relative risk models, which is introduced in Section 3.5.

we specify that the log relative hazard for either death or transplantation depends additively on treatment, age, and sex of the patients. In the last line, the `summary()` method is invoked to summarize the fit of the Cox model. Column `coef` in the output contains the estimated regression coefficients $\hat{\gamma}$. More easily interpretable are the exponentiated coefficients, provided by the column `exp(coef)`, that denote the multiplicative change in the risk due to each covariate. We observe that the active treatment reduces the risk for the composite event by about 12.9%, though not statistically significantly. On the other hand, one year increase in the baseline age is associated with a 2.2% increase in the risk, and males have 63.8% higher risk for an event compared to females.

3.4   Time-Dependent Covariates

In the relative risk model introduced in Section 3.3 we assumed that the hazard depends only on covariates whose value is constant during follow-up, such as age at baseline, sex, randomized treatment, etc. However, in many studies it may also be of interest to investigate whether time-dependent covariates are associated with the risk for an event. These could include, among others, environmental factors, biochemical and clinical parameters measured during follow-up, and adjustments to treatment dose.

Before we explain how such covariates are handled in practice, we should first distinguish between two different categories of time-dependent covariates, namely, *external* or *exogenous* covariates and *internal* or *endogenous* covariates. The reason why it is important to distinguish between time-varying covariates is that an endogenous covariate requires special treatment compared to an exogenous one. To introduce these two types of covariates, let $y_i(t)$ denote the covariate vector at time t for subject i, and $\mathcal{Y}_i(t) = \{y_i(s), 0 \le s < t\}$ denote the covariate history up to t. Following Kalbfleisch and Prentice (2002, Section 6.3), the formal definition of exogenous covariates requires such covariates to satisfy the relation:

$$\Pr\{s \le T_i^* < s + ds \mid T_i^* \ge s, \mathcal{Y}_i(s)\}$$
$$= \Pr\{s \le T_i^* < s + ds \mid T_i^* \ge s, \mathcal{Y}_i(t)\}, \tag{3.8}$$

for all s, t such that $0 < s \le t$, and $ds \to 0$. An equivalent definition is

$$\Pr\{\mathcal{Y}_i(t) \mid \mathcal{Y}_i(s), T_i^* \ge s\} = \Pr\{\mathcal{Y}_i(t) \mid \mathcal{Y}_i(s), T_i^* = s\}, \quad s \le t, \tag{3.9}$$

which formalizes the idea that $y_i(\cdot)$ is associated with the rate of failures over time, but its future path up to any time $t > s$ is not affected by the occurrence of failure at time s. In particular, an exogenous covariate is a predictable process, meaning that its value at any time t is known infinitesimally before

t. On the other hand, endogenous time-varying covariates are the ones that do not satisfy (3.8) or equivalently (3.9), and they are also not predictable.

A standard example of an exogenous covariate is the time of the day or the season of the year. For instance, seasonal patterns have been recognized in suicides attempts, with higher occurrence rates encountered during the winter months. Another example of exogenous covariates are those whose complete path is predetermined from the beginning of the study. For example, in some studies there is interest in comparing treatment strategies in which the treatment dose is adjusted according to predetermined criteria. Yet another type of exogenous covariates are stochastic processes that are external to the subjects under study. For instance, the levels of environmental factors, such as air pollution, may be associated with the frequency of asthma attacks. In all of these examples it is clear that the value of these covariates at any time point t is not affected by the true failure time, and therefore (3.9) is satisfied. For external covariates, and under condition (3.8) or (3.9), we can directly define the survival function conditional on the covariate path, using its relation to the hazard function, i.e.,

$$S_i(t \mid \mathcal{Y}_i(t)) = \Pr(T_i^* > t \mid \mathcal{Y}_i(t))$$

$$= \exp\left\{ -\int_0^t h_i(s \mid \mathcal{Y}_i(s)) \, ds \right\}.$$

Endogenous covariates, on the other hand typically arise as time-dependent measurements taken on the subjects under study. These include biomarkers and clinical parameters, such as the serum bilirubin levels for patients with primary biliary cirrhosis, CD4 cell counts for HIV-infected patients, the prothrombin index for patient with liver cirrhosis, and aortic gradient level for patients with aortic stenosis (see Section 1.2). There are several important features that complicate statistical analysis with such covariates. The first important characteristic of endogenous covariates is that they typically require the survival of the subject for their existence. Thus, when failure is defined as the death of the subject, their path carries direct information about the failure time. More specifically, provided that $y_i(t-ds)$ with $ds \to 0$ exists, the survival function satisfies

$$S_i(t \mid \mathcal{Y}_i(t)) - \Pr(T_i^* > t \mid \mathcal{Y}_i(t)) - 1. \tag{3.10}$$

On the other hand, failure of the subject at time s corresponds to nonexistence of the covariate at $t \geq s$, which has as a direct implication the violation of the endogeneity condition (3.9). Moreover, a consequence of identity (3.10) is that, contrary to exogenous covariates, the hazard function, defined before as

$$h_i(t \mid \mathcal{Y}_i(t)) = \lim_{dt \to 0} \Pr\{t \leq T^* < t + dt \mid T^* \geq t, \mathcal{Y}_i(t)\}/dt,$$

is not directly related to a survival function. That is, the functions

$$\mathcal{S}_i(t \mid \mathcal{Y}_i(t)) = \exp\left\{-\int_0^t h_i(s \mid \mathcal{Y}_i(s)) \, ds\right\} \quad \text{and}$$

$$p(t \mid \mathcal{Y}_i(t)) = h_i(t \mid \mathcal{Y}_i(t))\mathcal{S}_i(t \mid \mathcal{Y}_i(t)),$$

do not have the usual survival and density function interpretations. Due to this feature, the log-likelihood construction (3.4) based on $p(\cdot)$ and $\mathcal{S}(\cdot)$ is not meaningful for endogenous covariates. Another feature of endogenous covariates is that they are typically measured with error. This measurement error primarily refers to the biological variation induced by the patient herself rather than to the error induced by the procedure/machinery that determines the value of this covariate. In particular, measuring the same patient twice, even on the same day, we do not expect to observe exactly the same value for an endogenous covariate, such as a biomarker. Thus, for such covariates, it would be more reasonable to assume that the observed marker levels are actually a contaminated with biological variation version of the true marker levels. Nonetheless, it should be mentioned that the measurement error is not a distinguishing feature of endogenous covariates, because some exogenous covariates are also measured with error (e.g., air pollution). The final important implication with endogenous covariates is that their complete path up to any time t is not fully observed. That is, the levels of a biomarker or any other clinical parameter for a patient are only known for the specific occasions that this patient visited the study center to provide measurements, and not in between these visit times.

3.5   Extended Cox Model

The Cox model presented in Section 3.3 can be extended to handle exogenous time-dependent covariates using the counting process formulation investigated in detail by Andersen and Gill (1982) and presented in greater detail in Fleming and Harrington (1991) and Andersen et al. (1993). The intuitive idea behind this formulation of the Cox model is to think occurrence of events as the realization of a very slow Poisson process. In counting process notation, the event process for subject i is written as $\{N_i(t), R_i(t)\}$, with $N_i(t)$ denoting the number of events for subject i by time t, and $R_i(t)$ is a left continuous at risk process with $R_i(t) = 1$ if subject i is at risk at time t, and $R_i(t) = 0$ otherwise. The extended Cox model (also known as the Andersen-Gill model) is written as

$$h_i(t \mid \mathcal{Y}_i(t), w_i) = h_0(t)R_i(t)\exp\{\gamma^\top w_i + \alpha y_i(t)\}, \qquad (3.11)$$

where, as in (3.6), w_i denotes a vector of baseline covariates, such as sex or randomized treatment, and $y_i(t)$ denotes a vector of time-dependent covariates. The interpretation of the regression coefficients vector α is exactly the same as for γ. In particular, assuming for simplicity that there is only a single time-dependent covariate, then at any particular time point t, $\exp(\alpha)$ denotes the relative increase in the risk for an event at time t that results from one unit increase in $y_i(t)$ at the same time point. Moreover, note that since $y_i(t)$ is time-dependent, model (3.11) no longer assumes that the hazard ratio is constant in time.

Estimation of γ and α is again based on the corresponding partial log-likelihood function that can be written as

$$
p\ell(\gamma) \;=\; \sum_{i=1}^{n} \int_{0}^{\infty} \Big\{ R_i(t) \exp\{\gamma^\top w_i + \alpha y_i(t)\}
$$
$$
- \log\Big[\sum_{j} R_j(t) \exp\{\gamma^\top w_j + \alpha y_j(t)\}\Big] \Big\} \, dN_i(t),
$$

in which the counting processes integral notation is used (Fleming and Harrington, 1991; Andersen et al., 1993). As an illustration, we fit a Cox model for the Liver Cirrhosis dataset that postulates that the risk for death depends on the prothrombin index and on randomized treatment. The model has the form

$$
h_i(t) = h_0(t) \exp\{\gamma \mathtt{Predns}_i + \alpha y_i(t)\},
$$

where **Predns** is the indicator variable for prednisone treatment group, and $y_i(t)$ denotes the level of the prothrombin index at time t. In the extended Cox model time-dependent covariates are usually encoded using the (start, stop] notation. In particular, each subject is represented by multiple rows, each one holding the information on $y_i(t)$ for a specific time interval. The rows for the first patient in the Liver Cirrhosis dataset are

```
> head(prothro[c("id", "pro", "start", "stop", "event")], n = 3)
  id pro    start       stop event
1  1  38 0.0000000 0.2436754     0
2  1  31 0.2436754 0.3805717     0
3  1  27 0.3805717 0.4134268     1
```

The **start** and **stop** variables denote the limits of the time intervals during which the prothrombin index is recorded. In particular, for Patient 1 prothrombin equals 38 at baseline, 31 at 0.24 years, and 27 at 0.38 years. Variable **event** equals 1 if an event occurred at the end of the corresponding time interval. The **treat** denotes the randomized treatment variable, which is fixed throughout the follow-up period for each patient. The corresponding extended Cox model is fitted using the syntax:

```
> tdCox.pro <- coxph(Surv(start, stop, event) ~ pro + treat,
      data = prothro)

> summary(tdCox.pro)
```

```
Call:
coxph(formula = Surv(start, stop, event) ~ pro + treat, data = prothro)

  n= 2968, number of events= 292

                    coef exp(coef)  se(coef)       z Pr(>|z|)
pro             -0.034985  0.965620 0.002494 -14.03   <2e-16
treatprednisone -0.137770  0.871299 0.118738  -1.16    0.246

                exp(coef) exp(-coef) lower .95 upper .95
pro                0.9656      1.036    0.9609    0.9704
treatprednisone    0.8713      1.148    0.6904    1.0996

Concordance= 0.725  (se = 0.019 )
Rsquare= 0.067    (max possible= 0.657 )
Likelihood ratio test= 207.1  on 2 df,    p=0
Wald test             = 197.2  on 2 df,    p=0
Score (logrank) test = 203.2  on 2 df,    p=0
```

The only difference compared to the syntax used to fit the standard Cox model in Section 3.3, is in the specification of the Surv() function in which the first two arguments denote the limits of the interval, and the last argument is the corresponding event indicator. Moreover, in the data argument the data should be supplied in the long format. From the results we observe that, after correcting for treatment differences, the prothrombin index is strongly associated with the risk for death, with each one unit decrease in prothrombin resulting in 1.036-fold increase in the risk (95% CI: 1.031; 1.041).

The counting process formulation of the Cox model is a quite general formulation that not only allows for time-dependent covariates but also for left truncation, multiple time scales, multiple events per subject and various forms of case-cohort models, among others (Therneau and Grambsch, 2000). However, despite this flexibility the extended Cox model is not appropriate when the time-dependent covariates are of endogenous nature. This is because the extended Cox model assumes that time-dependent covariates are predictable processes, measured without error, and have their complete path fully specified. The particular way the Cox model handles time-dependent covariates under the counting processes formulation is illustrated in Figure 3.2. More specifically, time-dependent covariates are assumed to change value at the follow-up visits and remain constant in the time interval in between these visits. Then the model postulates that the hazard for an event, at any time point t, is associated with the extrapolated value of the covariate at the same time point. It is evident that this step-function approximation is unrealistic for many endogenous covariates, such as biomarkers. For example, in the analysis for Liver Cirrhosis dataset presented above, it is not reasonable to assume that the prothrombin index remains constant between follow-up visits, especially because these can be several months apart. This in fact implies that this analysis based on the extended Cox model for the Liver Cirrhosis dataset is

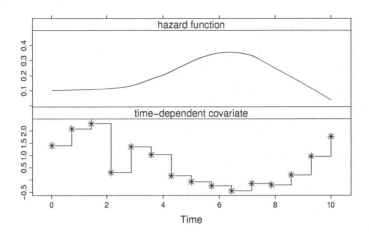

FIGURE 3.2: Time-dependent covariates in the extended Cox model.

not an optimal analysis. In particular, the problem that arises from this "Last Value Carried Forward" approach is that parameter estimates and standard errors can be severely biased (Prentice, 1982). In the rest of this book we will introduce a modeling framework especially designed to account for the special features of endogenous time-dependent covariates.

3.6 Further Reading

The aim of this chapter is to present a brief introduction in the special characteristics of failure time data, and the basic statistical tools that have been developed in the literature for their analysis. However, this introduction was not intended to be at any case exhaustive. There are many excellent texts in the literature that go into more depth regarding different aspects of the analysis of survival data. In particular, Cox and Oakes (1984), Kalbfleisch and Prentice (2002), Lawless (2002), and Klein and Moeschberger (2003) explain in detail the special features of event time data, such as censoring and truncation, and present in detail and with examples the different statistical tools that are currently available for their analyses. A more theoretical treatment of the Cox model using point processes and martingales is given by Fleming and Harrington (1991), Andersen et al. (1993), and Aalen et al. (2008), while a more practical point of view with primary focus in model building and model testing techniques, and their implementation in standard software is taken by Therneau and Grambsch (2000), Harrell (2001, Chapters 16–20), and Tableman and Kim (2003). Hougaard (2000) presents several methods for multivariate survival data, including frailty and marginal models. Frailty models are presented in greater detail by Duchateau and Janssen (2008), and Wienke (2011). An overview of the available methods for the analysis of interval censored failure is presented by Sun (2006). Finally, Ibrahim et al. (2001) illustrate how the standard survival models presented in the previous texts can be fitted under the Bayesian paradigm.

Chapter 4

Joint Models for Longitudinal and Time-to-Event Data

Based on the linear mixed-effects and relative risk models presented in the previous two chapters, we introduce here the standard joint model for longitudinal and time-to-event data. We discuss maximum likelihood estimation of the model's parameter, including optimization and numerical integration algorithms, inference for the regression coefficients and the random effects, and we present a tool for investigating the sensitivity of inferences for the longitudinal outcome to the assumptions for the dropout process.

4.1   The Basic Joint Model

As we have seen in Section 3.5, the extended Cox model is only appropriate for exogenous time-dependent covariates and therefore cannot handle longitudinal biomarkers. When primary interest is in the association between such endogenous time-dependent covariates and survival, an alternative modeling framework has been introduced in the literature, known as the joint modeling framework for longitudinal and time-to-event data (Faucett and Thomas, 1996; Wulfsohn and Tsiatis, 1997; Henderson et al., 2000; Tsiatis and Davidian, 2004). The motivating idea behind these joint models is to couple the survival model, which is of primary interest, with a suitable model for the repeated measurements of the endogenous covariate that will account for its special features, elucidated in Section 3.4. To introduce this modeling framework, we will use similar notation as in Chapters 2 and 3. In particular, we denote by T_i^* the true event time for the ith subject, T_i the observed event time, defined as the minimum of the potential censoring time C_i and T_i^*, and by $\delta_i = I(T_i^* \leq C_i)$ the event indicator. For the endogenous time-dependent covariate (e.g., a biomarker) we let $y_i(t)$ denote its observed value at time point t for the ith subject. We should note that we do not actually observe $y_i(t)$ for any time t, but rather only at the very specific occasions t_{ij} at which measurements were taken. Thus, the observed longitudinal data consist of the measurements $y_{ij} = \{y_i(t_{ij}), j = 1, \ldots, n_i\}$.

4.1.1   The Survival Submodel

Our aim is to measure the association between the longitudinal marker level and the risk for an event, while accounting for the special features of the former. To achieve this we introduce the term $m_i(t)$ that denotes the *true* and *unobserved* value of the longitudinal outcome at time t. Note that $m_i(t)$ is different from $y_i(t)$, with the latter being the contaminated with measurement error value of the longitudinal outcome at time t. To quantify the strength of the association between $m_i(t)$ and the risk for an event, a straightforward approach is to postulate a relative risk model of the form:

$$
\begin{aligned}
h_i(t \mid \mathcal{M}_i(t), w_i) &= \lim_{dt \to 0} \Pr\{t \leq T_i^* < t + dt \mid T_i^* \geq t, \mathcal{M}_i(t), w_i\}/dt \\
&= h_0(t) \exp\{\gamma^\top w_i + \alpha m_i(t)\}, \quad t > 0, \tag{4.1}
\end{aligned}
$$

where $\mathcal{M}_i(t) = \{m_i(s), 0 \leq s < t\}$ denotes the history of the true unobserved longitudinal process up to time point t, $h_0(\cdot)$ denotes the baseline risk function, and w_i is a vector of baseline covariates (such as a treatment indicator, history of diseases, etc.) with a corresponding vector of regression coefficients γ. Similarly, parameter α quantifies the effect of the underlying longitudinal outcome to the risk for an event. The interpretation of γ and α is exactly the same as we have seen in Section 3.5. In particular, $\exp(\gamma_j)$ denotes the ratio of hazards for one unit change in w_{ij} at any time t, whereas $\exp(\alpha)$ denotes the relative increase in the risk for an event at time t that results from one unit increase in $m_i(t)$ at the same time point. Moreover, note that the relative risk model (4.1) postulates that the risk for an event at time t depends only on the current value of the time-dependent marker $m_i(t)$. However, this does not hold for the survival function. In particular, using the known relation between the survival function and the cumulative hazard function, we obtain that:

$$
\begin{aligned}
S_i(t \mid \mathcal{M}_i(t), w_i) &= \Pr(T_i^* > t \mid \mathcal{M}_i(t), w_i) \\
&= \exp\left(-\int_0^t h_0(s) \exp\{\gamma^\top w_i + \alpha m_i(s)\} \, ds\right), \tag{4.2}
\end{aligned}
$$

which implies that the corresponding survival function depends on the whole covariate history $\mathcal{M}_i(t)$. As we will see later in Section 4.3, this feature becomes of practical importance in the estimation of joint models, because the survival function is a part of the likelihood of the model.

To complete the specification of (4.1) we need to discuss the choice for the baseline risk function $h_0(\cdot)$. As we have seen in Chapter 3, in standard survival analysis it is customary to leave $h_0(\cdot)$ completely unspecified in order to avoid the impact of misspecifying the distribution of survival times. However, within the joint modeling framework and as we will explain later in Section 4.3.3, it turns out that following such a route may lead to an underestimation of the standard errors of the parameter estimates (Hsieh et al., 2006). To avoid such problems we will need to explicitly define $h_0(\cdot)$. A standard option is to use a risk function corresponding to a known parametric distribution. In the survival analysis context, typically used distributions include the Weibull, the log-normal and the Gamma. Alternatively, and even more preferably, we can opt for a parametric but flexible specification of the baseline risk function. Several approaches have been proposed in the literature to flexibly model the baseline risk function. For instance, Whittemore and Killer (1986) used step-functions and linear splines to obtain a non-parametric estimate of the risk function, Rosenberg (1995) utilized a B-splines approximation, and Herndon and Harrell (1996) used restricted cubic splines. Two simple options that often work quite satisfactorily in practice are the piecewise-constant and regression splines approaches. Under the piecewise-constant model, the baseline risk function takes the form:

$$h_0(t) = \sum_{q=1}^{Q} \xi_q I(v_{q-1} < t \le v_q),\qquad(4.3)$$

where $0 = v_0 < v_1 < \cdots < v_Q$ denotes a split of the time scale, with v_Q being larger than the largest observed time, and ξ_q denotes the value of the hazard in the interval $(v_{q-1}, v_q]$. As the number of knots increases the specification of the baseline hazard becomes more flexible. In the limiting case where each interval $(v_{q-1}, v_q]$ contains only a single true event time (assuming no ties), this model is equivalent to leaving $h_0(\cdot)$ completely unspecified and estimating it using nonparametric maximum likelihood. For the regression splines model the log baseline risk function $\log h_0(t)$ is expanded into B-spline basis functions for cubic splines as follows:

$$\log h_0(t) = \kappa_0 + \sum_{d=1}^{m} \kappa_d B_d(t, q),\qquad(4.4)$$

where $\kappa^\top = (\kappa_0, \kappa_1, \ldots, \kappa_m)$ are the spline coefficients, q denotes the degree of the B-splines basis functions $B(\cdot)$, and $m = \ddot{m} + q - 1$, with $\ddot{m}$ denoting the number of interior knots. Similarly to the piecewise-constant model, increasing the number of knots increases the flexibility in approximating $h_0(\cdot)$. However in both approaches, we should keep a balance between bias and variance and avoid overfitting. A standard rule of thumb is to keep the total number of

parameters, including the parameters in the linear predictor in (4.1) and in
the model for $h_0(\cdot)$, between 1/10 and 1/20 of the total number of events
in the sample (Harrell, 2001, Section 4.4). After the number of knots has
been decided, their location is typically based on percentiles of either the
observed event times $T_i = \min(T_i^*, C_i)$ or only the true event times $\{T_i :
T_i^* \leq C_i, i = 1, \ldots, n\}$, such that to allow for more flexibility in the region of
greatest density.

4.1.2   The Longitudinal Submodel

In the definitions of the survival models presented above we used $m_i(t)$ to
denote the true value of the underlying longitudinal covariate at time point
t. However, and as mentioned earlier, longitudinal information is actually collected intermittently and with error at a set of a few time points t_{ij} for each
subject. Therefore, to measure the effect of the longitudinal covariate to the
risk for an event, we need to estimate $m_i(t)$ and successfully reconstruct the
complete longitudinal history $\mathcal{M}_i(t)$ for each subject. To achieve this we postulate a suitable mixed-effects model to describe the subject-specific time evolutions. For now we will focus on normally distributed longitudinal outcomes
and use a linear mixed-effects model. In particular, following similar notation
as in Section 2.2, we have

$$\begin{cases} y_i(t) & = & m_i(t) + \varepsilon_i(t), \\\\ m_i(t) & = & x_i^\top(t)\beta + z_i^\top(t)b_i, \\\\ b_i & \sim & \mathcal{N}(0, D), \quad \varepsilon_i(t) \sim \mathcal{N}(0, \sigma^2), \end{cases} \qquad (4.5)$$

where we explicitly note that the design vectors $x_i(t)$ for the fixed effects β,
and $z_i(t)$ for the random effects b_i, as well as the error terms $\varepsilon_i(t)$, are time-
dependent. Moreover, and similarly to Section 2.2, we assume that error terms
are mutually independent, independent of the random effects, and normally
distributed with mean zero and variance σ^2.

The mixed model accounts for the measurement error problem by postulating that the observed level of the longitudinal outcome $y_i(t)$ equals the
true level $m_i(t)$ plus a random error term. Moreover, the time structure in the
definitions of $x_i(t)$ and $z_i(t)$, and the use of subject-specific random effects
allows to reconstruct the complete path of the time-dependent process $\mathcal{M}_i(t)$
for each subject. In particular, the intuitive idea behind joint models is presented in Figure 4.1, where at each time point we want to associate the true
level of the marker (bottom panel) with the risk for an event (top panel). The
dashed line represents the step function assumed by the extended Cox model
when handling time-varying covariates, which in many cases is not a realistic
description of the subject-specific longitudinal trajectory.

As noted earlier, the survival function (4.2) depends on the whole history
of the true marker levels, and therefore, for an accurate estimation of $\mathcal{S}_i(t)$ it

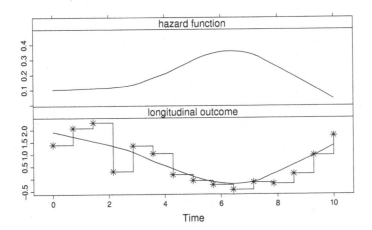

FIGURE 4.1: Intuitive representation of joint models. In the top panel the solid line illustrates how the hazard function evolves in time. In the bottom panel the dashed line corresponds to the extended Cox approximation of the longitudinal trajectory, and the solid line to the joint model approximation $m_i(t)$.

is important to obtain a good estimate of $\mathcal{M}_i(t)$. This entails considering an elaborate specification of the time structure in $x_i(t)$ and $z_i(t)$, and possibly interactions terms between the postulated time structure and baseline covariates. For instance, in applications in which subjects show highly non-linear longitudinal trajectories, it is advisable to consider flexible representations for $x_i(t)$ and $z_i(t)$ using a possibly high-dimensional vector of functions of time t, expressed in terms of high-order polynomials or splines. Compared to polynomials, splines are usually preferred due to their local nature and better numerical properties (Ruppert et al., 2003). In the joint modeling framework several authors have considered spline-based approaches to model flexibly the subject-specific longitudinal profiles. For example, Rizopoulos et al. (2009) and Brown et al. (2005) have utilized B-splines with multidimensional random effects, Ding and Wang (2008) proposed the use of B-spines with a single multiplicative random effect, and Rizopoulos and Ghosh (2011) have considered natural cubic splines. An alternative approach to model highly nonlinear shapes of subject-specific evolutions is to incorporate in the linear mixed model an additional stochastic term that aims to capture the remaining serial correlation in the observed measurements not captured by the random effects. In this framework the linear mixed model takes the form

$$y_i(t) = m_i(t) + u_i(t) + \varepsilon_i(t), \qquad (4.6)$$

where $u_i(t)$ is a mean-zero stochastic process, independent of b_i and $\varepsilon_i(t)$, and

$m_i(t)$ has the same mixed-effects model structure as in (4.5). Joint models with such terms have been considered by Wang and Taylor (2001), who postulated an integrated Ornstein-Uhlenbeck process, and by Henderson et al. (2000), who considered a latent stationary Gaussian process shared by both the longitudinal and event processes. The choice between the two approaches is to a large extent a philosophical issue dictated in part by the analyst's belief about the "true" underlying biological mechanism that generates the data. In particular, model (4.5) posits that the trajectory followed by a subject throughout time is dictated by the time-independent random effects b_i alone. This implies that the shape of the longitudinal profile of each subject is an inherent characteristic of this subject that is constant in time. On the other hand, model (4.6) that includes both a serial correlation stochastic term and random effects attempts to more precisely capture the features of the longitudinal trajectory by allowing the subject-specific trends to vary in time. We should note that because both the random-effects and a stochastic serial correlation process attempt to appropriately model the marginal correlation in the data, there is a contest for information between the two approaches. For instance, if we have postulated a linear mixed model with a random-intercepts and random-slopes structure and there is excess serial correlation that the random effects have not adequately captured, then extending this model by either including the serial correlation term $u_i(t)$ or by considering a more elaborate random-effects structure (using e.g., splines in the design matrix $Z_i(t)$) could produce practically indistinguishable fits to the data. Therefore, even though it might seem intuitively appealing to use both elaborate random-effects and serial correlation structures, it is advisable to opt for either of those. Computationally the random-effects approach is easier to implement in practice because it only requires an appropriate specification of the random-effects design matrix $Z_i(t)$.

4.2   Joint Modeling in R: A Comparison with the Extended Cox Model

To illustrate the virtues of the joint modeling approach we will compare it with the extended Cox model for the AIDS dataset. In particular, we would like to assess the strength of the association between the square root CD4 cell count at time t and the risk for death at the same time point. The AIDS dataset is available in R as the data frame `aids` in package **JM** (Rizopoulos, 2010, 2012b). To load this package we use the command `library("JM")`. The `aids` dataset contains in the long format both the longitudinal information and the survival information for each patient. The recorded information for the first two patients is

```
> head(aids[c("patient", "start", "stop", "event",
    "CD4", "obstime", "drug")], 7)
  patient start  stop event      CD4 obstime drug
1       1     0  6.00     0 10.677078       0  ddC
2       1     6 12.00     0  8.426150       6  ddC
3       1    12 16.97     0  9.433981      12  ddC
4       2     0  6.00     0  6.324555       0  ddI
5       2     6 12.00     0  8.124038       6  ddI
6       2    12 18.00     0  4.582576      12  ddI
7       2    18 19.00     0  5.000000      18  ddI
```

where start, stop, and event denote the risk interval and event status indicator, using the counting process formulation introduced in Section 3.5, column CD4 contains the square root CD4 cell count measurements, and obstime the time points at which these measurements were recorded (in fact it is a copy of the start column). We start our analysis by fitting the extended Cox model, in which the square root CD4 cell count is taken as an exogenous time-dependent covariate, and we additionally control for treatment. In model terms we have

$$h_i(t) = h_0(t) \exp\{\gamma \mathtt{ddI}_i + \alpha y_i(t)\},$$

where $\mathtt{ddI}_i$ is the dummy variable for the ddI group, and $y_i(t)$ denotes the observed level of the square root CD4 cell count. As we have seen in Section 3.5, to fit this model in R we use the syntax

```
> td.Cox <- coxph(Surv(start, stop, event) ~ drug + CD4,
    data = aids)

> td.Cox
Call:
coxph(formula = Surv(start, stop, event) ~ drug + CD4, data = aids)


          coef exp(coef) se(coef)     z       p
drugddI  0.309     1.363   0.1465  2.11 3.5e-02
CD4     -0.193     0.824   0.0244 -7.94 2.1e-15

Likelihood ratio test=94.6  on 2 df, p=0  n= 1405, number of events= 188
```

We observe that the CD4 cell count has indeed a strong association with the risk for death. In particular, a unit decrease in the square root CD4 cell count corresponds to a $\exp(-\alpha) = 1.2$-fold increase in the risk for death (95% CI: 1.16; 1.27).

We proceed by specifying and fitting a joint model that explicitly accounts for the endogeneity of the CD4 cell count marker. In particular, taking advantage of the randomization setup of the study, we fit the linear mixed model

$$
\begin{aligned}
y_i(t) &= m_i(t) + \varepsilon_i(t) \\
&= \beta_0 + \beta_1 t + \beta_2\{t \times \mathtt{ddI}_i\} + b_{i0} + b_{i1}t + \varepsilon_i(t),
\end{aligned}
$$

where in the fixed-effects part we include the main effect of time and the interaction of treatment with time, and in the random-effects design matrix we include an intercept and a time term. For the survival submodel and similarly to the Cox model above, we include as a time-independent covariate the treatment, and as a time-dependent one the true underlying profile of the CD4 cell count as estimated from the longitudinal model, i.e.,

$$
h_i(t) = h_0(t)\exp\{\gamma \mathtt{ddI}_i + \alpha m_i(t)\}.
$$

Contrary to the Cox model where $h_0(t)$ is unspecified, here the baseline risk function is assumed piecewise-constant with six knots placed at equally spaced percentiles of the observed event times. In order to fit this joint model using package **JM**, we need first to fit separately the linear mixed-effects and Cox models, and then supply the returned objects as main arguments in function `jointModel()`. More specifically, in the default specification, the joint model fitted by `jointModel()` has exactly the same structure for the longitudinal and survival submodels as these two separately fitted models, with the addition that in the survival submodel the effect of the estimated 'true' longitudinal outcome $m_i(t)$ is included in the linear predictor. The Cox model needs to be fitted in the dataset containing only the survival information (i.e., single row per patient). For the AIDS dataset this is available as the data.frame `aids.id`, which was constructed using the syntax

```
> aids.id <- aids[!duplicated(aids$patient), ]
```

Function `jointModel()` uses the fitted linear mixed and Cox models (supplied as the first two arguments) to extract all the required information (e.g., response vectors, design matrices, the event indicator, etc.) to fit the joint model; for this reason, in the call to `coxph()` we need to specify x = TRUE, such that the design matrix of the Cox model is included in the returned object.[1] The following code illustrates how to fit the joint model for the AIDS dataset:

```
> lmeFit.aids <- lme(CD4 ~ obstime + obstime:drug,
      random = ~ obstime | patient, data = aids)
```

---

[1]In addition to setting x = TRUE in the call to `coxph()`, it is also advisable (but not required) to set the option model = TRUE, such that the whole model frame (and not only the design matrix) is included in the returned object.

```
> coxFit.aids <- coxph(Surv(Time, death) ~ drug,
      data = aids.id, x = TRUE)

> jointFit.aids <- jointModel(lmeFit.aids, coxFit.aids,
      timeVar = "obstime", method = "piecewise-PH-aGH")

> summary(jointFit.aids)

Call:
jointModel(lmeObject = lmeFit.aids, survObject = coxFit.aids,
      timeVar = "obstime", method = "piecewise-PH-aGH")

Data Descriptives:
Longitudinal Process                Event Process
Number of Observations: 1405        Number of Events: 188 (40.3%)
Number of Groups: 467


Joint Model Summary:
Longitudinal Process: Linear mixed-effects model
Event Process: Relative risk model with piecewise-constant
                baseline risk function
Parameterization: Time-dependent

   log.Lik      AIC       BIC
 -4328.261 8688.523 8754.864


Variance Components:
            StdDev    Corr
(Intercept) 4.5839   (Intr)
obstime     0.1822 -0.0468
Residual    1.7377


Coefficients:
Longitudinal Process
                 Value Std.Err z-value p-value
(Intercept)     7.2203  0.2218 32.5537 <0.0001
obstime        -0.1917  0.0217 -8.8374 <0.0001
obstime:drugddI 0.0116  0.0302  0.3834  0.7014


Event Process
           Value Std.Err  z-value p-value
drugddI    0.3348  0.1565   2.1397  0.0324
Assoct    -0.2875  0.0359  -8.0141 <0.0001
log(xi.1) -2.5438  0.1913 -13.2953
log(xi.2) -2.2722  0.1784 -12.7328
log(xi.3) -1.9554  0.2403  -8.1357
log(xi.4) -2.5011  0.3412  -7.3297
log(xi.5) -2.4152  0.3156  -7.6531
```

```
log(xi.6) -2.4018  0.4007  -5.9941
log(xi.7) -2.4239  0.5301  -4.5725
```

```
Integration:
method: (pseudo) adaptive Gauss-Hermite
quadrature points: 5
```

```
Optimization:
Convergence: 0
```

The main argument `timeVar` of `jointModel()` is used to specify the name of the time variable in the linear mixed-effects model, which is required in internal computations of $m_i(t)$. The `method` argument specifies the type of baseline risk function, which here is assumed to be piecewise-constant, and the numerical integration approach (for more information regarding the numerical integration options, the reader is referred to Section 4.3.5). A detailed output of the fitted joint model is produced by function `summary()` that returns, among others, the parameter estimates, their standard errors, and asymptotic Wald tests for both the longitudinal and survival submodels. In the results for the event process, the parameter labeled 'Assoct' is, in fact, parameter α in (4.1) that measures the association between $m_i(t)$ (i.e., in our case of the true square root CD4 cell count) and the risk for death. The parameters `xi.1`, ..., `xi.7` are the ξ_q ($q = 1, \ldots, 7$) parameters for the piecewise-constant baseline risk function in (4.3). The joint model also finds a strong association between the square root CD4 cell count and the risk for death, with a unit decrease in the marker corresponding to a $\exp(-\alpha) = 1.3$-fold increase in the risk for death (95% CI: 1.24; 1.43). Comparing the point estimates and the corresponding 95% confidence intervals from the extended Cox model and the joint model, we clearly observe non-negligible differences. In particular, the log hazard ratio for the square root CD4 cell count in the joint model is about 49% larger than in the extended Cox model, and the upper bound of the 95% confidence interval for the hazard ratio from the Cox model is just above the lower bound of the same confidence interval from the joint model. These findings convincingly demonstrate the degree of attenuation in the regression coefficients of the standard Cox analysis due to the measurement error in the CD4 cell count levels.

Package **JM** follows the random-effects paradigm and currently only works with linear mixed-effects submodels with iid error terms and no serial correlation structure as in (4.6). Therefore, in the call to `lme()` to produce the object supplied as first argument to `jointModel()`, users should not specify a correlation structure (`correlation` argument) or a variance function (`weights` argument). Regarding the covariance matrix of the random effects, by default `jointModel()` assumes it to be unstructured and estimates all of its free parameters. However, it also allows for a diagonal covariance matrix, which can be specified using function `pdDiag()` in the `random` argument of `lme()`. This option is particularly useful when high-dimensional random-effects structures are considered. Moreover, in addition to the piecewise-constant baseline risk function assumed in the joint model fitted to the AIDS data, `jointModel()` also allows for alternative formulations of the survival submodel. These are specified by the `method` argument, and available options are

`method = "piecewise-PH-GH"`: the relative risk model (4.1) with a piecewise-constant baseline risk function (4.3). By default six internal knots are used placed at equally spaced percentiles of the observed event times. To change the default number of internal knots, the control argument `lng.in.kn` can be used, whereas to directly specify the positions of the knots, one can use the control argument `knots`.

`method = "spline-PH-GH"`: the relative risk model (4.1) with a spline-approximation of the log baseline risk function (4.4). Similar to the piecewise-constant, by default five internal knots are used placed at equally spaced percentiles of the observed event times, and again argument `lng.in.kn` and `knots` may be used for finer control.

`method = "Cox-PH-GH"`: the relative risk model (4.1) with an unspecified baseline risk function. This assumption turns out to be equivalent to assuming that $h_0(\cdot)$ is discrete with point-masses at the unique event times, i.e.,

$$h_0(t) = \begin{cases} \xi_q, & t = T_q^* \\ 0, & t \neq T_q^*, \end{cases}$$

where T_q^* denotes the qth unique true event time. This option corresponds to the joint model proposed by Wulfsohn and Tsiatis (1997).

`method = "weibull-PH-GH"`: the relative risk model (4.1) with a Weibull baseline risk function. In this case $h_0(t) = \sigma_t t^{\sigma_t - 1}$ and the design matrix W for the baseline covariates in (4.1) also contains the intercept term.[2]

`method = "weibull-AFT-GH"`: an accelerated failure time model with a Weibull baseline risk function. More details regarding this formulation are given in Section 5.6.

4.3   Estimation of Joint Models

4.3.1   Two-Stage Approaches

Due to complexities (as it will be explained in the following sections) in the numerical computation of the likelihood of joint models, initial approaches to

---

[2]Note that the standard formulation of the Weibull baseline risk function has the form $h_0(t) = \phi \sigma_t t^{\sigma_t - 1}$, and therefore the intercept term corresponds to $\log(\phi)$.

fit these models have focused on two-stage methods. In particular, Self and Pawitan (1992) proposed a joint model with a relative risk submodel of the form (4.1) with an unspecified baseline risk function $h_0(t)$, and with the term $\exp\{\alpha m_i(t)\}$ replaced by $\{1 + \alpha m_i(t)\}$, such that the model would be linear in the random effects b_i. The authors proposed to estimate this joint model using a two-step inferential approach, in which at step one the random effects are estimated using a least-squares approach, and at step two these estimates are used to impute appropriate values of $m_i(t)$ that are substituted in the classical partial likelihood of the Cox model. Tsiatis et al. (1995) also developed a two-stage approach to estimate the joint model that combines (4.1) with (4.5), but without linearizing the hazard function. In particular, for each unique event time they proposed to replace in the partial likelihood contribution the term $m_i(t)$ with the estimate $E\{m_i(t) \mid \mathcal{Y}_i(t), T_i \geq t\}$. For any event time t, this estimate can be obtained by fitting the corresponding mixed model using the observed responses up to time t from all the subjects still at risk at t, and using the empirical Bayes estimates of the random effect b_i to calculate the best linear unbiased predictor of $m_i(t)$.

Even though these approaches are relatively easy to implement with standard software, in many instances they produce biased results. This has been shown with a series of simulations studies by Dafni and Tsiatis (1998), Tsiatis and Davidian (2001), Ye et al. (2008b), and Sweeting and Thompson (2011). For this reason and instead of relying on approximations, the literature for this type of joint models has primarily focused on full likelihood approaches that eliminate this bias.

4.3.2 Joint Likelihood Formulation

The main estimation method that has been proposed for joint models is (semiparametric) maximum likelihood (Wulfsohn and Tsiatis, 1997; Henderson et al., 2000; Hsieh et al., 2006). The asymptotic properties of the semiparametric maximum likelihood estimators under an unspecified baseline risk function have been investigated by Zeng and Cai (2005). Bayesian estimation of joint models using MCMC techniques has been considered by Hanson et al. (2011), Chi and Ibrahim (2006), Brown and Ibrahim (2003), Xu and Zeger (2001), and Wang and Taylor (2001), among others. Moreover, Tsiatis and Davidian (2001) have proposed a conditional score approach in which the random effects are treated as nuisance parameters, and they developed a set of unbiased estimating equations that yields consistent and asymptotically normal estimators.

We give here the basics of the maximum likelihood method for joint models as one of the more traditional approaches. The maximum likelihood estimates are derived as the modes of the log-likelihood function corresponding to the joint distribution of the observed outcomes $\{T_i, \delta_i, y_i\}$. To define this joint distribution we will assume that the vector of time-independent random effects b_i underlies both the longitudinal and survival processes. This means that these random effects account for both the association between the longitudinal and event outcomes, and the correlation between the repeated measurements in the longitudinal process (conditional independence). Formally, we have that

$$p(T_i, \delta_i, y_i \mid b_i; \theta) \;=\; p(T_i, \delta_i \mid b_i; \theta)\, p(y_i \mid b_i; \theta), \quad \text{and} \qquad (4.7)$$

$$p(y_i \mid b_i; \theta) \;=\; \prod_j p\{y_i(t_{ij}) \mid b_i; \theta\}, \qquad (4.8)$$

where $\theta = (\theta_t^\top, \theta_y^\top, \theta_b^\top)^\top$ denotes the full parameter vector, with θ_t denoting the parameters for the event time outcome, θ_y the parameters for the longitudinal outcomes and θ_b the unique parameters of the random-effects covariance matrix, and y_i is the $n_i \times 1$ vector of longitudinal responses of the ith subject. In addition, we assume that given the observed history, the censoring mechanism and the visiting process are independent of the true event times and future longitudinal measurements. As defined earlier, the visiting process is the mechanism (stochastic or deterministic) that generates the time points at which longitudinal measurements are collected (Lipsitz et al., 2002), and for any time point t, we define as observed history all available information for the longitudinal process prior to t. Practically speaking, these assumptions imply the belief that decisions on whether a subject withdraws from the study or appears at the clinic for a longitudinal measurement depend on the observed past history (longitudinal measurements and baseline covariates), but there is no additional dependence on underlying, latent subject characteristics associated with prognosis. A setting in which these assumptions are violated is when either of the two processes depends on the random effects. This is because such a dependence implicitly corresponds to a dependence to future longitudinal measurements. Evaluating the plausibility of the non-informativeness for the visiting and censoring processes usually requires external information from subject-matter experts, since the observed data do not contain enough information to suggest otherwise.

Under these assumptions the log-likelihood contribution for the ith subject can be formulated as follows

$$\log p(T_i, \delta_i, y_i; \theta) = \log \int p(T_i, \delta_i, y_i, b_i; \theta)\, db_i \qquad (4.9)$$

$$= \log \int p(T_i, \delta_i \mid b_i; \theta_t, \beta) \Big[\prod_j p\{y_i(t_{ij}) \mid b_i; \theta_y\}\Big] p(b_i; \theta_b)\, db_i,$$

with the conditional density for the survival part $p(T_i, \delta_i \mid b_i; \theta_t, \beta)$ taking the form

$$p(T_i, \delta_i \mid b_i; \theta_t, \beta) \;=\; h_i(T_i \mid \mathcal{M}_i(T_i); \theta_t, \beta)^{\delta_i} \mathcal{S}_i(T_i \mid \mathcal{M}_i(T_i); \theta_t, \beta) \quad (4.10)$$

$$= \left[h_0(T_i) \exp\{\gamma^\top w_i + \alpha m_i(T_i)\} \right]^{\delta_i}$$
$$\times \exp\left(-\int_0^{T_i} h_0(s) \exp\{\gamma^\top w_i + \alpha m_i(s)\} \, ds \right),$$

where $h_0(\cdot)$ can be any positive function of time, such as the piecewise-constant model (4.3), or the B-spline model (4.4) or the hazard function of any known distribution, and the survival function is given by (4.2). The joint density for the longitudinal responses together with the random effects is given by

$$p(y_i \mid b_i; \theta)p(b_i; \theta) \;=\; \prod_j p\{y_i(t_{ij}) \mid b_i; \theta_y\}p(b_i; \theta_b) \qquad (4.11)$$

$$= (2\pi\sigma^2)^{-n_i/2} \exp\{- \parallel y_i - X_i\beta - Z_i b_i \parallel^2 / 2\sigma^2\}$$
$$\times (2\pi)^{-q_b/2} \det(D)^{-1/2} \exp\left(-b_i^\top D^{-1} b_i / 2\right),$$

where q_b denotes the dimensionality of the random-effects vector, and $\parallel x \parallel = \{\sum_i x_i^2\}^{1/2}$ denotes the Euclidean vector norm.

Maximization of the log-likelihood function $\ell(\theta) = \sum_i \log p(T_i, \delta_i, y_i; \theta)$ with respect to θ can be achieved using standard algorithms, such as the Expectation-Maximization (EM; Dempster et al., 1977) algorithm or the Newton-Raphson algorithm or any of its variants (Lange, 2004). In the joint modeling literature the EM algorithm has been traditionally preferred (treating the random effects as 'missing data'), mainly due to the fact that in the M-step some of the parameters have closed-form updates. However, a serious drawback of the EM algorithm is its linear convergence rate that results in slow convergence especially near the maximum. Nonetheless, Rizopoulos et al. (2009) have noted that the score vector corresponding to $\ell(\theta)$ is, in fact, the key function required either in the EM or a Newton-type algorithm. In particular, it is useful to note that this score vector can be rewritten in the form

$$
\begin{aligned}
S(\theta) \;&=\; \sum_i \frac{\partial}{\partial \theta^\top} \log \int p(T_i, \delta_i \mid b_i; \theta)\, p(y_i \mid b_i; \theta)\, p(b_i; \theta)\, db_i \\[4pt]
&=\; \sum_i \frac{1}{p(T_i, \delta_i, y_i; \theta)} \frac{\partial}{\partial \theta^\top} \int p(T_i, \delta_i \mid b_i; \theta)\, p(y_i \mid b_i; \theta)\, p(b_i; \theta)\, db_i \\[4pt]
&=\; \sum_i \frac{1}{p(T_i, \delta_i, y_i; \theta)} \int \frac{\partial}{\partial \theta^\top} \{ p(T_i, \delta_i \mid b_i; \theta)\, p(y_i \mid b_i; \theta)\, p(b_i; \theta) \}\, db_i \\[4pt]
&=\; \sum_i \int \left[\frac{\partial}{\partial \theta^\top} \log\{ p(T_i, \delta_i \mid b_i; \theta)\, p(y_i \mid b_i; \theta)\, p(b_i; \theta) \} \right] \\[4pt]
&\qquad\qquad\qquad \times \frac{p(T_i, \delta_i \mid b_i; \theta)\, p(y_i \mid b_i; \theta)\, p(b_i; \theta)}{p(T_i, \delta_i, y_i; \theta)}\, db_i \\[4pt]
&=\; \sum_i \int A(\theta, b_i)\, p(b_i \mid T_i, \delta_i, y_i; \theta)\, db_i, \qquad\qquad\qquad (4.12)
\end{aligned}
$$

where $A(\cdot)$ denotes the complete data score vector, given by $A(\theta, b_i) = \partial\{\log p(T_i, \delta_i \mid b_i; \theta) + \log p(y_i \mid b_i; \theta) + \log p(b_i; \theta)\}/\partial\theta^\top$. Note that the observed data score vector is expressed as the expected value of the complete data score vector with respect to the posterior distribution of the random effects. This implies that (4.12) can play a double role. In particular, if the score equations corresponding to (4.12) are solved with respect to θ, with $p(b_i \mid T_i, \delta_i, y_i; \theta)$ fixed at the θ value of the previous iteration, then this corresponds to an EM algorithm, whereas if the score equations are solved with respect to θ considering $p(b_i \mid T_i, \delta_i, y_i; \theta)$, also a function of θ, then this corresponds to a direct maximization of the observed data log-likelihood $\ell(\theta)$. More details regarding the specification of the steps of the EM algorithm for joint models are given in Appendix B.

This last fact also facilitates a straightforward calculation of the standard errors for the parameter estimates. In particular, even if we have estimated the joint model using the EM algorithm, we can easily make use of the observed data score vector (4.12) to calculate the Hessian matrix and subsequently standard errors using the observed information matrix (i.e., the negative of the inverse Hessian matrix). Using similar computations as in the derivation of the score vector above, we can rewrite the Hessian matrix in the following form:

$$
\begin{aligned}
\frac{\partial S_i(\theta)}{\partial \theta} \;&=\; \frac{\partial}{\partial \theta} \int A(\theta, b_i) p(b_i \mid T_i, \delta_i, y_i; \theta)\, db_i \\[4pt]
&=\; \int \frac{\partial A(\theta, b_i)}{\partial \theta} p(b_i \mid T_i, \delta_i, y_i; \theta)\, db_i \\[4pt]
&\qquad + \underbrace{\int A(\theta, b_i) \frac{\partial p(b_i \mid T_i, \delta_i, y_i; \theta)}{\partial \theta}\, db_i}_{I_1},
\end{aligned}
$$

where

$$
\begin{aligned}
I_1 &= \int A(\theta, b_i) \left\{ \frac{\partial \log p(b_i \mid T_i, \delta_i, y_i; \theta)}{\partial \theta} \right\}^{\top} p(b_i \mid T_i, \delta_i, y_i; \theta) \, db_i \\
&= \int A(\theta, b_i) \left\{ \frac{\partial \{\log p(T_i, \delta_i \mid b_i; \theta) + \log p(y_i \mid b_i; \theta) + \log p(b_i; \theta)\}}{\partial \theta} \right. \\
&\qquad\qquad \left. - \frac{\partial \log p(T_i, \delta_i, y_i; \theta)}{\partial \theta} \right\}^{\top} p(b_i \mid T_i, \delta_i, y_i; \theta) \, db_i \\
&= \int A(\theta, b_i) \left\{ A(\theta, b_i) - S_i(\theta) \right\}^{\top} p(b_i \mid T_i, \delta_i, y_i; \theta) \, db_i.
\end{aligned}
$$

However, in practice, it is typically easier to employ a numerical derivative routine, such as the forward or the central difference approximation (Press et al., 2007), and calculate the Hessian using only the function that computes the score vector. After having estimated $\mathcal{I}(\theta)$, standard errors for the parameter estimates can be based on the estimated observed information matrix, i.e.,

$$
\mathrm{v\hat{a}r}(\hat{\theta}) = \{\mathcal{I}(\hat{\theta})\}^{-1}, \quad \text{with} \quad \mathcal{I}(\hat{\theta}) = - \sum_{i=1}^{n} \frac{\partial S_i(\theta)}{\partial \theta} \bigg|_{\theta = \hat{\theta}}.
$$

We should note that because of the dropout caused by the occurrence of events, the observed information matrix is preferable to the expected one for the calculation of standard errors; for more details, we refer to Section 4.6, and Kenward and Molenberghs (1998).

4.3.3 Standard Errors with an Unspecified Baseline Risk Function

As we have discussed in Chapter 3, the great advantage of the Cox model in standard survival analysis is that the partial likelihood can be used to estimate the regression coefficients of a relative risk model. This in practice means that standard errors and inference for the regression coefficients of the (extended) Cox model enjoy nice asymptotic properties similar to those of asymptotic maximum likelihood theory, without having to specify an appropriate baseline risk function (Andersen and Gill, 1982).

Unfortunately, under the joint modeling framework this nice feature is not carried over (Hsieh et al., 2006). In particular, due to the use of random effects, and, as we have seen in Section 4.3.2, estimation of joint models can no longer be based on the partial likelihood alone and full likelihood approach must be employed instead. When we define a joint model with an unspecified baseline risk function for the survival submodel, the calculation of the likelihood is based on nonparametric maximum likelihood arguments under which the unspecified cumulative incidence function $H_0(t) = \int_0^t h_0(s) ds$ is replaced by a step function with jumps at the unique event times (van der Vaart, 1998). Under this setting it is evident that the parameter vector θ is typically of very high dimension because it also contains the high-dimensional subvector $h_0(t)$.

From a practical point of view the high dimensionality of the parameter vector may result in numerical complications in the calculation and inversion of the Hessian matrix required to produce standard errors. For this reason estimation of standard errors is typically based on a profile likelihood approach. That is, $\ell_p(\beta, \sigma, \gamma, \alpha, \hat{h}_0(\beta, \sigma, \gamma, \alpha))$, where $\hat{h}_0(\beta, \sigma, \gamma, \alpha)$ denotes the nonparametric maximum likelihood estimator of $h_0(t)$ as a function of the remaining parameters. In order for profile likelihood asymptotics to work, this nonparametric maximum likelihood estimator should not depend on $h_0(t)$ (Hsieh et al., 2006). Unfortunately, however, this is not the case under joint models because this estimator has no closed-form solution due to the use of random effects. In practice, the following estimator from the M-step of the EM algorithm is typically used:

$$\hat{h}_0(t) = \sum_{i=1}^{n} \frac{\delta_i I(T_i = t)}{\sum_{j=1}^{n} I(T_i \geq t) \int \exp\{\hat{\gamma}^\top w_j + \hat{\alpha} m_j(t, b)\} \, p(b_i \mid T_i, \delta_i, y_i; \hat{\theta}) \, db_i},$$

which, as it can be seen, remains a function of $h_0(t)$ through the posterior distribution of the random effects $p(b_i \mid T_i, \delta_i, y_i; \hat{\theta})$. For this reason, standard errors for the remaining parameter estimates $\hat{\theta}_{-h} = (\beta, \sigma, \gamma, \alpha)$ that are based on the profile score vector,

$$S(\theta_{-h}, \hat{h}_0(\theta_{-h})) = \frac{\partial}{\partial \theta_{-h}^\top} \ell_p(\theta_{-h}, \hat{h}_0(\theta_{-h})),$$

will be generally underestimated. To overcome this problem, Hsieh et al. (2006) proposed to use Bootstrapping (Efron and Tibshirani, 1994) to estimate standard errors when an unspecified baseline risk function is used. However, it is evident that such an approach renders joint models of this type rather computationally demanding. A feasible alternative is to postulate a flexible but parametric model for $h_0(t)$. As we have seen in Section 4.1.1, two options are to use cubic splines or a piecewise-constant model. The advantages of these parametric models are twofold: first, they can be made arbitrarily flexible by increasing the number of internal knots, and thus capture various shapes of $h_0(t)$, and second, under such models, estimation of standard errors directly follows from asymptotic maximum likelihood theory (Cox and Hinkley, 1974).

In function jointModel() standard errors for joint models with an unspecified baseline risk function (i.e., option "Cox-PH-GH" for the method argument) are calculated based on the profile score vector introduced above, and therefore users should expect these to be underestimated.

4.3.4 *Optimization Control in JM*

Function jointModel() implements a hybrid optimization procedure to locate the maximum likelihood estimates. In particular, this procedure starts with the EM algorithm for a fixed number of iterations, and if convergence is not achieved switches to a quasi-Newton algorithm until convergence is attained. Available quasi-Newton algorithms are the BFGS of `optim()` (Nash, 1990), and the PORT routines of `nlminb()` (Gay, 1990). Initial values for the parameters are taken from the linear mixed and survival models that are supplied as the first two arguments in `jointModel()`. During the EM iterations convergence is declared whenever either of the following two commonly used criteria is satisfied:

$$\max\{|\theta^{(it)} - \theta^{(it-1)}|/(|\theta^{(it-1)}| + \epsilon_1)\} < \epsilon_2,$$
$$\ell(\theta^{(it)}) - \ell(\theta^{(it-1)}) < \epsilon_3\{|\ell(\theta^{(it-1)})| + \epsilon_3\},$$

where $\theta^{(it)}$ denotes the parameters values at the itth iteration, $\ell(\theta) = \sum_i \log p(T_i, \delta_i, y_i; \theta)$. Commonly used values for ϵ_1 and ϵ_2 are about 10^{-3} or 10^{-4}, and ϵ_3 is by default set to `sqrt(.Machine$double.eps)`, which is about 10^{-8}. During the quasi-Newton iterations, typically only the latter criterion is used. A finer control of the optimization procedure is provided via the `control` argument of `jointModel()`. This specifies, among others, the number of EM (argument `iter.EM`) and quasi-Newton iterations (argument `iter.qN`), the type of quasi-Newton algorithm (argument `optimizer`), the tolerance values for the convergence criteria (arguments `tol1`, `tol2` and `tol3` corresponding to ϵ_1, ϵ_2 and ϵ_3, respectively), and the type of numerical derivative that calculates the Hessian matrix based on the score vector (i.e., forward or central difference approximation – arguments `numeriDeriv` and `eps.Hes`).

Changing the default values for these arguments can be easily achieved by directly including the control arguments of interest in the call to `jointModel()`. For example, to refit the joint model to the AIDS dataset, presented in Section 4.2, using 80 EM iterations, with a stricter convergence tolerance, and using the central difference approximation to calculate standard errors, the following syntax can be used:

```
> jointFit.aids <- jointModel(lmeFit.aids, coxFit.aids,
    timeVar = "obstime", method = "piecewise-PH-aGH", iter.EM = 80,
    tol3 = 1e-09, numeriDeriv = "cd", eps.Hes = 1e-04)
```

The last argument `eps.Hes` controls the step-size length in the central difference approximation.

4.3.5 *Numerical Integration*

A key computational difficulty in fitting joint models for longitudinal and survival data is that the integral with respect to time in the definition of the survival function (4.2), as well as the integral with respect to the random effects in the specification of the score vector (4.12), do not have an analytical solution, except in very special cases. This implies that a numerical approach is typically employed to approximate these integrals for each subject in the calculation of the log-likelihood and the score vector. This feature combined with the requirement for numerical optimization makes the fitting of joint models a computationally intensive task.

From the two integrals involved in the specification of a joint model, the one with respect to the random effects is the main computational bottleneck. In particular, the integral in the definition of the survival function is always a unidimensional one, and it can be relatively efficiently approximated using the 7-point or 15-point Gauss-Kronrod rule (Press et al., 2007). However, the integral with respect to the random effects becomes computationally demanding to approximate as its dimensionality increases. Standard numerical integration techniques to evaluate such multidimensional integrals include Gaussian quadrature rules and Monte Carlo sampling, and have been routinely utilized in fitting joint models in the literature (Wulfsohn and Tsiatis, 1997; Henderson et al., 2000; Song et al., 2002). Furthermore, Rizopoulos et al. (2009) and Ye et al. (2008a) have discussed the use of Laplace approximations for joint models that are more computationally efficient compared to the Gaussian quadrature and Monte Carlo, in settings where a high-dimensional random-effects vector is posited (e.g., to capture nonlinearities as explained in Section 4.1). Nonetheless, all of these approaches still remain relatively computationally demanding and constitute the main reason why joint models have not yet found their rightful place in the toolbox of modern applied statisticians.

An alternative approach that decreases the computational burden to some degree has been proposed by Rizopoulos (2012a). The idea behind this approach is to first fit the mixed-effects model for the longitudinal outcome and extract information regarding the location and scale of the posterior distribution of the random effects given the longitudinal responses for each subject. This information is then used to appropriately rescale the subject-specific integrands in the definitions of the log-likelihood and score vector of the joint model. To motivate this approach, we first introduce the standard and adaptive Gauss-Hermite rules for the calculation of the score vector of a joint model. Under the standard Gauss-Hermite rule, and for any form of the $A(\cdot)$ function of the random effects, the integral in the definition of the score vector is approximated by a weighted sum of integrand evaluations at prespecified abscissas:

$$E\{A(\theta, b_i) \mid T_i, \delta_i, y_i; \theta\} = \int A(\theta, b_i) p(b_i \mid T_i, \delta_i, y_i; \theta) \, db_i$$

$$\approx 2^{q_b/2} \sum_{t_1 \cdots t_q} \pi_t A(\theta, b_t \sqrt{2}) \, p(b_t \sqrt{2} \mid T_i, \delta_i, y_i; \theta) \exp(\|b_t\|^2),$$

where $\sum_{t_1 \cdots t_q}$ is used as shorthand for $\sum_{t_1=1}^{K} \cdots \sum_{t_q=1}^{K}$ with K denoting the number of quadrature points, and $b_t^\top = (b_{t_1}, \ldots, b_{t_q})$ are the abscissas with corresponding weights π_t. The location of the abscissas and the weights are designed to provide an exact solution to the integral if the integrand can be expressed in the form $\exp(-b^{\top}b)l(b)$, with $l(b)$ denoting any polynomial of degree $2K - 1$ or less that interpolates the abscissas. Thus, the quality of the approximation is improved as the number of quadrature points K is increased. However, due to the fact that the Gauss-Hermite rule requires evaluating the integrand over the cartesian product of the abscissas for each random effect, the computational burden increases exponentially with q_b. Another critical aspect that also greatly influences the quality of the Gauss-Hermite approximation is the locations of the quadrature points with respect to the location of the main mass of the integrand. That is, if $g(b) = A(\theta, b)p(b \mid T_i, \delta_i, y_i; \theta)$ is concentrated around a point far from zero, or if the spread in $g(b)$ is quite different from the weight function $\exp(-b^2)$, then applying the standard Gaussian-Hermite rule directly to $g(b)$ can give a very poor approximation, even for large K, because the abscissas in the quadrature rule will not be located where most of the mass of $g(b)$ is located (Pinheiro and Bates, 1995). To solve this problem, the adaptive Gauss-Hermite rule has been proposed that appropriately centers and scales the integrand in each iteration. More specifically,

$$E\{A(\theta, b_i) \mid T_i, \delta_i, y_i; \theta\}$$
$$\approx 2^{q_b/2}|\widehat{B}_i|^{-1} \sum_{t_1 \cdots t_q} \pi_t A(\theta, \hat{r}_t) \, p(\hat{r}_t \mid T_i, \delta_i, y_i; \theta) \exp(\|b_t\|^2), \quad (4.13)$$

where $\hat{r}_t = \hat{b}_i + \sqrt{2}\widehat{B}_i^{-1} b_t$, $\hat{b}_i = \arg\max_b\{\log p(T_i, \delta_i, y_i, b; \theta)\}$, and $\widehat{B}_i$ denotes the Choleski factor of $\widehat{H}_i$, with $\widehat{H}_i = -\partial^2 \log p(T_i, \delta_i, y_i, b; \theta)/\partial b \partial b^{\top}\big|_{b=\hat{b}_i}$. Using this transformation, the integrand approximately behaves like the density of a $\mathcal{N}(0, 2^{-1}\mathrm{I})$ distribution, and since the Gauss-Hermite weight function is proportional to this density, we achieve the optimal approximation. Thus, the adaptive Gauss-Hermite rule typically requires much less quadrature to obtain an approximation error of the same magnitude compared to the standard Gauss-Hermite. Nevertheless, the requirement for the location of the mode $\hat{b}_i$ and the calculation of the second order derivative matrix $\widehat{H}_i$ for each subject in each iteration dramatically increases the computational burden.

Fortunately, however, the computational burden behind the adaptive Gauss-Hermite rule can be considerably decreased by exploiting the properties of the posterior distribution of the random effects $p(b_i \mid T_i, \delta_i, y_i; \theta)$, whose mode $\hat{b}_i$ and second order derivative matrix $\widehat{H}_i$ we need to determine (Rizopoulos, 2012a). More specifically, if we write this density in the log-scale, then it is found to be proportional to

$$\log p(b_i \mid T_i, \delta_i, y_i; \theta)$$
$$\propto \sum_{j=1}^{n_i} \log p\{y_i(t_{ij}) \mid b_i; \theta_y\} + \log p(b_i; \theta_b) + \log p(T_i, \delta_i \mid b_i; \theta_t, \beta).$$

Thus, we observe that as n_i increases, the leading term in the log posterior density is the logarithm of the density of the linear mixed model, namely $\log p(y_i \mid b_i; \theta_y) = \sum_j \log p\{y_i(t_{ij}) \mid b_i; \theta_y\}$, which is quadratic in b_i and will resemble the shape of a multivariate normal distribution. In particular, using a variant of the Bayesian central limit theorem (Cox and Hinkley, 1974, pp. 399–400) and under general regularity conditions, we obtain that as $n_i \rightarrow \infty$,

$$p(b_i \mid T_i, \delta_i, y_i; \theta) \xrightarrow{P} \mathcal{N}(\tilde{b}_i, \tilde{H}_i^{-1}), \qquad (4.14)$$

where $\tilde{b}_i$ denotes the mode of $\log p(y_i \mid b; \theta_y)$ with respect to b, and $\tilde{H}_i = -\partial^2 \log p(y_i \mid b; \theta_y)/\partial b \partial b^\top \big|_{b=\tilde{b}_i}$. In practice, this suggests that as n_i increases, it is sufficient to re-center and re-scale the integrand for each subject by utilizing only the information that comes from the mixed-effects model for the longitudinal outcome. Thus, instead of the standard transformation used in the adaptive Gauss-Hermite rule (4.13), we can first fit the linear mixed-effects model, extract the empirical Bayes estimates $\tilde{b}_i = \arg\max_b \{\log p(y_i, b; \tilde{\theta}_y)\}$ and their covariance matrix $\tilde{H}_i^{-1}$ with $\tilde{H}_i = -\partial^2 \log p(y_i, b; \tilde{\theta}_y)/\partial b \partial b^\top \big|_{b=\tilde{b}_i}$, and use the transformation

$$
\begin{aligned}
&E\{A(\theta, b_i) \mid T_i, \delta_i, y_i; \theta\} \\
&\approx \ 2^{q/2} |\tilde{B}_i|^{-1} \sum_{t_1 \cdots t_q} \pi_t A(\theta, \tilde{r}_t) \, p(\tilde{r}_t \mid T_i, \delta_i, y_i; \theta) \exp(\|b_t\|^2), \quad (4.15)
\end{aligned}
$$

where $\tilde{r}_t = \tilde{b}_i + \sqrt{2}\tilde{B}^{-1} b_t$, $\tilde{B}_i$ denotes the Choleski factor of $\tilde{H}_i$, and $\tilde{\theta}_y$ are the maximum likelihood estimates from the linear mixed model fit. This procedure is very similar with the adaptive Gauss-Hermite rule, but we implement it only once, at the start of the optimization, and we do not further update the quadrature points afterwards. The computational advantages are twofold: first, we can use fewer quadrature points than we would have used in the standard Gauss-Hermite rule, and second, we can avoid the computationally demanding relocation of the quadrature points at each iteration of the adaptive Gauss-Hermite rule.

To illustrate the effectiveness of the pseudo-adaptive rule compared with the standard Gauss-Hermite rule, we refitted the joint model fitted to the AIDS dataset (Section 4.2) with various choices for the number of quadrature points, and compare the parameter estimates and the corresponding standard errors. The results are presented in Tables 4.1 and 4.2. We observe that the standard Gauss-Hermite rule needs about 13 to 15 quadrature points to provide more stable parameter estimates. On the contrary, the results from the pseudo-adaptive even with three points are very close to the ones using 15 points. The last line of Table 4.1 contains the time in sec required to fit the joint model under the different Gaussian quadrature settings, from which we clearly observe that the pseudo-adaptive rule with three points is considerably faster than the other options. Additional numerical studies (Rizopoulos, 2012a) have shown that the pseudo-adaptive rule performs excellent in practice for both the parameters of longitudinal and event time submodels, and, moreover, its performance did not seem to be compromised by the fact that the average n_i was quite small. Nevertheless, as it is the case for all types of

TABLE 4.1: A comparison of point estimates between the standard Gauss-Hermite quadrature rule and the pseudo-adaptive Gauss-Hermite quadrature rule for different numbers of quadrature points

	standard GH			pseudo-adaptive GH		
	9	13	15	3	5	15
ddI	0.30	0.35	0.35	0.33	0.33	0.33
α	−0.25	−0.29	−0.30	−0.29	−0.29	−0.29
$\log(\xi_1)$	−2.66	−2.53	−2.49	−2.54	−2.54	−2.54
$\log(\xi_2)$	−2.36	−2.24	−2.20	−2.27	−2.27	−2.27
$\log(\xi_3)$	−2.04	−1.93	−1.90	−1.95	−1.96	−1.96
$\log(\xi_4)$	−2.56	−2.47	−2.44	−2.50	−2.50	−2.50
$\log(\xi_5)$	−2.47	−2.39	−2.36	−2.41	−2.42	−2.42
$\log(\xi_6)$	−2.46	−2.38	−2.36	−2.40	−2.40	−2.40
$\log(\xi_7)$	−2.44	−2.37	−2.35	−2.42	−2.42	−2.42
Intercept	7.69	7.26	7.21	7.22	7.22	7.22
Time	−0.16	−0.19	−0.19	−0.19	−0.19	−0.19
Time:ddI	−0.02	0.02	0.02	0.01	0.01	0.01
$\log(\sigma)$	0.70	0.63	0.63	0.55	0.55	0.55
D_{11}	21.86	21.14	20.51	21.01	21.01	21.01
D_{12}	−0.05	−0.06	−0.04	−0.04	−0.04	−0.04
D_{22}	0.02	0.03	0.03	0.03	0.03	0.03
Time (sec)	113.67	143.39	178.62	15.10	33.76	290.18

mixed models that require numerical integration, it is advisable (especially in difficult datasets) to check the stability of the maximum likelihood estimates with an increasing number of Gauss-Hermite quadrature points.

4.3.6   Numerical Integration Control in **JM**

Function jointModel() provides three control arguments that allow for a fine control of the numerical integration algorithms. In particular, for the integral in the definition of the survival function (4.2), argument GKk controls the number of Gauss-Kronrod quadrature points, whereas for the integral with respect to the random effects, arguments method and GHk control the type of numerical integration and the number of Gauss-Hermite quadrature points. For the latter case, and as we have already seen in Section 4.2, the first two parts of the character string supplied in the method argument specify the baseline risk function and the type of survival model. The last part, however,

TABLE 4.2: A comparison of standard error estimates between the standard Gauss-Hermite quadrature rule and the pseudo-adaptive Gauss-Hermite quadrature rule for different numbers of quadrature points. D^*_{ij} denotes the ij-element of the Choleski factor of the random effects covariance matrix D

	standard GH			pseudo-adaptive GH		
	9	13	15	3	5	15
ddI	0.154	0.157	0.158	0.156	0.156	0.156
α	0.031	0.036	0.038	0.036	0.036	0.036
$\log(\xi_1)$	0.184	0.192	0.197	0.191	0.191	0.191
$\log(\xi_2)$	0.173	0.181	0.186	0.179	0.178	0.178
$\log(\xi_3)$	0.236	0.241	0.244	0.240	0.240	0.240
$\log(\xi_4)$	0.339	0.342	0.344	0.341	0.341	0.341
$\log(\xi_5)$	0.313	0.316	0.318	0.316	0.316	0.316
$\log(\xi_6)$	0.398	0.401	0.403	0.401	0.401	0.401
$\log(\xi_7)$	0.527	0.533	0.535	0.530	0.530	0.530
Intercept	0.123	0.122	0.134	0.222	0.222	0.222
Time	0.021	0.021	0.021	0.021	0.022	0.022
Time:ddI	0.027	0.027	0.027	0.030	0.030	0.030
$\log(\sigma)$	0.024	0.024	0.024	0.027	0.027	0.028
$\tilde{D}_{11}$	0.036	0.036	0.036	0.036	0.036	0.036
$\tilde{D}_{12}$	0.015	0.015	0.016	0.015	0.016	0.016
$\tilde{D}_{22}$	0.132	0.112	0.111	0.076	0.096	0.097

specifies the type of numerical integration, where GH stands for the standard Gauss-Hermite rule, and aGH for the pseudo-adaptive one. For instance, the joint model fitted in Section 4.2 was based on the pseudo-adaptive rule with the default number of quadrature points (i.e., five in this case). To refit the same model with 15 points, we should use the syntax

```
> jointFit.aids <- jointModel(lmeFit.aids, coxFit.aids,
      timeVar = "obstime", method = "piecewise-PH-aGH", GHk = 15)
```

whereas to fit a joint model with the standard Gauss-Hermite rule and 21 points for the random effects and the 15-point Gauss-Kronrod rule, we can use

```
> jointModel(..., method = "piecewise-PH-GH", GHk = 21, GKk = 15)
```

4.3.7   Convergence Problems

We have seen in the previous two sections that fitting joint models for longitudinal and survival data requires a combination of a double numerical integration and optimization. These requirements make joint models computationally and numerically much more demanding compared to a separate analysis per outcome. This implies that in some occasions we may experience convergence problems. Function `jointModel()` attempts to make reasonable choices for default control arguments (e.g., number of quadrature points, number of iterations, convergence tolerances, etc.), but these are not guaranteed to work in all datasets. Thus, joint modelers should also develop a general intuition on how to fine-tune the optimization procedure, by suitably changing the default values of the control arguments, in order to succeed in fitting the joint model(s) of interest in 'difficult' datasets. To aid in that respect, `jointModel()` has the control argument `verbose`, which, if set to `TRUE`, the optimization path towards the maximum is printed on the screen. This argument can be used to spot a possible divergence of the algorithm early on, and therefore stop it and re-initiate with different defaults. In the majority of the cases, the most helpful changes are changing the stating values (using argument `init` of `jointModel()`), increasing the number of EM iterations, and choosing other locations for the knots in the piecewise-constant or spline-based baseline hazard functions.

As an example of the usefulness of the `verbose` argument, we fit an elaborate joint model to the Aortic Valve data. In particular, as it can be seen from Figure 4.2, some of the patients in this dataset showed nonlinear evolutions in their aortic gradient values. Following the recommendations of Section 4.1.2 and in order to capture the nonlinear subject-specific evolutions, we postulate a flexible linear mixed-effects model that expands the time effect into a B-splines basis matrix. The specification of this model is as follows:

$$y_i(t) = m_i(t) + \varepsilon_i(t)$$

$$= (\beta_0 + b_{i0}) + (\beta_1 + b_{i1})B_n(t, \lambda_1) + (\beta_2 + b_{i2})B_n(t, \lambda_2)$$

$$+ (\beta_3 + b_{i3})B_n(t, \lambda_3) + \beta_4\{B_n(t, \lambda_1) \times \texttt{TypeOpRR}_i\}$$

$$+ \beta_5\{B_n(t, \lambda_2) \times \texttt{TypeOpRR}_i\} + \beta_6\{B_n(t, \lambda_3) \times \texttt{TypeOpRR}_i\}$$

$$+ \beta_7\texttt{Age}_i + \beta_8\texttt{TypeOpRR}_i + \varepsilon_i(t),$$

where $\{B_n(t, \lambda_k); k = 1, 2, 3\}$ denotes a B-spline basis matrix for a natural cubic spline of time with two internal knots placed at the 33.3% and 66.7%

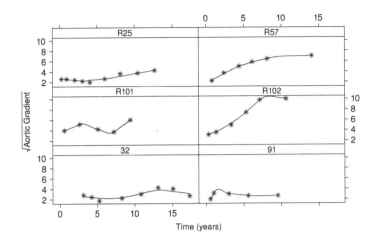

FIGURE 4.2: Subject-specific longitudinal profiles for six patients from the Aortic Valve study.

percentiles of the follow-up times, `TypeOpRR` denotes the dummy variable for the root replacement type of operation, and we also control for the age of the patients at baseline. To fit this model in R we use function **ns()** from package **splines** that generates the basis matrix for the natural cubic splines. The corresponding syntax is

```
> lmeFit.av <- lme(sqrt(AoGradient) ~ ns(time, 3) * TypeOp + Age,
    data = AoValv, random = list(id = pdDiag(form = ~ ns(time, 3))))
```

The formulation in the **random** argument in the call to **lme()** specifies a diagonal covariance matrix for the random effects $b_i^\top = (b_{i0}, \ldots, b_{i3})$. For the survival part we fit a simple Cox model in which we only include the type of operation as a covariate, i.e.,

$$h_i(t \mid \mathcal{M}_i(t), w_i) = h_0(t) \exp\{\gamma \texttt{TypeOpRR}_i + \alpha m_i(t)\},$$

and we fit it in R using

```
> coxFit.av <- coxph(Surv(Time, death) ~ TypeOp, data = AoValv.id,
    x = TRUE)
```

Based on the fitted linear mixed and Cox models we fit the corresponding joint model, setting also the **verbose** argument to TRUE,

```
> jointFit.av <- jointModel(lmeFit.av, coxFit.av, timeVar = "time",
    method = "piecewise-PH-aGH", verbose = TRUE)
```

```
iter: 1
log-likelihood: -2107.672
betas: 4.275 1.4198 2.4489 2.4651 -0.4827
       -0.0201 -0.1128 -0.5105 -1.1762
sigma: 0.6148
gammas: -0.0336
alpha: -0.3875
xi: 0.2721 0.3413 0.431 0.3953 0.9664 0.838 0
D: 0.453 4.4725 1.973 1.2492
```

.
.
.

```
iter: 4
log-likelihood: 0
betas: 1377.697 427.4287 -3691.91 -2033.504
       -1791.215 1.443 -1806.379 5975.356 5294.583
sigma: 8.516
gammas: 0.1557
alpha: -0.6494
xi: 0.1113 0.143 0.2657 0.3479 0.9492 0.7238 0
D: 0.7401 7.0717 2.7674 2.039
```

The printed output is rather self-explanatory. Iteration 1 corresponds to the initial values taken from the two separately fitted submodels, and seems to produce a quite reasonable value for the log-likelihood of the joint model. However, by iteration 4 we observe that the algorithm has diverged producing a log-likelihood value of zero, and huge values for the parameters of the longitudinal submodel. A divergence occurring so early on is, in the majority of the cases, attributed to a failure of the numerical integration rule or to a parameter scaling problem. For this example, it turns out to be the latter. In particular, for optimization algorithms it is often important that the optimization problem (i.e., finding the maximum) is well scaled, in the sense that a unit change in any of the parameters results in a change of similar magnitude in the log-likelihood. However, from the output of the longitudinal submodel we observe that the coefficient for Age is several orders of the magnitude smaller compared to the other parameters:

```
> summary(lmeFit.av)
```

. . .

	Value	Std.Error	DF	t-value	p-value
(Intercept)	4.274976	0.2444552	980	17.487764	0.0000
ns(time, 3)1	1.419787	0.3136259	980	4.527007	0.0000

```
ns(time, 3)2                2.448946 0.3903572 980  6.273602 0.0000
ns(time, 3)3                2.465096 0.2942019 980  8.378925 0.0000
TypeOpRR                   -0.482702 0.1881059 286 -2.566121 0.0108
Age                        -0.020102 0.0038463 286 -5.226250 0.0000
ns(time, 3)1:TypeOpRR -0.112810 0.4052867 980 -0.278345 0.7808
ns(time, 3)2:TypeOpRR -0.510547 0.5304223 980 -0.962529 0.3360
ns(time, 3)3:TypeOpRR -1.176218 0.6369125 980 -1.846749 0.0651
 . . .
```

This indicates that if we would like to avoid the 'overshooting' of the log-likelihood during the optimization procedure, we should scale the coefficient for Age such that it changes in smaller steps than the coefficients of the other parameters. In jointModel() this can be achieved by setting the **parscale** control argument, which is in fact a control argument of optim(). This should be a vector of scaling values for all the parameters in the optimization, which means that we should specify the scaling vector for all the parameters of the joint model. A simpler alternative approach to overcome this problem is to refit the linear mixed model but with Age scaled by its sample standard deviation:

```
> lmeFit2.av <- lme(sqrt(AoGradient) ~ ns(time, 3) * TypeOp + I(Age/15),
    data = AoValv, random = list(id = pdDiag(form = ~ ns(time, 3))))

> jointFit2.av <- jointModel(lmeFit2.av, coxFit.av, timeVar = "time",
    method = "piecewise-PH-aGH", verbose = TRUE)

> summary(jointFit2.av)

 . . .

Variance Components:
              StdDev
(Intercept)   0.6584
ns(time, 3)1  2.1192
ns(time, 3)2  1.3661
ns(time, 3)3  0.3175
Residual      0.6289

Coefficients:
Longitudinal Process
              Value Std.Err z-value p-value
(Intercept)   4.3392 0.2422 17.9142 <0.0001
ns(time, 3)1  1.4735 0.3112  4.7342 <0.0001
ns(time, 3)2  2.2797 0.3831  5.9507 <0.0001
ns(time, 3)3  2.2362 0.2277  9.8193 <0.0001
TypeOpRR     -0.4845 0.1886 -2.5683  0.0102
I(Age/15)    -0.3174 0.0566 -5.6086 <0.0001
```

```
ns(time, 3)1:TypeOpRR -0.0965  0.4015 -0.2405  0.8100
ns(time, 3)2:TypeOpRR -0.5994  0.5066 -1.1831  0.2368
ns(time, 3)3:TypeOpRR -1.3934  0.5537 -2.5164  0.0119
```

```
Event Process
                Value   Std.Err  z-value  p-value
TypeOpRR       0.0964    0.3041   0.3170   0.7512
Assoct        -0.3580    0.1521  -2.3533   0.0186
log(xi.1)     -3.1443    0.6225  -5.0509
log(xi.2)     -2.7835    0.7187  -3.8731
log(xi.3)     -2.5458    0.7633  -3.3352
log(xi.4)     -2.6127    0.8070  -3.2373
log(xi.5)     -1.7131    0.7661  -2.2361
log(xi.6)     -1.8092    0.8593  -2.1054
log(xi.7)    -14.8215  516.6937  -0.0287
```

. . .

We observe that after this transformation the joint model converges happily without any problems, and produces reasonable parameter estimates.

4.4   Asymptotic Inference for Joint Models

4.4.1   Hypothesis Testing

Having fitted the joint model under a maximum likelihood framework, the standard asymptotic likelihood inference tests are directly available. In general, if we are interested in testing the null hypothesis

$$H_0 : \theta = \theta_0 \quad \text{versus} \quad H_a : \theta \neq \theta_0, \tag{4.16}$$

we could use:

a **Likelihood Ratio Test**, with the test statistic defined as:

$$LRT = -2\{\ell(\hat{\theta}_0) - \ell(\hat{\theta})\},$$

where $\hat{\theta}_0$ and $\hat{\theta}$ denote the maximum likelihood estimates under the null and alternative hypothesis, respectively;

a **Score Test**, with the test statistic defined as:

$$U = S^\top(\hat{\theta}_0) \left\{ \mathcal{I}(\hat{\theta}_0) \right\}^{-1} S(\hat{\theta}_0),$$

where $S(\cdot)$ and $\mathcal{I}(\cdot)$ denotes the score function and the observed information matrix of the model under the alternative hypothesis;

or a **Wald Test**, with the test statistic defined as

$$W = (\hat{\theta} - \theta_0)^\top \mathcal{I}(\hat{\theta})(\hat{\theta} - \theta_0).$$

Under the null hypothesis, the asymptotic distribution of each of these tests is a chi-squared distribution on p degrees of freedom, with p denoting the number of parameters being tested. For a single parameter θ_j the Wald test is equivalent to $(\hat{\theta}_j - \theta_{0j})/\widehat{s.e.}(\hat{\theta}_j)$, which under the null follows an asymptotic standard normal distribution. These test statistics are approximately low-order Taylor series expansion of each other, and they are asymptotically equivalent. However, in practice, when we are dealing with finite samples, they usually differ. In this case, the likelihood ratio test is generally considered the most reliable and the Wald test the least reliable. The score and Wald test require fitting the model only under the null and alternative hypotheses, respectively, whereas the likelihood ratio test requires to fit the joint model under both hypothesis, and thus it is a bit more computationally expensive. If there are missing data in the variable we are interested to test for, then the score test will be more efficient since it requires fitting the model only under the null and therefore, avoids a case-wise deletion of missing values (i.e., excluding subjects who have a missing value in the variable of interest).

In the joint modeling analysis of the AIDS presented in Section 4.2, the output of the `summary()` function also contains the univariate Wald tests for testing whether each of the fixed effects β in the longitudinal submodel, and the regression coefficients γ and the association parameter α in the survival submodel are statistically different from zero. If a general hypothesis is of interest, then the multivariate Wald test defined above could be used. For instance, for the joint model fitted to the AIDS dataset, we would like to test whether the overall time effect in the longitudinal process is different from zero. This corresponds to the following set of hypotheses:

$$H_0: \qquad \beta_1 = \beta_2 = 0$$
$$H_a: \qquad \beta_1 \neq 0 \ \text{ or } \ \beta_2 \neq 0,$$

where β_1 is the coefficient of the time effect, and β_2 the coefficient of the interaction effect between time and treatment. Wald tests for joint models are performed using function `anova()`. In the call to this function we specify that we only need the Wald tests for the parameters of the longitudinal submodel.

```
> anova(jointFit.aids, process = "Longitudinal")
Marginal Wald Tests Table

Longitudinal Process
              Chisq df Pr(>|Chi|)
obstime     126.3887  2    <1e-04
drug          0.1470  1    0.7014
obstime:drug  0.1470  1    0.7014
```

Each row in the output table corresponds to a Wald test for all the parameters involving that specific term. Thus, the first row that contains the results for the time variable, corresponds to testing whether all terms involving time are significantly different from zero, which in turn corresponds to the set of hypotheses given above. The result indicates a quite strong overall time effect. For testing more general set of hypotheses, we can restate (4.16) as:

$$H_0 : L\theta = 0 \quad \text{versus} \quad H_a : L\theta \neq 0,$$

where L specifies the linear combination of coefficients we would like to test. For instance, to test whether the covariates in the survival submodel contribute something in explaining the variability in the risk for death of the advanced AIDS patients, i.e., to test the global null hypothesis:

$$H_0 : \quad \gamma = \alpha = 0$$
$$H_a : \quad \gamma \neq 0 \text{ or } \alpha \neq 0,$$

we specify that we are interested only in the parameters of the survival submodel, and that L is the identity matrix of appropriate dimensions:

```
> anova(jointFit.aids, process = "Event", L = diag(2))
Marginal Wald Tests Table

User-defined Contrasts Matrix
    Chisq df Pr(>|Chi|)
L 67.3251  2    < 1e-04
```

A problem with the Wald test for testing the fixed effects in the classical linear mixed model is that it is based on standard errors which underestimate the true variability in $\hat{\beta}$ because they do not take into account the variability introduced by estimating the variance components, i.e., the covariance matrix for the random effects (Dempster et al., 1981). For this reason, typically an approximate F distribution with appropriate degrees of freedom is used in place of the standard chi-squared distribution that the Wald test assumes. In joint models this problem could be exaggerated because we do not only ignore the fact that we estimate the variance components, but also that we need to estimate the survival process. Asymptotically, we expect that the Wald statistic will follow the claimed chi-squared distribution, but in finite samples there has not been much work in the joint modeling literature to investigate its properties. Therefore, it is generally advisable to prefer likelihood ratio tests even though they are more computationally expensive.

The likelihood ratio test is also implemented by function anova() by supplying as arguments two fitted joint models, with the first one always being the model under the null hypothesis. As an illustration we are testing for the treatment effect in the risk for death. The Wald test included in the output of the summary() function indicated that there is non-negligible difference between the two treatments ($W = 0.3$, d.f. $= 1$, p-value $= 0.0324$). As we mentioned above, in order to implement the likelihood ratio test we need first to fit the joint model under the null hypothesis, that is, a joint model with no treatment in the survival submodel (we also include again the linear mixed model fit for completeness):

```
> lmeFit.aids <- lme(CD4 ~ obstime + obstime:drug,
     random = ~ obstime | patient, data = aids)

> coxFit2.aids <- coxph(Surv(Time, death) ~ 1, data = aids.id, x = TRUE)

> jointFit2.aids <- jointModel(lmeFit.aids, coxFit2.aids,
     timeVar = "obstime", method = "piecewise-PH-aGH")

> anova(jointFit2.aids, jointFit.aids)


               AIC     BIC   log.Lik  LRT df p.value
jointFit2.aids 8691.10 8753.30 -4330.55
jointFit.aids  8688.52 8754.86 -4328.26 4.58  1  0.0323
```

We arrive at the same conclusion with an identical p-value to the Wald test.

Contrary to the Wald and likelihood ratio test, the implementation of a score test requires a few extra steps. This is mainly due to the fact that the calculation of the score test statistic entails the evaluation of the score vector and the Hessian matrix of the joint model under the alternative hypothesis, but at the parameter values under the null. As an illustration of how this test can be performed in R, we test the null hypothesis of no association between the square root CD4 cell count and the risk for death, i.e.,

$$H_0 : \alpha = 0 \quad \text{versus} \quad H_a : \alpha \neq 0,$$

for the advanced HIV infected patients of the AIDS dataset. To perform this test we take advantage of the flexibility offered by the arguments of jointModel(), and use this function to calculate the required components of the score test statistic. As a first step we need to extract the maximum likelihood estimates for the longitudinal and survival submodels under the null. For the former, these can be easily obtained from the fitted linear mixed-effects models provided as first argument to jointModel(). More specifically, we extract the estimated fixed-effect coefficients β using function fixef(), and the estimated covariance matrix of the random effects D using function getVarCov(). The estimated residual standard error is directly extracted as the "sigma" component of the returned "lme" object fit. Before proceeding in extracting these estimates from object lmeFit.aids, we should note that, by default, function lme() computes the REML estimates of the parameters of the mixed model (for more information on restricted maximum likelihood estimation, the reader is referred to Section 2.2.1). Therefore, before extracting the estimated parameters we should first re-fit under maximum likelihood; the updated model fit is produced in R with the syntax:

```
> lmeFitML.aids <- update(lmeFit.aids, method = "ML")
```

For the survival submodel we cannot repeat the same procedure to extract the parameter estimates under the null, because the survival submodel `coxFit.aids` is a Cox model with an unspecified baseline hazard function, whereas in the joint model fitted to the AIDS dataset we have assumed a piecewise-constant baseline hazard function. To obtain the coefficients under the piecewise-constant model we use the utility function `piecewiseExp.ph()`. This takes a fitted Cox model and fits the corresponding relative risk model with a piecewise constant baseline hazard using the Poisson regression equivalence (Hougaard, 2000, Section 2.2.4). The algorithm used to determine the internal knots is exactly the same as the one used by `jointModel()`.

```
> pwc <- piecewiseExp.ph(coxFit.aids)

> coef(pwc)
        X         xi1        xi2        xi3        xi4        xi5
 0.2059221 -3.8393612 -3.4105302 -3.0497646 -3.5896874 -3.4312411
       xi6        xi7
-3.3413437 -3.1331363
```

The output of this function is a `"glm"` object in which the first part of the coefficients vector corresponds to the covariates entered in the Cox model, and the remaining part to the logarithm of the ξ_q, $q = 1, \ldots, Q$ parameters of the baseline risk function (4.3).

To perform the score test we collect all parameter estimates in a named list and call `jointModel()` with these as initial values:

```
> init <- list(
      betas = fixef(lmeFitML.aids),
      sigma = lmeFitML.aids$sigma,
      D = getVarCov(lmeFitML.aids),
      gammas = coef(pwc)[1],
      alpha = 0,
      xi = exp(coef(pwc)[-1]) # piecewiseExp.ph() returns log(xi)
  )

> JMScoreTest <- jointModel(lmeFitML.aids, coxFit.aids,
      timeVar = "obstime", method = "piecewise-PH-aGH", init = init,
      only.EM = TRUE, iter.EM = 0)
```

Argument `init` accepts the named list with initial values for the parameters of the joint model, the control argument `only.EM = TRUE` specifies that we want to use only the EM algorithm (i.e., do not proceed to the quasi-Newton algorithm if converge is not attained), and the control argument `iter.EM` sets the number of EM iterations; here we set it to zero, which corresponds to performing all remaining calculations (i.e., computing the Hessian matrix and the score vector) only for the initial values and not proceeding in the maximization of the log-likelihood. Then we extract the score vector from the returned joint model fit, the Hessian matrix using function `vcov()`, and we calculate the score test statistic and the corresponding p-value:

```
> score.vector <- JMScoreTest$Score

> inv.Hessian <- vcov(JMScoreTest)

> ScoreStat <- c(t(score.vector) %*% inv.Hessian %*% score.vector)

> c("Statistic" = ScoreStat, "df" = 1,
    "p-value" = pchisq(ScoreStat, df = 1, lower.tail = FALSE))
    Statistic            df        p-value
8.845084e+01 1.000000e+00 5.211407e-21
```

Similar to the result of the Wald test provided by the `summary()` method in Section 4.2, the score test also indicates that there is strong association between the CD4 cell count and the risk for death.

The three standard tests we have seen so far are only appropriate for the comparison of two nested models, in the sense that the model under the null hypothesis is a special case of the model under the alternative. When interest lies in comparing non-nested models, information criteria are typically used. The main idea behind these criteria is to compare two models based on their maximized log-likelihood value, but to penalize for the use of too many parameters. The two most commonly used information criteria are the Akaike's Information Criterion (AIC; Akaike, 1974) and the Bayesian Information Criterion (BIC; Schwarz, 1978). These are included in the output of the `anova()` and `summary()` functions, and are defined as:

$$AIC = -2\ell(\hat{\theta}) + 2n_{par}$$
$$BIC = -2\ell(\hat{\theta}) + n_{par}\log(n),$$

where n_{par} denotes the number of parameters in the model. Under these definitions 'smaller is better'. That is, if we are using either AIC or BIC to compare two models for the same data, we prefer the model with the lowest value for the corresponding criterion. The choice between the two criteria can be an issue since they do not always agree in practice. AIC tends to select more elaborate models than BIC due to the fact that the latter penalizes much more heavily for the complexity of the model. Note that this is also the case for the test for a treatment effect in the survival process in the AIDS dataset presented above. In particular, both the AIC and the likelihood ratio test indicate that there is a small but significant difference in the risk for death between the two treatments, whereas the BIC chooses the more parsimonious joint model with no treatment effect in the survival submodel. Therefore, these criteria should be considered as rules of thumb to discriminate between two (non-nested) statistical models.

An additional important issue arises when we are interested in testing whether an extra random effect should be included in the joint model. This in fact corresponds to increasing the dimensionality of the random effects design matrix D with extra variance components. In this case the model under the null hypothesis is obtained by setting some of the elements of D to zero in the full model. At least one of these elements is always an element in the diagonal of D (i.e., a variance parameter), meaning that under the null some parameters are set to a value on the boundary of their parameter space. The problem under this setting is that the classical maximum likelihood asymptotic arguments do not apply to boundary cases. In particular, some work on this topic in the linear mixed models framework by Stram and Lee (1994) following the results of Self and Liang (1987), and later by Verbeke and Molenberghs (2003) and Molenberghs and Verbeke (2007) has shown that all three tests statistics we have seen above do not follow the claimed χ_p^2 distribution under the null. As an alternative, it has been suggested to use mixtures of chi-squared distributions with appropriately chosen degrees of freedom. However, Greven et al. (2008) have demonstrated that even this choice could be rather conservative in some settings, and they have instead proposed a simulation-based approach to approximate the distribution of the likelihood ratio test statistic under the null. Within the joint modeling framework there has not been much work about this issue. As a practical guideline we would suggest using a higher type I error rate, e.g., 10 to 15%, to guarantee that we do not oversimplify the random-effects structure of the posited joint model.

4.4.2 Confidence Intervals

Asymptotic 95% confidence intervals for the parameter of interest can be based on Wald statistics, that is $\hat{\theta} \pm 1.96 \widehat{s.e.}(\hat{\theta})$. In R these are produced by the confint() function. For example, from the joint model fitted to the Aortic Valve dataset in Section 4.3.7, the 95% confidence intervals for the parameters in the longitudinal process are obtained via

```
> confint(jointFit2.av, parm = "Longitudinal")
                  2.5 %         est.       97.5 %
(Intercept)      3.8644755   4.33922289   4.8139703
ns(time, 3)1     0.8634598   1.47347658   2.0834934
ns(time, 3)2     1.5288204   2.27966532   3.0305103
ns(time, 3)3     1.7898180   2.23616498   2.6825120
TypeOpRR        -0.8542210  -0.48448673  -0.1147525
I(Age/15)       -0.4283111  -0.31739557  -0.2064800
```

```
ns(time, 3)1:TypeOpRR -0.8834019 -0.09654611  0.6903097
ns(time, 3)2:TypeOpRR -1.5924389 -0.59943345  0.3935720
ns(time, 3)3:TypeOpRR -2.4787575 -1.39343219 -0.3081069
```

whereas for the survival process, 95% confidence intervals for the hazard ratios are obtained via

```
> exp(confint(jointFit2.av, parm = "Event"))
            2.5 %      est.    97.5 %
TypeOpRR 0.6067633 1.1012094 1.9985752
Assoct   0.5188071 0.6990497 0.9419118
```

Similarly, asymptotic confidence intervals for the fitted values can be based on the asymptotic normal distribution of the MLEs. For example, for the average longitudinal evolutions $\mu = X\beta$ in the longitudinal process we can construct a 95% pointwise confidence interval of the form

$$\hat{\mu} \quad \pm \quad 1.96\widehat{s.e.}(\hat{\mu}) \Rightarrow$$
$$X\hat{\beta} \quad \pm \quad 1.96\left[\text{diag}\{X\text{vâr}(\hat{\beta})X^{\top}\}\right]^{1/2},$$

where X denotes the design matrix of interest, and $\text{vâr}(\hat{\beta})$ the block of the observed Hessian matrix corresponding to $\hat{\beta}$. To calculate the fitted values $\hat{\mu} = X\hat{\beta}$, their standard errors and the corresponding 95% pointwise confidence intervals in R, we use the predict() function. As an initial step, and before calling this function, we need to construct the data frame that contains the covariates values of interest based on which the design matrix X is to be derived. As an illustration, we produce the fitted average longitudinal evolutions of the two types of operation for a patient with the median age (i.e., 47.3 years old), with associated 95% pointwise confidence intervals, based on the joint model fitted to the Aortic Valve dataset. The following R code constructs a data frame with a regular sequence of 30 time points from the minimum to the maximum observed follow-up time, for each of the two types of operation, and with age set to the median age in the sample at hand.

```
> DF <- with(AoValv, expand.grid(
    time = seq(min(time), max(time), length = 30),
    TypeOp = levels(TypeOp),
    Age = median(AoValv.id$Age)))
```

Next, we supply the fitted joint model jointFit2.av and the above data frame as main arguments to the predict() function. In addition, we specify that we would like to compute confidence intervals for μ (i.e., argument interval), and that the results should be returned within the input data frame (i.e., argument return)

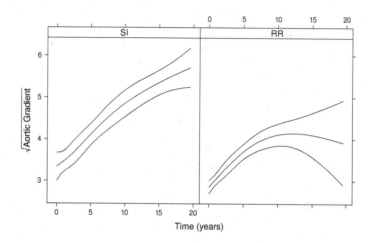

FIGURE 4.3: Fitted average longitudinal profiles for aortic gradient for the two types of operation for a patient with the median age.

```
> Ps <- predict(jointFit2.av, newdata = DF, interval = "confidence",
    return = TRUE)

> xyplot(pred + low + upp ~ time | TypeOp, data = Ps,
    type = "l", col = 1, lty = c(1,2,2), lwd = 2,
    ylab = expression(sqrt("Aortic Gradient")), xlab = "Time (years)")
```

The object `Ps` will in fact be the input data frame `DF` augmented with four extra columns with the fitted values $\hat{\mu}$, their standard errors and the limits of the asymptotic 95% pointwise confidence intervals. The plot of the resulting estimates is produced using function `xyplot()` from package **lattice** (Sarkar, 2008), and is shown in Figure 4.3.

4.4.3 Design Considerations

When the longitudinal and survival outcomes are considered separately, there have been several proposals in the literature regarding design consideration. For linear mixed models we refer to Verbeke and Molenberghs (2000, Chapter 23) and Fitzmaurice et al. (2004, Chapter 15), whereas for survival models to Therneau and Grambsch (2000, Section 3.6). Unfortunately, there has not yet been much work in the joint modeling framework regarding power and sample size calculations, and general design considerations. Due to the fact that joint models are quite complex models they do not lend themselves to easy derivations of power formulas, unless restrictive assumptions are made. In that respect, the only viable solution is to employ a simulation based approach, under which data are simulated from a joint model with the desired effect sizes.

An additional important point that is usually overlooked when designing a study in which a joint model is to be used has to do with choice of the follow-up times. In particular, it is customary to ask from *all* patients to come back to the study center to provide longitudinal measurements at a set of prespecified time points $t_1, \ldots, t_q$. Assuming that all patients will be compliant, it is evident that we only record information for the longitudinal marker at those specific time points and not in between them. However, we have already seen that the survival function, which is one of the parts of the likelihood of the joint model, requires an estimate of the complete path $\mathcal{M}_i(t) = \{m_i(s), 0 \le s < t\}$ of the true marker levels for each subject. Thus, since we will only have information at $t_1, \ldots, t_q$, we will have to interpolate to estimate $\mathcal{M}_i(t)$ in between these time points where we have no recorded information. To avoid this interpolation, when designing a study with Q planned follow-up measurements per subject, it would be generally advisable to span the follow-up period in $Q' > Q$ time points, create several random groups of patients, and ask each group to report for a visit at different sets of Q time points.

4.5 Estimation of the Random Effects

Until now we have primarily focused on estimation and inference for the joint model's parameters θ. The random effects b_i were used as a construct to describe heterogeneity in the patient longitudinal evolutions and to build the association between the longitudinal and event time processes. Nonetheless, in many settings interest may lie in deriving patient-specific predictions for either of the outcomes. To derive such predictions, an estimate of the random effects vector b_i is required. Since the random effects are assumed to be random variables, it is natural to estimate them using the Bayesian paradigm. In particular, assuming that $p(b_i; \theta)$ is the prior distribution, and that $p(T_i, \delta_i \mid b_i; \theta) \, p(y_i \mid b_i; \theta)$ is the conditional likelihood part, we can derive the corresponding posterior distribution:

$$p(b_i \mid T_i, \delta_i, y_i; \theta) = \frac{p(T_i, \delta_i \mid b_i; \theta) p(y_i \mid b_i; \theta) p(b_i; \theta)}{p(T_i, \delta_i, y_i; \theta)}$$

$$\propto p(T_i, \delta_i \mid b_i; \theta) p(y_i \mid b_i; \theta) p(b_i; \theta). \qquad (4.17)$$

Contrary to the linear mixed models framework where this posterior distribution is a multivariate normal distribution, in joint models it does not have a closed-form solution and it has to be numerically computed. However, as it was argued in Section 4.3.5, as the number of longitudinal measurements n_i increases, this distribution will converge to a normal distribution.

To describe this posterior distribution, standard summary measures are often utilized. For its location the mean or the mode are typically used, defined as

$$\begin{cases} \bar{b}_i = \int b_i \, p(b_i \mid T_i, \delta_i, y_i; \theta) \, db_i, & \text{and} \\ \hat{b}_i = \arg\max_b \{\log p(b \mid T_i, \delta_i, y_i; \theta)\}, \end{cases} \tag{4.18}$$

respectively, and as a measure of dispersion we may use the posterior variance or the inverse Hessian matrix of the random effects, i.e.,

$$\begin{cases} \mathrm{var}(b_i) = \int (b_i - \bar{b}_i)^2 \, p(b_i \mid T_i, \delta_i, y_i; \theta) \, db_i, \\ H_i = \left\{ -\frac{\partial^2 \log p(b \mid T_i, \delta_i, y_i; \theta)}{\partial b^\top \partial b} \Big|_{b=\hat{b}_i} \right\}^{-1}. \end{cases} \tag{4.19}$$

For the estimation of (4.18) and (4.19), an empirical Bayes approach is employed in which we replace θ by $\hat{\theta}$. In R these empirical Bayes estimates are produced by function `ranef()`. The choice between computing the mean $\bar{b}_i$ or the mode $\hat{b}_i$ of the posterior distribution of the random effects is controlled by the `type` argument, with the default being the mean. The following code compares the two estimates for the first six patients in the Aortic Valve dataset, using the joint model fitted in Section 4.3.7.

```
> head(ranef(jointFit2.av))
```

```
   (Intercept) ns(time, 3)1 ns(time, 3)2 ns(time, 3)3
1   -1.1623809   -0.8068030   -1.02519836   -0.3556301
12  -0.1321869   -2.8733450    0.12983730   -0.1927253
17   0.6676618    6.3404689   -0.05272436   -0.4205397
22  -1.0028832   -0.2602472   -0.80103372   -0.4455364
30   0.3022234    1.1862843    0.58932015   -0.1061563
32  -0.2307416   -1.1798982   -0.20725047   -0.4421050
```

```
> head(ranef(jointFit2.av, type = "mode"))
```

```
   (Intercept) ns(time, 3)1 ns(time, 3)2 ns(time, 3)3
1   -1.1843751   -0.7924597   -1.00020579   -0.31466724
12  -0.1233876   -2.9351389    0.19557269   -0.01697451
17   0.7093392    6.1951976    0.11981311    0.12332890
22  -1.0470046   -0.2106992   -0.74552794   -0.31381140
30   0.3084187    1.1835448    0.60205282   -0.01085677
32  -0.2491193   -1.3722186   -0.05329907   -0.07602029
```

The corresponding dispersion estimates of the posterior distribution are calculated by employing the extra optional argument `postVar`. Again, the `type` argument specifies which of the two estimators is computed. In particular, when `type = "mean"` and `postVar = TRUE`, `ranef()` returns the posterior variance, whereas for option `type = "mode"` it returns the inverse Hessian matrix. We display for the first patient in the Aortic Valve dataset

```
> attr(ranef(jointFit2.av, postVar = TRUE),
    "postVar")[[1]]


              (Intercept) ns(time, 3)1 ns(time, 3)2 ns(time, 3)3
(Intercept)    0.191306871 -0.132015303 -0.322848727 -0.001335748
ns(time, 3)1  -0.132015303  0.765628082 -0.042482949  0.001492416
ns(time, 3)2  -0.322848727 -0.042482949  0.804884199  0.001927672
ns(time, 3)3  -0.001335748  0.001492416  0.001927672  0.003195026
```

```
> attr(ranef(jointFit2.av, type = "mode", postVar = TRUE),
    "postVar")[[1]]


              (Intercept) ns(time, 3)1 ns(time, 3)2 ns(time, 3)3
(Intercept)    0.20482469  -0.14697481  -0.34151558  -0.03213124
ns(time, 3)1  -0.14697481   0.78573758  -0.02209749   0.03603327
ns(time, 3)2  -0.34151558  -0.02209749   0.83216730   0.04631669
ns(time, 3)3  -0.03213124   0.03603327   0.04631669   0.07689786
```

In general we observe very small differences between the two types of estimators, i.e., mean versus mode, and variance versus inverse Hessian matrix. As also explained in Section 4.3.5, this is to be expected because the leading term of the posterior distribution of the random effects under a joint model is the density of the longitudinal model, and therefore this posterior will be well approximated by a normal distribution for which the two types of estimators coincide.

4.6   Connection with the Missing Data Framework

So far we have motivated joint models from a survival point of view, namely as a modeling framework to handle error-prone time-dependent covariates. We now turn our attention to the setting where the longitudinal outcome is of primary interest. In this case, occurrence of an event for a patient usually corresponds to a discontinuation of her longitudinal process. This is because either follow-up measurements can no longer be collected or their distribution changes after the event occurred and therefore are considered non-relevant. Thus, under this setting it is evident that we can draw a direct connection between joint models and the missing data framework introduced in Section 2.3.

We should mention here that in some clinical studies in which the terminating event is death, it may not be conceptually reasonable to consider the values of the longitudinal outcome after the event time (Kurland and Heagerty, 2005; Kurland et al., 2009). However, we should also note that even though we have defined a mixed model (4.5) for the observed longitudinal responses, the joint model implicitly makes assumptions for the 'complete' longitudinal response vector, including observations that would have been collected after the event or censoring. To illustrate this more clearly, we define for each subject the observed and missing part of the longitudinal response vector. The observed part $y_i^o = \{y_i(t_{ij}) : t_{ij} < T_i^*, j = 1, \ldots, n_i\}$ consists of all observed longitudinal measurements of the ith subject before the event time, whereas the missing part $y_i^m = \{y_i(t_{ij}) : t_{ij} \geq T_i^*, j = 1, \ldots, n_i'\}$ contains the longitudinal measurements that would have been taken until the end of the study, had the event not occurred. Under these definitions, we can derive the dropout mechanism, which is the conditional distribution of the time-to-dropout given the complete vector of longitudinal responses (y_i^o, y_i^m). In particular, we obtain

$$
\begin{aligned}
p(T_i^* \mid y_i^o, y_i^m; \theta) &= \int p(T_i^*, b_i \mid y_i^o, y_i^m; \theta)\, db_i \\
&= \int p(T_i^* \mid b_i, y_i^o, y_i^m; \theta)\, p(b_i \mid y_i^o, y_i^m; \theta)\, db_i \\
&= \int p(T_i^* \mid b_i; \theta)\, p(b_i \mid y_i^o, y_i^m; \theta)\, db_i,
\end{aligned}
\tag{4.20}
$$

where the simplification in the last line is due to the conditional independence assumption (4.7). We observe that the time-to-dropout depends on y_i^m through the posterior distribution of the random effects $p(b_i \mid y_i^o, y_i^m; \theta)$, which means that joint models correspond to a MNAR missing data mechanism. A closer inspection of (4.20) reveals that the key component behind the attrition mechanism in joint models is the random effects b_i. More specifically, and as we have already seen, under the joint model

$$
\left\{
\begin{aligned}
y_i(t) &= x_i^\top(t)\beta + z_i^\top(t)b_i + \varepsilon_i(t) \\
h_i(t) &= h_0(t)\exp\left[\gamma^\top w_i + \alpha\{x_i^\top(t)\beta + z_i^\top(t)b_i\}\right],
\end{aligned}
\right.
$$

the survival and longitudinal submodels *share* the same random effects. Due to this feature joint models belong to the class of shared-parameter models, introduced in Section 2.3.2 (Wu and Carroll, 1988; Wu and Bailey, 1989; Follmann and Wu, 1995; Vonesh et al., 2006). Under a simple random-effects structure (i.e., random intercepts and random slopes), this missing data mechanism implies that subjects which show steep increases in their longitudinal profiles may be more (or less) likely to drop out.

A relevant issue here is the connection of the association parameter α with the type of the missing data mechanism. In particular, a null value for α corresponds to a MCAR missing data mechanism, because once conditioned upon available covariates, the dropout process does not depend on either missing or observed longitudinal responses. Moreover, since under $\alpha = 0$ the parameters in the two submodels are distinct, the joint probability of the dropout and longitudinal processes can be factorized as follows:

$$
\begin{aligned}
p(T_i, \delta_i, y_i; \theta) &= p(T_i, \delta_i; \theta_t)\, p(y_i; \theta_y, \theta_b) \\
&= p(T_i, \delta_i; \theta_t) \int p(y_i \mid b_i; \theta_y) p(b_i; \theta_b)\, db_i,
\end{aligned}
$$

implying that the parameters in the two submodels can be separately estimated. Nonetheless, because we have adopted a full likelihood approach, the estimated parameters derived from maximizing the log-likelihood of the longitudinal process $\ell(\theta_y) = \sum_i \log p(y_i; \theta_y)$, will also be valid under a MAR missing data mechanism, i.e., under the hypothesis that dropout depends on the observed responses only. Thus, while strictly speaking $\alpha = 0$ corresponds to a MCAR mechanism, the parameter estimates that we will obtain will be still valid under MAR. As a side note, we should also mention that, in practice, a discontinuation of the data collection for the longitudinal process also occurs when a subject leaves the study because of censoring. However, in the formulation of the likelihood function of joint models, we have assumed that the censoring mechanism may depend on the observed history of longitudinal responses and covariates, but is independent of future longitudinal outcomes. Hence, under this assumption, censoring corresponds to a MAR missing data mechanism.

An additional nice feature of the shared-parameter models framework is that these models can very easily handle both intermittent missingness and attrition. To see how this is achieved, we write the observed data log-likelihood under the complete data model $\{y_i^o, y_i^m\}$ for the longitudinal outcome:

$$
\begin{aligned}
\ell(\theta) &= \sum_{i=1}^{n} \log \int p(T_i, \delta_i, y_i^o, y_i^m; \theta)\, dy_i^m \\
&= \sum_{i=1}^{n} \log \int \int p(T_i, \delta_i, y_i^o, y_i^m \mid b_i; \theta)\, p(b_i; \theta)\, dy_i^m db_i \\
&= \sum_{i=1}^{n} \log \int p(T_i, \delta_i \mid b_i; \theta) \left\{ \int p(y_i^o, y_i^m \mid b_i; \theta)\, dy_i^m \right\} p(b_i; \theta)\, db_i \\
&= \sum_{i=1}^{n} \log \int p(T_i, \delta_i \mid b_i; \theta)\, p(y_i^o \mid b_i; \theta)\, p(b_i; \theta)\, db_i.
\end{aligned}
$$

Under the first conditional independence assumption (4.7) we obtain that the missing longitudinal responses y_i^m are only involved in the density of the longitudinal submodel. Moreover, under the second conditional independence assumption (4.8) the longitudinal responses conditionally on the random effects are independent with each other, and therefore, the integral with respect to

y_i^m is easily dropped. Thus, even if some subjects have intermittently missing responses, the likelihood of a joint model is easily obtained without requiring integration with respect to the missing responses. This is in fact in contrast to the other two standard modeling frameworks for handling missing data. In particular, in the case of intermittent missing data and under both the selection and pattern mixture models framework cumbersome computations are required to evaluate the likelihood (Jansen and Molenberghs, 2008; Troxel et al., 1998, Troxel et al., 1998).

4.7 Sensitivity Analysis under Joint Models

A practical problem in the handling of missing data in longitudinal outcomes is the fact that the observed data alone cannot distinguish between a MAR and a MNAR dropout mechanism. In fact, Molenberghs et al. (2008) have shown that every MNAR model has a MAR counterpart that provides exactly the same fit to the data (i.e., the same likelihood value), though inferences may be substantially different between the two models. This in practice means that identification of the non-ignorability parameter(s) in any MNAR model primarily is implicitly provided through modeling assumptions. Therefore, the only pragmatic approach to investigate the impact of violation of any of these assumptions is only via a sensitivity analysis (Diggle et al., 2007; Jansen et al., 2006; Little and Rubin, 2002; Kenward, 1998; Copas and Li, 1997; Diggle and Kenward, 1994).

Traditionally, the first step of a sensitivity analysis in the missing data context is to compare the results of the postulated MNAR model with the results under the corresponding MAR model. In our setting this means comparing the results of the joint model with the results of the longitudinal submodel (that are valid under MAR). We illustrate this first step of the sensitivity analysis for the AIDS dataset used in Section 4.2. The results under the linear mixed model that we used to fit the joint model are

```
> summary(lmeFit.aids)

. . .

Random effects:
 Formula: ~obstime | patient
 Structure: General positive-definite, Log-Cholesky parametrization
             StdDev    Corr
(Intercept) 4.5901583 (Intr)
obstime     0.1738082 -0.155
Residual    1.7497905
```

```
Fixed effects: CD4 ~ obstime + obstime:drug
                  Value   Std.Error  DF  t-value  p-value
(Intercept)       7.188833 0.22215874 936 32.35899  0.0000
obstime          -0.163451 0.02080804 936 -7.85519  0.0000
obstime:drugddI   0.028272 0.02970929 936  0.95162  0.3415
 . . .
```

and the corresponding results from the joint model are

```
> summary(jointFit.aids)
```

```
 . . .
```

```
Variance Components:
             StdDev   Corr
(Intercept)  4.5839   (Intr)
obstime      0.1822  -0.0468
Residual     1.7377
```

```
Coefficients:
Longitudinal Process
                 Value  Std.Err  z-value  p-value
(Intercept)      7.2203  0.2218  32.5537  <0.0001
obstime         -0.1917  0.0217  -8.8374  <0.0001
obstime:drugddI  0.0116  0.0302   0.3834   0.7014
 . . .
```

We should note that a potential misspecification of the missing data mechanism (e.g., assuming MAR whereas the true one is MNAR) could affect both the parameter estimates and the standard error estimates. With this in mind, we observe some small sensitivity in the fixed effects estimates, which is more easily noticeable by comparing the parameter estimates divided by their corresponding standard errors (i.e., `z-value` column in the results of the joint model fit and `t-value` column in the results of the linear mixed model fit).

To continue our sensitivity analysis we should decide between staying within the shared-parameter / joint models framework or opting for another type of MNAR model, such as a selection or a pattern mixture model. In the missing data context, the majority of the statistical literature has focused on sensitivity analysis for selection and pattern mixture models (Ibrahim and Molenberghs, 2009; Molenberghs and Kenward, 2007; Little and Rubin, 2002; Little, 1995; Diggle and Kenward, 1994; Little, 1993, 1994) with very little work in the shared-parameter models framework (Creemers et al., 2010; Tsonaka et al., 2010, 2009). Since our focus here is in joint models, we will opt to stay within this modeling framework. Again we can now choose between a global and local sensitivity analysis approach. The former entails fitting several joint models in which we make several alternations in the survival submodel (4.1). These could include correcting for additional baseline covariates or positing alternative parameterizations for the longitudinal marker. We will elaborate further on this topic in Section 5.1. In the case of local sensitivity we focus on a MNAR model and assess how inferences may be affected by the nonrandom dropout under this specific model. A nice tool to investigate such sensitivity issues is the index of local sensitivity to non-ignorability (ISNI) proposed by Troxel et al. (2004) and Ma et al. (2004) for selection models, and an adaptation of this tool for shared-parameter models has been presented by Viviani et al. (2012). The aim of this index is to investigate how much the maximum likelihood estimates for the longitudinal process are influenced by the hypothesis about the ignorability of the dropout mechanism. To introduce this index and for a fixed value of the association parameter α, let $\hat{\beta}(\alpha)$ and $\hat{\theta}_{-\beta}(\alpha)$ denote the maximum likelihood estimates of the fixed effects in the longitudinal submodel, and all other parameters of a joint model except β, respectively. The ISNI is a measure of the local behavior of $\hat{\beta}(\alpha)$ at $\alpha = 0$, i.e.,

$$\text{ISNI} = \frac{\partial}{\partial \alpha} \hat{\beta}(\alpha) \Big|_{\alpha=0}, \tag{4.21}$$

which quantifies how fast $\hat{\beta}(\alpha)$ is expected to change as $|\alpha|$ moves away from zero. Since (4.21) cannot be derived analytically Troxel et al. (2004) proposed to approximate it using a second-order Taylor series expansion of the log-likelihood of the MNAR model. In particular, let $\beta^{(0)} = \hat{\beta}(0)$ and $\hat{\theta}_{-\beta}^{(0)} = \hat{\theta}_{-\beta}(0)$ denote the maximum likelihood estimates under $\alpha = 0$. A second order approximation of the log-likelihood of the joint model around $\theta^{(0)} = \{\beta^{(0)}, \hat{\theta}_{-\beta}^{(0)}, \alpha = 0\}$ gives

$$\ell(\theta) \approx \ell(\theta^{(0)}) + (\theta - \theta^{(0)})^\top \left\{ \frac{\partial}{\partial \theta^\top} \ell(\theta) \Big|_{\theta=\theta^{(0)}} \right\}$$
$$+ \frac{1}{2}(\theta - \theta^{(0)})^\top \left\{ \frac{\partial^2}{\partial \theta^\top \partial \theta} \ell(\theta) \Big|_{\theta=\theta^{(0)}} \right\} (\theta - \theta^{(0)}),$$

which leads to the following approximation for (4.21):

$$\text{ISNI} \approx -\left\{ \frac{\partial^2}{\partial \beta^\top \partial \beta} \ell(\theta) \Big|_{\theta=\theta^{(0)}} \right\}^{-1} \left\{ \frac{\partial^2}{\partial \beta^\top \partial \alpha} \ell(\theta) \Big|_{\theta=\theta^{(0)}} \right\}. \tag{4.22}$$

We observe that calculation of the approximate ISNI (4.22) entails only the calculation of the Hessian matrix of a joint model under $\alpha = 0$. This computation can be performed by function `jointModel()` using suitable control arguments, and a post-manipulation of the results. Continuing the sensitivity analysis for AIDS dataset, we will calculate the ISNI for the fixed effects parameters β of the linear mixed model. For the sake of simplicity, we will assume a joint model with a Weibull relative risk submodel for the event time outcome. As an initial step, we need to compute the MLEs for the longitudinal and survival submodels under $\alpha = 0$. For the former these are already available from the fitted model object `lmeFit.aids` used in Section 4.2. For the survival submodel, we use the `survreg()` function from the **survival** package as follows:

```
> WeibFit.aids <- survreg(Surv(Time, death) ~ drug, data = aids.id,
      x = TRUE)

> WeibFit.aids
Call:
survreg(formula = Surv(Time, death) ~ drug, data = aids.id, x = TRUE)

Coefficients:
(Intercept)      drugddI
  3.3107850   -0.1535739

Scale= 0.7323405

Loglik(model)= -825.4   Loglik(intercept only)= -826.5
        Chisq= 2.06 on 1 degrees of freedom, p= 0.15
n= 467
```

We should note that `survreg()` fits (by default) the Weibull model, but under the accelerated failure time parameterization. This corresponds to the following log-linear model for the true event times:

$$\log T_i^* = \tilde{\gamma}_0 + \tilde{\gamma}\mathrm{ddI}_i + \sigma_t \epsilon_i,$$

where ddI is the dummy variable for the ddI group, ϵ_i is an error term following the extreme value distribution, and σ_t is a scale parameter. Because we want the MLEs of the Weibull model under the relative risk parameterization, we need to use the transformation $\gamma = -\tilde{\gamma}/\sigma_t$, with γ denoting the parameters under (4.1) with $h_0(t) = \sigma_t t^{\sigma_t-1}$. As we have seen in Section 4.4.1, to calculate the Hessian matrix of the joint models at the MLEs of the two submodels under $\alpha = 0$, we will supply these, and specify that we do not want `jointModel()` to proceed with the optimization of the log-likelihood; we achieve this with the syntax:

```
> init.list <- list(betas = fixef(lmeFit.aids),
    sigma = lmeFit.aids$sigma,
    D = getVarCov(lmeFit.aids),
    gammas = -coef(WeibFit.aids2)/WeibFit.aids2$scale,
    sigma.t = WeibFit.aids$scale, alpha = 0)

> ISNI.aids <- jointModel(lmeFit.aids, WeibFit.aids, timeVar = "obstime",
    method = "weibull-PH-aGH", only.EM = TRUE, iter.EM = 0,
    init = init.list)
```

In argument `init` we provide the named list with initial values for the parameters of the joint model, we set the control argument `only.EM` to `TRUE` in order to specify that we want to use only the EM algorithm (i.e., do not proceed to the quasi-Newton algorithm if converge is not attained), and we also set the control argument `iter.EM` to zero. To extract the corresponding blocks of the Hessian matrix and calculate the ISNI, we use the commands:

```
> H <- ISNI.aids$Hessian
> H.inv <- solve(H)
> pBetas <- head(grep("Y.", colnames(H), fixed = TRUE), -1)
> pAlpha <- which(colnames(H) == "T.alpha")
> isni <- - c(H.inv[pBetas, pBetas] %*% H[pBetas, pAlpha])
> se.betas <- sqrt(diag(vcov(lmeFit.aids)))
> round(cbind(ISNI = isni, rISNI = isni/se.betas), 3)
                  ISNI   rISNI
(Intercept)      0.096   0.433
obstime         -0.207  -9.965
obstime:drugddI -0.064  -2.168
```

The first two lines extract the Hessian matrix from the joint model and compute its inverse, the third and fourth lines compute vectors with position indexes for the rows of the Hessian matrix that correspond to β and α, respectively, and the fifth line computes the ISNI according to its definition. The second column in the output is the relative ISNI, which is the ISNI divided by the estimated standard error for $\hat{\beta}(0)$ under the linear mixed model, i.e., under MAR. This relative index has been proposed by Troxel et al. (2004) in order to allow for an easy comparison of the magnitude of the expected sensitivity for each parameter. These authors have considered values greater than one indicative for increased sensitivity in the estimates of the corresponding parameter under nonrandom dropout. Thus, for the AIDS dataset and as $|\alpha|$ moves away from zero, we would expect more sensitivity in the estimates of the slopes for the two treatment groups.

We should close this sensitivity analysis with a word of caution. Namely, note that we have investigated the sensitivity of the reported results only towards the MNAR mechanism implied by joint models (4.20). However, and as we have mentioned, the observed data cannot discern between missing data mechanisms, and therefore, if the true attrition mechanism was of another type, then the sensitivity in the results could be much greater.

Chapter 5

Extensions of the Standard Joint Model

This chapter presents several extensions of the standard joint model introduced in Chapter 4. These include several families of parameterizations for the association structure between the longitudinal and event outcomes, incorporating exogenous time-dependent covariates and stratification factors (either observed or latent), replacing relative risk models by accelerated failure time models, and joint models for multiple failure times and multiple longitudinal responses. Even though we attempt to provide a comprehensive presentation of most of the extensions that have been proposed in the literature for joint models, we should mention that we only present in greater detail the developments that are currently available in R.

5.1 Parameterizations

In the standard joint model, introduced in the previous chapter, it is assumed that the risk for an event at a particular time point t depends on the true level of the longitudinal marker at the same time point. The strength of the association between the current level of the marker and the risk is captured by the parameter α. Even though this is a very intuitively appealing parameterization with a clear interpretation for α, it is not realistic to expect that this parameterization will always be the most appropriate in expressing the correct relationship between the two processes. This is enforced by the fact that, in general, time-dependent covariates can be much more challenging to handle than baseline covariates. In particular, the choice of the functional form of a time-dependent covariate is usually not self-evident, and it may substantially influence the derived results. For instance, considering only the current value of a time-varying covariate to be associated with the risk for an event, may miss more complex forms of association between the longitudinal marker and the survival outcome or lead to etiologically incorrect conclusions (Vacek, 1997). For a more detailed discussion of these issues, we refer to Fisher and Lin (1999) and Wolkewitz et al. (2010).

In this section we present several alternative parameterizations that extend the standard parameterization (4.1) in different ways. These different parameterizations can be seen as special cases of the following general formulation of the association structure between the longitudinal marker and the risk for an event:

$$h_i(t) = h_0(t) \exp\left[\gamma^\top w_{i1} + f\{m_i(t - c), b_i, w_{i2}; \alpha\}\right], \tag{5.1}$$

where $f(\cdot)$ is a function of the true level of the marker $m_i(\cdot)$, of the random effects b_i and extra covariates w_{i2}. Under this general formulation α can potentially denote a vector of association parameters rather than a simple scalar as in (4.1).

5.1.1 Interaction Effects

The standard parameterization (4.1) assumes that the effect of the true level of the marker is the same in all subgroups of the target population. This is evidently a strong assumption that may not be true when the marker behaves differently for different subgroups of subjects. A straightforward extension to handle such situations is to include in the linear predictor of the relative risk model interaction terms of the marker with baseline covariates of interest, i.e.,

$$h_i(t) = h_0(t) \exp\left[\gamma^\top w_{i1} + \alpha^\top \{w_{i2} \times m_i(t)\}\right], \tag{5.2}$$

where, as before, w_{i1} is used to accommodate the direct effects of baseline covariate to the risk for an event, and w_{i2} contains interaction terms that expand the association of $m_i(t)$ in different subgroups in the data. When w_{i2} contains only the constant term, i.e., $w_{i2} = 1$, then (5.2) reduces to the standard parameterization (4.1).

To illustrate how such a joint model can be fitted in R, we investigate for the PBC dataset whether the strength of the association between the true level of serum bilirubin and the risk for death is different for patients with and without hepatomegaly. In particular, for the longitudinal outcome we assume a linear mixed model with quadratic evolutions in time for each patient with different average effects per treatment group:

$$\begin{aligned} y_i(t) &= \beta_0 + \beta_1 \text{D-pnc}_i + \beta_2 t + \beta_3 t^2 + \beta_4 \{\text{D-pnc}_i \times t\} + \beta_5 \{\text{D-pnc}_i \times t^2\} \\ &\quad + b_{i0} + b_{i1} t + b_{i2} t^2 + \varepsilon_i(t), \end{aligned}$$

with $y_i(t)$ denoting the logarithm of the observed levels of serum bilirubin, and D-pnc$_i$ the dummy for the D-penicillamine group. For the survival part we included the effects of treatment, hepatomegaly and the true level of log serum bilirubin, and in addition, we allow for a different association strength of bilirubin with the risk for death for patients with and without hepatomegaly:

$$h_i(t) = h_0(t) \exp\left[\gamma_1 \text{D-pnc}_i + \gamma_2 \text{HepMeg}_i + \alpha_1 m_i(t) + \alpha_2\{\text{HepMeg}_i \times m_i(t)\}\right],$$

where HepMeg$_i$ is the dummy variable for patients with hepatomegaly. The baseline risk function $h_0(\cdot)$ is assumed piecewise-constant. The longitudinal information for the patients in the PBC dataset is available in package **JM** as the data frame pbc2, and the survival information as the data frame pbc2.id. To fit the joint model, and as we have seen before, we first need to fit separately the linear mixed and Cox models with the corresponding covariate structures. For the latter we only need to include the $\gamma^\top w_{i1}$ of the linear predictor, i.e.,

```
> lmeFit.pbc <- lme(log(serBilir) ~ drug * (year + I(year^2)),
      random = ~ year + I(year^2) | id, data = pbc2)

> coxFit.pbc <- coxph(Surv(years, status2) ~ drug + hepatomegaly,
      data = pbc2.id, x = TRUE)
```

As in Section 3.3, status2 is the indicator for the composite event, i.e., either transplantation or death. To include the interaction part $\alpha^\top\{w_{i2} \times m_i(t)\}$ in the linear predictor of the corresponding joint model, we exploit the interFact argument of jointModel(). This argument should be a named list with a component named value that provides an R formula specifying the form of the W_2 design matrix, and a component named data specifying the data frame into which the formula is to be applied. For our particular example we use the syntax:

```
> jointFit.pbc <- jointModel(lmeFit.pbc, coxFit.pbc, timeVar = "year",
      method = "piecewise-PH-aGH",
      interFact = list(value = ~ hepatomegaly, data = pbc2.id))

> summary(jointFit.pbc)
```

. . .

```
Event Process
                        Value Std.Err  z-value p-value
drugD-penicil          0.0882  0.1677   0.5263  0.5987
hepatomegalyYes        0.2288  0.4112   0.5566  0.5778
Assoct                 1.1562  0.1286   8.9900 <0.0001
Assoct:hepatomegalyYes 0.2353  0.1850   1.2722  0.2033
```

log(xi.1)	-4.7939 0.3297	-14.5386
log(xi.2)	-4.4271 0.3326	-13.3117
log(xi.3)	-4.3962 0.3543	-12.4092
log(xi.4)	-4.2151 0.3794	-11.1102
log(xi.5)	-4.2400 0.3824	-11.0890
log(xi.6)	-4.0540 0.4018	-10.0905
log(xi.7)	-4.6011 0.5146	-8.9419

. . .

We observe that indeed serum bilirubin is strongly related with the risk for death. Each one unit increase of the current value of log serum bilirubin is associated with a $\exp(1.1562) = 3.2$-fold increase (95% CI: 2.5; 4.1) in a patient's risk without hepatomegaly, and a $\exp(1.1562 + 0.2353) = 4$-fold increase (95% CI: 3.1; 5.2) in a patient's risk with hepatomegaly.

5.1.2   Lagged Effects

In some occasions the typical assumption that the current value of the time-dependent covariate affects the current risk for an event may lead to medically illogical conclusions. For example, this has been observed by Cavender et al. (1992) who in a study on patients with coronary artery disease noted that the current smoking status decreased the risk for death (although not statistically significantly). The reason behind this surprising result was that most of those who died were smokers, but many had stopped smoking at the last follow-up before their death. Thus, many of the patients who died had just quit smoking, whereas some of the patients who were still alive were still smoking, leading to the surprising result.

One approach to tackle such situations is to use time-lagged covariates. In particular, we use the following formulation of the relative risk model:

$$h_i(t) = h_0(t) \exp\left[\gamma^\top w_i + \alpha m_i\{\max(t - c, 0)\}\right], \tag{5.3}$$

which postulates that the risk at time t depends on the true value of the longitudinal marker at time $t-c$, where c specifies the time lag of interest. Such lagged effects are easily incorporated in the specification of the joint model in R using the `lag` argument of function `jointModel()`. As an illustration, we fit two joint models to the Liver Cirrhosis dataset. For the longitudinal part and in order to allow for a flexible specification of the subject-specific longitudinal trajectories, we assume a linear mixed model with a natural cubic spline effect for time, with different average profiles per treatment group. In addition, to capture sudden changes in the prothrombin index in the very early part of follow-up in each treatment group, we also include a separate indicator variable of the baseline measurement. The model takes the form

$$y_i(t) \;=\; m_i(t) + \varepsilon_i(t)$$

$$= \;(\beta_0 + b_{i0}) + (\beta_1 + b_{i1})B_n(t, \lambda_1) + (\beta_2 + b_{i2})B_n(t, \lambda_2)$$

$$+ (\beta_3 + b_{i3})B_n(t, \lambda_3) + \beta_4\{B_n(t, \lambda_1) \times \text{Predns}_i\}$$

$$+ \beta_5\{B_n(t, \lambda_2) \times \text{Predns}_i\} + \beta_6\{B_n(t, \lambda_3) \times \text{Predns}_i\}$$

$$+ \beta_7\text{Predns}_i + \beta_8\text{T0}_i + \beta_9\{\text{Predns}_i \times \text{T0}_i\} + \varepsilon_i(t),$$

with $y_i(t)$ denoting the prothrombin index, $\{B_n(t, \lambda_k); k = 1, 2, 3\}$ the B-spline basis matrix for a natural cubic spline of time with two internal knots placed at the 33.3% and 66.7% percentiles of the follow-up times, **Predns** the indicator variable for prednisone, and **T0** is the indicator variable for the baseline time. The random effects are assumed to have a diagonal covariance matrix. The longitudinal responses of the prothrombin index are available in the data frame **prothro**; we fit the model using the syntax:

```
> prothro$t0 <- as.numeric(prothro$time == 0)

> lmeFit.pro <- lme(pro ~ treat * (ns(time, 3) + t0),
      random = list(id = pdDiag(form = ~ ns(time, 3))),
      data = prothro)
```

In the survival submodel, we correct for treatment and compare two formulations for the time-dependent prothrombin index, namely, in the first, we posit that the risk for death depends on the current value of prothrombin, while in the second one we posit that it depends on the two-year earlier prothrombin value, i.e.,

$$h_i(t) \;=\; h_0(t)\exp\{\gamma\text{Predns}_i + \alpha m_i(t)\}$$

$$h_i(t) \;=\; h_0(t)\exp\left[\gamma\text{Predns}_i + \alpha m_i\{\max(t - 2, 0)\}\right].$$

As before, and before fitting the two joint models, we need first to fit the Cox model that only contains the baseline covariates part, in this case, treatment; the relevant syntax is

```
> coxFit.pro <- coxph(Surv(Time, death) ~ treat, data = prothros,
      x = TRUE)
```

where **prothros** is the data frame holding the survival information. The first joint model is fitted by a standard call to `jointModel()`, as we have used so far

```
> jointFit.pro <- jointModel(lmeFit.pro, coxFit.pro, timeVar = "time",
      method = "piecewise-PH-aGH")
```

To fit the second joint model, we use argument **lag** to specify the lag of interest. Moreover, since the only difference from the previous call to `jointModel()` is the extra specification of the **lag** argument, we can easily fit the new joint model by updating the previous fit using the **update()** function:

```
> jointFit2.pro <- update(jointFit.pro, lag = 2)
```

We focus on the parameters of main interest, that is the parameters of the survival submodel γ and α, and we compare the asymptotic 95% confidence intervals under the two parameterizations.

```
> confint(jointFit.pro, parm = "Event")
                 2.5 %        est.        97.5 %
treatpredns  0.10149967  0.42367774  0.74585581
Assoct      -0.04775799 -0.04059136 -0.03342473

> confint(jointFit2.pro, parm = "Event")
                   2.5 %        est.       97.5 %
treatpredns    -0.06517853  0.20906811  0.48331474
Assoct(lag=2) -0.04621767 -0.03842666 -0.03063565
```

For the association parameter we observe relatively small differences between the two formulations for the time-dependent prothrombin index. However, the treatment effect with no lag effect $c = 0$ is about double than that with $c = 2$, though under both parameterizations nonsignificant. To statistically compare the two models we will need to use the information criteria introduced in Section 4.4, since the two models are not nested. We perform this comparison using the **anova()** function, in which we explicitly specify, using the **test** argument, that we do not wish to perform a likelihood ratio test

```
> anova(jointFit.pro, jointFit2.pro, test = FALSE)
                  AIC       BIC    log.Lik df
jointFit.pro  27918.33  28018.90 -13935.17
jointFit2.pro 27407.40  27507.97 -13679.70  0
```

Both AIC and BIC agree that the joint model with the lagged time-dependent prothrombin index has a better predictive ability than the model that assumes that the current value of the index is associated with the risk for death.

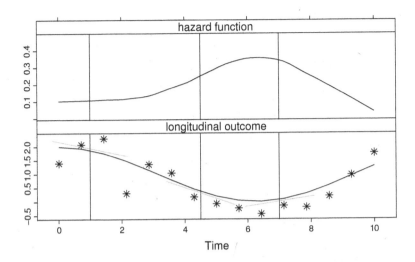

FIGURE 5.1: Graphical representation of the time-dependent slopes parameterization. The top panel illustrates the evolution of the hazard function in time, and the bottom panel shows that at each time point the value and/or the slope of the longitudinal trajectory (grey segments) is associated with the hazard.

5.1.3   Time-Dependent Slopes Parameterization

In the previous parameterizations we have assumed that the risk for an event depends on either the current or a previous value of the longitudinal marker. However, since for each patient the marker follows a trajectory in time, it is also reasonable to consider parameterizations that allow the risk for an event to also depend on other features of this trajectory. A parameterization of this type has been considered by Ye et al. (2008b) who postulated a joint model in which the risk depends on both the current true value of the trajectory and the slope of the true trajectory at time t. A graphical representation of this parameterization is given in Figure 5.1. More specifically, the relative risk survival submodel takes the form

$$h_i(t) = h_0(t) \exp\{\gamma^\top w_i + \alpha_1 m_i(t) + \alpha_2 m_i'(t)\}, \tag{5.4}$$

where

$$m_i'(t) = \frac{d}{dt} m_i(t) = \frac{d}{dt}\{x_i^\top(t)\beta + z_i^\top(t)b_i\}.$$

The interpretation of parameter α_1 remains the same as in the standard parameterization (4.1). Parameter α_2 measures how strongly associated is the value of the slope of the true longitudinal trajectory at time t with the risk for an event at the same time point, provided that $m_i(t)$ remains constant. This parameterization could capture situations where, for instance, at a specific time point two patients show similar true marker levels, but they may differ in the rate of change of the marker.

To investigate the added value of this parameterization for the PBC dataset presented in Section 5.1.1, we refit the joint model with an updated survival submodel of the form:

$$h_i(t) = h_0(t) \exp\{\gamma_1 \text{D-pnc}_i + \gamma_2 \text{HepMeg}_i + \alpha_1 m_i(t) + \alpha_2 m_i'(t)\},$$

where we have excluded the interaction term of serum bilirubin with hepatomegaly, and we included the time-dependent slopes term. We first refit the joint model presented in Section 5.1.1, excluding the interaction term, i.e.,

```
> jointFit2.pbc <- update(jointFit.pbc, interFact = NULL)
```

To include the time-dependent slopes term we use the **parameterization** and **derivForm** arguments of **jointModel()**. In particular, the **parameterization** argument specifies the type of parameterization we are interested in with the current value of the marker being the default. Here we want both the current value and the slope, and therefore we specify the option "both". In the **derivForm** argument we must specify the functional form of the derivative of the trajectory using the formula interface of R. Under the linear mixed-effects submodel fitted to the PBC data, $m_i(t)$ has the form

$$
\begin{aligned}
m_i(t) \;=\; & \beta_0 + \beta_1 \text{D-pnc}_i + \beta_2 t + \beta_3 t^2 + \beta_4 \{\text{D-pnc}_i \times t\} + \beta_5 \{\text{D-pnc}_i \times t^2\} \\
& + b_{i0} + b_{i1} t + b_{i2} t^2,
\end{aligned}
$$

which, after taking the derivative with respect to t, reduces to

$$m_i'(t) = \beta_2 + 2\beta_3 t + \beta_4 \text{D-pnc}_i + 2\beta_5 \{\text{D-pnc}_i \times t\} + b_{i1} + 2b_{i2}t.$$

To explain how argument **derivForm** should be invoked, we first rewrite $m_i'(t)$ under the mixed-effects model structure, that is,

$$m_i'(t) = [x_i^{sl}(t)]^\top \beta^{sl} + [z_i^{sl}(t)]^\top b_i^{sl},$$

with $x_i^{sl}(t) = [1, 2t, \text{D-pnc}_i, 2(t \times \text{D-pnc}_i)]$, $z_i^{sl}(t) = [1, 2t]$, $\beta^{sl} = (\beta_2, \beta_3, \beta_4, \beta_5)^\top$, and $b_i^{sl} = (b_{i1}, b_{i2})^\top$. Using this formulation, argument **derivForm** is specified as a named list with four components, namely, two R formulas, named **fixed** and **random**, used to construct the fixed- and random-effects design matrices in the definition of $m_i'(t)$, respectively, and two numeric vectors, named **indFixed** and **indRandom**, specifying which of the fixed effects parameters β and random effects b_i of the original $m_i(t)$ are involved in the specification of $m_i'(t)$. Therefore, for our example, the **derivForm** list takes the form

```
> dform <- list(fixed = ~ I(2*year) + drug + I(2*year):drug,
      indFixed = 3:6, random = ~ I(2*year), indRandom = 2:3)
```

where indFixed = 3:6 because in the definition of $m_i'(t)$ above, the third to
sixth fixed effects parameters of $m_i(t)$ are used, and similarly for component
indRandom. Note that, by default, R formulas used to construct design matrices
include the intercept term. The corresponding joint model is fitted by:

```
> jointFit3.pbc <- update(jointFit2.pbc, parameterization = "both",
      derivForm = dform)

> summary(jointFit3.pbc)
```

```
. . .

Event Process
                   Value Std.Err  z-value p-value
drugD-penicil     0.1036  0.1786   0.5801  0.5619
hepatomegalyYes   0.6233  0.1899   3.2824  0.0010
Assoct            1.1933  0.1043  11.4404 <0.0001
Assoct.s          2.5407  0.5934   4.2819 <0.0001
log(xi.1)        -5.7767  0.4080 -14.1595
log(xi.2)        -5.2080  0.3629 -14.3515
log(xi.3)        -5.1169  0.3640 -14.0590
log(xi.4)        -4.9142  0.3838 -12.8027
log(xi.5)        -4.9285  0.3773 -13.0642
log(xi.6)        -4.8102  0.4207 -11.4345
log(xi.7)        -4.9366  0.5115  -9.6516

. . .
```

We observe that the slope of the trajectory, labeled in the output 'Assoct.s',
is highly associated with the risk for death. In particular, for patients having
the same level of log serum bilirubin, the log hazard ratio for a unit increase
in the current slope of the bilirubin trajectory is 2.5 (95% CI: 1.4; 3.7). To
statistically test for the overall effect of the marker, we can perform a multivariate Wald test using the anova() function. As we have seen in Section 4.4,
by default this function will provide marginal Wald tests for all parameters in
the model. Here we focus on the event process

```
> anova(jointFit3.pbc, process = "Event")
Marginal Wald Tests Table

Event Process
              Chisq df Pr(>|Chi|)
drug         0.3365  1    0.5619
hepatomegaly 10.7744  1    0.0010
```

Assoct(all)	168.6603	2	<1e-04
Assoct	130.8826	1	<1e-04
Assoct.s	18.3347	1	<1e-04

The p-value associated with the entry `Assoct(all)` corresponds to testing the following set of hypotheses:

$$H_0: \qquad \alpha_1 = \alpha_2 = 0$$
$$H_a: \quad \alpha_1 \neq 0 \ \text{ or } \ \alpha_2 \neq 0,$$

under model (5.4). The result validates the hypothesis that for PBC patients, the current value of log serum bilirubin and the slope of the bilirubin trajectory are highly associated with the hazard for the composite event (death or transplantation).

5.1.4   Cumulative Effects Parameterization

A common characteristic of all parameterizations we have seen so far is that they assume that the risk for an event at a specific time depends on features of the longitudinal trajectory at only a single time point. That is, from the entire history of the true marker levels $\mathcal{M}_i(t) = \{m_i(s), 0 \leq s < t\}$, the risk at time t is typically assumed to depend on either the marker level on the same time point $m_i(t)$ or in a previous time point $m_i(t - c)$, if lagged effects are considered as in Section 5.1.2. However, several authors have argued that this assumption is not always realistic, and in many cases we may benefit by allowing the risk to depend on a more elaborate function of the longitudinal marker history (Sylvestre and Abrahamowicz, 2009; Hauptmann et al., 2000; Vacek, 1997).

One approach that allows the whole history of the marker to be associated with the hazard for an event is to include in the linear predictor of the relative risk submodel the integral of the longitudinal trajectory, representing the cumulative effect of the longitudinal outcome up to time point t. A graphical representation of this parameterization is given in Figure 5.2. More specifically, the survival submodel takes the form

$$h_i(t) = h_0(t) \exp\left\{\gamma^\top w_i + \alpha \int_0^t m_i(s)\, ds\right\}, \tag{5.5}$$

where for any particular time point t, α measures the strength of the association between the risk for an event at time point t and the area under the longitudinal trajectory up to the same time t, with the area under the longitudinal trajectory regarded as a suitable summary of the whole trajectory.

To fit a joint model under this parameterization, we can exploit the flexibility provided by the `derivForm` argument of `jointModel()` for the specification of an extra marker term to be added in the linear predictor of the survival submodel. In particular, instead of specifying the R formulas to define the

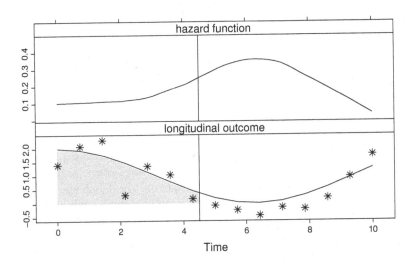

FIGURE 5.2: Graphical representation of the cumulative effects parameterization. The top panel illustrates the evolution of the hazard function in time, and the bottom panel shows that at each time point the entire area under the longitudinal trajectory is associated with the hazard.

time-dependent slope term $m_i'(t)$, as we have done in Section 5.1.3, we specify the corresponding R formulas for the fixed- and random-effects parts required to calculate the integral of $m_i(t)$. We illustrate how this can be achieved continuing on the same example with the PBC dataset from the previous section, where now we fit a joint model with a survival submodel of the form:

$$h_i(t) = h_0(t) \exp\left\{\gamma_1 \texttt{D-pnc}_i + \gamma_2 \texttt{HepMeg}_i + \alpha \int_0^t m_i(s)\,ds\right\}.$$

Under the formulation of $m_i(t)$ presented in Section 5.1.3, it can be easily seen that its integral has the following closed-form solution:

$$\int_0^t m_i(s)\,ds = \beta_0 t + \beta_1 \{\texttt{D-pnc}_i \times t\} + \beta_2 t^2/2 + \beta_3 t^3/3$$
$$+ \beta_4\{\texttt{D-pnc}_i \times t^2/2\} + \beta_5\{\texttt{D-pnc}_i \times t^3/3\} + b_{i0}t + b_{i1}t^2/2 + b_{i2}t^3/3.$$

We translate this equation to a pair of R formulas for the fixed- and random-effects parts. Moreover, we also specify in the `indFixed` and `indRandom` components which fixed- and random-effects parameters of the original linear mixed model correspond to the columns of the design matrices that calculate the integral of $m_i(t)$:

```
> iform <- list(fixed = ~ -1 + year + I(year * (drug == "D-penicil"))
    + I(year^2/2) + I(year^3/3) + I(year^2/2 * (drug == "D-penicil"))
    + I(year^3/3 * (drug == "D-penicil")),
    indFixed = 1:6,
    random = ~ -1 + year + I(year^2/2) + I(year^3/3),
    indRandom = 1:3)
```

The "`-1`" added in the definitions of the formulas for the fixed- and random-effects parts is used to exclude the intercept term, which is by default included in the construction of design matrices in R. The corresponding joint model is simply fitted by supplying the `iform` list in the `derivForm` argument. Moreover, option "`slope`" in the `parameterization` argument specifies that we only want to include in the linear predictor of the survival submodel the term created by the `derivForm` argument, and not the current value term $m_i(t)$.

```
> jointFit4.pbc <- update(jointFit3.pbc, parameterization = "slope",
    derivForm = iform)

> summary(jointFit4.pbc)

. . .

Event Process
```

	Value	Std.Err	z-value	p-value
drugD-penicil	-0.0191	0.1604	-0.1191	0.9052
hepatomegalyYes	0.9375	0.1736	5.3993	<0.0001
Assoct.s	0.2064	0.0199	10.3471	<0.0001
log(xi.1)	-3.4572	0.2203	-15.6920	
log(xi.2)	-3.3750	0.2328	-14.4993	
log(xi.3)	-3.6893	0.2715	-13.5882	
log(xi.4)	-3.7373	0.3124	-11.9623	
log(xi.5)	-4.0011	0.3319	-12.0562	
log(xi.6)	-4.1640	0.4058	-10.2607	
log(xi.7)	-5.9524	0.6261	-9.5074	

```
. . .
```

Similarly to the previous analyses, we observe that serum bilirubin remains strongly related with the risk for death. In particular, a unit increase in the area under the log serum bilirubin longitudinal profile corresponds to a 1.2-fold increase in the risk for death.

A restriction of parameterization (5.5) is that it places the same weight for all past values of the marker, which may not be reasonable in some situations. A straightforward extension to account for this issue is to adjust the integrand and multiply the $m_i(t)$ with an appropriately chosen weight function that places different weights at different time points:

$$h_i(t) = h_0(t) \exp\left\{\gamma^\top w_i + \alpha \int_0^t \varpi(t-s)m_i(s)\,ds\right\}, \qquad (5.6)$$

where $\varpi(\cdot)$ denotes the weight function. A desirable property of $\varpi(\cdot)$ would be to place smaller weights in points further in the past. One possible family of functions with this property are probability density functions of known parametric distributions, such as the normal, the Student's-t, and the logistic. The scale parameter in these densities and also the degrees of freedom parameter in the Student's-t density can be utilized to tune the relative weights of more recent marker values compared to older ones. Parameterization (5.6) has a direct connection with the concept of weight cumulative exposure discussed by Breslow et al. (1983) and Thomas (1988).

As an illustration, we update the cumulative effect analysis for the PBC dataset and use as weight function the standard normal density, i.e., $\varpi(x) = \exp(-x^2/2)/\sqrt{2\pi}$. By setting the variance of the normal density to one, we practically assume that the three most recent years of the log serum bilirubin history are associated with the risk for death. The specification of $m_i(t)$ in the longitudinal submodel assumes a second-order degree polynomial for the time effect, in both the fixed- and random-effects parts. Thus, in order to construct the weighted cumulative effect, we are required to evaluate integrals of the form:

$$\int_0^t s^j \varpi(t-s)\,ds = (1/\sqrt{2\pi}) \int_0^t s^j \exp\{-(t-s)^2/2\}\,ds,$$

for $j = 0, 1, 2$. Due to the fact that these integrals do not have closed-form solutions for $j > 0$, we will use the build-in function `integrate()` in R to approximate them numerically. This function is based on the Gauss-Kronrod rule we have seen earlier for the approximation of the integral in the definition of the survival function (4.2). Similar to the unweighted analysis, we will need to define appropriate formulas for the fixed- and random-effects part, which will be supplied in the `derivForm` argument of `jointModel()`. As an initial step, we define the function `g()` that calculates the required integrals using `integrate()`:

```
> g <- function (u, pow = 0) {
    f <- function (t)
        integrate(function (s) s^pow * dnorm(t - s), 0, t)$value
    sapply(u, f)
}
```

The `sapply()` statement in the last line is used to vectorize `g()` with respect to its first argument, i.e., to make `g()` work when `u` is a vector. Following, using `g()` we define the fixed and random parts of the weight cumulative effect and fit the corresponding joint model

```
> iformW <- list(fixed = ~ -1 + I(g(year)) +
    I(g(year) * (drug == "D-penicil")) +
    I(g(year, 1)) + I(g(year, 2)) +
    I(g(year, 1) * (drug == "D-penicil")) +
    I(g(year, 2) * (drug == "D-penicil")),
    indFixed = 1:6,
    random = ~ -1 + I(g(year)) + I(g(year, 1)) + I(g(year, 2)),
    indRandom = 1:3)

> jointFit5.pbc <- update(jointFit3.pbc, parameterization = "slope",
    derivForm = iformW)

> summary(jointFit5.pbc)

. . .

Event Process
                Value Std.Err  z-value p-value
drugD-penicil  0.0301  0.1629   0.1848  0.8534
hepatomegalyYes 0.7738 0.1769   4.3741 <0.0001
Assoct.s       2.4345  0.1746  13.9471 <0.0001
log(xi.1)     -4.2032  0.2543 -16.5290
log(xi.2)     -4.2729  0.2757 -15.4982
log(xi.3)     -4.2987  0.2919 -14.7253
log(xi.4)     -4.1447  0.3183 -13.0220
log(xi.5)     -4.2028  0.3219 -13.0579
log(xi.6)     -3.9873  0.3482 -11.4498
log(xi.7)     -4.6520  0.4801  -9.6895

. . .
```

We observe that the weighted cumulative effect is also strongly related to the hazard for death, with one unit increase in weighted area under the log serum bilirubin trajectory corresponding to 11.4-fold increase in the risk. Table 5.1 illustrates a comparison using information criteria of the three joint models fitted to the PBC dataset under the weighted cumulative effect, unweighted cumulative effect, and current value parameterizations. We observe that inclusion of the weight function clearly improves the fit under the cumulative effect parameterization. However, for this particular dataset it seems that using only the most recent value of the marker $m_i(t)$ in the hazard model provides better predictive ability than using cumulative effects. An additional comparison between these three parameterizations is given in Figure 5.3 that depicts the hazard functions for two patients from the PBC dataset. It is evident that the choice of the parameterization can have quite an impact on the shape of the subject-specific hazard functions, which demonstrates that choosing a parameterization not supported by the data may substantially affect the fit

TABLE 5.1: A comparison of three joint models fitted to the PBC dataset under the weighted cumulative effect, unweighted cumulative effect, and current value parameterizations

	logLik	AIC	BIC
weighted cum. (`jointFit5.pbc`)	−1878.94	3803.88	3889.96
unweighted cum. (`jointFit4.pbc`)	−1924.27	3894.54	3980.63
current value (`jointFit2.pbc`)	−1858.08	3762.15	3848.24

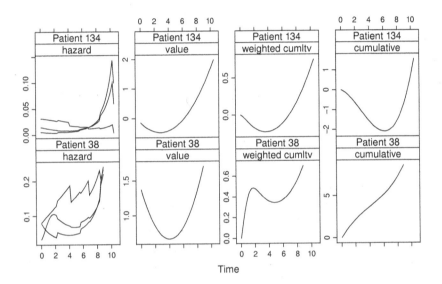

FIGURE 5.3: A comparison of the hazard functions of two patients in the PBC dataset under different parameterizations.

of the model. Thus, we should not always just rely on the standard formulation (4.1) but rather carefully consider the problem and investigate different parameterizations and possibly their combinations.

5.1.5 *Random-Effects Parameterization*

Another type of parameterization that is frequently used in joint models includes in the linear predictor of the risk model only the random effects of the longitudinal submodel, i.e.,

$$h_i(t) = h_0(t) \exp(\gamma^\top w_i + \alpha^\top b_i), \tag{5.7}$$

where α denotes a vector of association parameters each one measuring the association between the corresponding random effect and the hazard for an event. This parameterization is more meaningful when a simple random-intercepts and random-slopes structure is assumed for the longitudinal sub-model, in which case, the random effects express subject-specific deviations from the average intercept and average slope. Under this setting this param-eterization postulates that patients who have a lower/higher level for the longitudinal outcome at baseline (i.e., intercept) or who show a steeper in-crease/decrease in their longitudinal trajectories (i.e., slope) are more likely to experience the event (i.e., drop out). This interpretation has also motivated the use of this parameterization in joint models (i.e., shared-parameter mod-els) used in the missing data framework (Pulkstenis et al., 1998; Follmann and Wu, 1995; Wu and Bailey, 1989). This parameterization also shares similarities with the time-dependent slopes parameterization presented in Section 5.1.3. In particular, under a longitudinal submodel with a random-intercepts and random-slopes structure, i.e.,

$$y_i(t) = \beta_0 + \beta_1 t + b_{i0} + b_{i1} t + \varepsilon_i(t),$$

the relative risk submodel for the event process under the time-dependent slopes parameterization (5.4) with $\alpha_1 = 0$ takes the form

$$h_i(t) = h_0(t) \exp\{\gamma^\top w_i + \alpha_2(\beta_1 + b_{i1})\},$$

whereas the relative risk submodel under the same longitudinal submodel, but with parameterization (5.7) becomes

$$h_i(t) = h_0(t) \exp(\gamma^\top w_i + \alpha_1 b_{i0} + \alpha_2 b_{i1}).$$

If we set $\alpha_1 = 0$ in the latter formulation of the relative risk submodel, we ob-serve that this model also postulates that the risk depends only on the random-slopes component of the linear mixed model. It should be noted though that the interpretation of α_2 is different in the two parameterizations, because term $(\beta_1 + b_{i1})$ denotes the underlying slope of the longitudinal trajectory of the ith subject, whereas term b_{i1} denotes the deviation of the slope of subject i from the population average β_1.

A computational advantage of parameterization (5.7) is that it is time-independent, and therefore leads to a closed-form solution (under certain base-line risk functions) for the integral in the definition of the survival function (4.2). This facilitates computations because we do not have to numerically ap-proximate this integral. However, an important disadvantage of (5.7) emerges when an elaborate formulation of the subject-specific mean structure of lon-gitudinal submodel is assumed. In particular, when polynomials or splines are used to capture nonlinear subject-specific evolutions, the random effects do not have a straightforward interpretation. For instance, in the joint model fitted to the PBC dataset, in which we have assumed a second degree polyno-mial for the effect of time (see Section 5.1.1), we cannot interpret the linear subject-specific slopes b_{i1} independently from the quadratic subject-specific slopes b_{i2}. This evidently also affects the interpretability of the association parameters α. Due to this limitation package **JM** does not explicitly include this parameterization as an option. Nonetheless, as shown above, we can emulate a part of this parameterization under the simple random-intercepts and random-slopes setting, using the time-dependent slopes parameterization of Section 5.1.3. To illustrate this, we refit the joint model for the PBC dataset, assuming a simpler linear mixed model for serum bilirubin (i.e., we exclude the quadratic time trends):

$$y_i(t) = \beta_0 + \beta_1 \text{D-pnc}_i + \beta_2 t + \beta_3 \{\text{D-pnc}_i \times t\} + b_{i0} + b_{i1} t + \varepsilon_i(t),$$

and a relative hazard model for death including the patient-specific slopes as an extra covariate:

$$h_i(t) = h_0(t) \exp\{\gamma_1 \text{D-pnc}_i + \gamma_2 \text{HepMeg}_i + \alpha(\beta_2 + b_{i1})\}.$$

In the corresponding R syntax below, we first fit the simpler linear mixed model, next we define the list of formulas for the `derivForm` argument, and finally we update the previously fitted joint model, by specifying as parameterization that we only want to include the slope of the true trajectory in the hazard model:

```
> lmeFit2.pbc <- lme(log(serBilir) ~ year * drug,
      random = ~ year | id, data = pbc2)

> dform2 <- list(fixed = ~ 1, indFixed = 3,
      random = ~ 1, indRandom = 2)

> jointFit6.pbc <- update(jointFit3.pbc, lmeObject = lmeFit2.pbc,
      parameterization = "slope", derivForm = dform2)

> summary(jointFit6.pbc)
```

```
. . .

drugD-penicil    -0.0680  0.2203   -0.3087   0.7575
hepatomegalyYes   0.8409  0.2022    4.1586  <0.0001
Assoct.s          9.7530  1.1201    8.7070  <0.0001
log(xi.1)        -6.7693  0.5227  -12.9517
log(xi.2)        -5.3977  0.4295  -12.5686
log(xi.3)        -4.9452  0.3959  -12.4926
log(xi.4)        -4.4833  0.3943  -11.3707
log(xi.5)        -4.1852  0.3698  -11.3168
log(xi.6)        -3.5718  0.3652   -9.7797

. . .
```

We observe that the subject-specific slopes are strongly associated with the

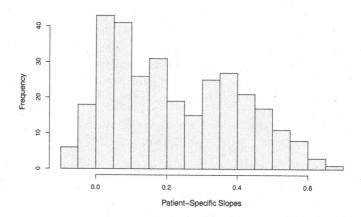

FIGURE 5.4: Empirical Bayes estimates of the subject-specific slopes β_2+b_{i1} for the PBC dataset.

instantaneous risk for death. As it can been in Figure 5.4, the very large value for the slopes' coefficients is explained by their rather small variability. Thus, it will not be meaningful to compute a hazard ratio for one unit increase in the slopes because an increase of such magnitude is not realistic. A more useful estimate for the subject-specific slopes can be obtained by dividing them with their estimated standard deviation from model `jointFit6.pbc` that equals 0.18. The updated joint model fit is produced with the syntax

```
> dform3 <- list(fixed = ~ -1 + I(rep(1/0.18, length(drug))),
     random = ~ -1 + I(rep(1/0.18, length(drug))),
     indFixed = 3, indRandom = 2)

> jointFit7.pbc <- update(jointFit6.pbc, derivForm = dform3)

> summary(jointFit7.pbc)
```

```
. . .
                 Value  Std.Err  z-value p-value
drugD-penicil  -0.0668  0.2207  -0.3028  0.7621
hepatomegalyYes 0.8443  0.2027   4.1655 <0.0001
Assoct.s        1.7617  0.2032   8.6689 <0.0001
log(xi.1)      -6.7889  0.5261 -12.9051
log(xi.2)      -5.4148  0.4326 -12.5158
log(xi.3)      -4.9596  0.3984 -12.4486
log(xi.4)      -4.4970  0.3966 -11.3394
log(xi.5)      -4.1969  0.3718 -11.2891
```

```
log(xi.6)        -3.5821  0.3668  -9.7653
log(xi.7)        -3.8953  0.4711  -8.2684
. . .
```

The results suggest that for patients receiving the same treatment and having the same hepatomegaly status, an increase of one standard deviation in the slope for log serum bilirubin is associated with a 5.82-fold increase (95% CI: 3.91; 8.67) in the hazard for death or transplantation.

5.2 Handling Exogenous Time-Dependent Covariates

In the previous section we saw several possible formulations of the association structure between an endogenous time-dependent covariates and risk for an event. However, in some cases it may also be of interest to incorporate in the linear predictor of the relative risk model additional exogenous time-dependent covariates. For example, in transplantation studies, we may want to examine the association between a biomarker recorded on the patient level and the risk for death, while accounting for the time-dependent effect of transplantation. With the standard current value parameterization (4.1) for the endogenous covariate, the relative risk model can be easily extended to handle exogenous covariates, as

$$h_i(t) = h_0(t) \exp\{\gamma^\top w_i(t) + \alpha m_i(t)\}, \qquad (5.8)$$

where the covariate vector $w_i(t)$ now contains both baseline and exogenous time-dependent covariates. Moreover, the alternative parameterizations of Section 5.1 can be considered for the endogenous covariate, and some of those for the exogenous one as well, such as, interaction effects with baseline covariates, lagged effects and cumulative effects, where for the latter the integral in (5.5) or (5.6) is replaced by a sum. The estimation of the joint model with both exogenous and endogenous time-dependent covariates proceeds in the same manner as with only endogenous covariates. The only practical difference is in the calculation of the integral in the definition of the survival function, which for computational reasons, is expanded as:

$$S_i(t \mid \mathcal{M}_i(t), w_i) = \exp\left(-\int_0^t h_i(s)\, ds\right)$$

$$= \exp\left(-\sum_{q=1}^{Q_i} \int_{\Omega_{iq}} h_0(s) \exp\{\gamma^\top w_{iq}(s) + \alpha m_i(s)\}\, ds\right),$$

where $\{\Omega_{iq}, q = 1, \ldots, Q_i\}$ denote the time intervals during which the exogenous time-dependent covariates $w_i(t)$ are assumed constant.

As an illustration, we fit a joint model to the PBC dataset with an updated relative risk submodel for the composite event (death or transplantation), that additional to the effect of treatment and log serum bilirubin, also includes the main effect of the existence of spiders (blood vessel malformations in the skin) during follow-up, and its interaction with treatment. We should note, however, that, in fact, the existence of spiders is an endogenous binary time-dependent covariate because its existence requires that the patient is still alive. This means that a correct analysis that incorporates the effects of both serum bilirubin and spiders should postulate a joint model with suitable mixed-effects submodels for each of the two longitudinal outcomes. For more information regarding the handling of categorical endogenous time-varying covariates, we refer to Section 5.7.2. Nevertheless, for the sake of illustration, we ignore this fact here and we treat spiders as an exogenous covariate.

As a first step, we need to construct a dataset in the long format, as illustrated in Section 3.5.

```
> pbc <- pbc2[c("id", "serBilir", "drug", "year", "years",
    "status2", "spiders")]

> pbc[pbc$id == "3", ]
   id serBilir      drug      year     years status2 spiders
12  3      1.4 D-penicil 0.0000000 2.770781       1      No
13  3      1.1 D-penicil 0.4818749 2.770781       1     Yes
14  3      1.5 D-penicil 0.9966050 2.770781       1      No
15  3      1.8 D-penicil 2.0342788 2.770781       1     Yes
```

For instance, we observe that Patient 3 had four follow-up measurements during which only in the second and fourth he had spiders. The start and stop variables denoting the limits of the time intervals during which the existence of spiders is recorded, and the event variable that equals 1 if an event occurred at the end of the corresponding time interval, are constructed using the code:

```
> pbc$start <- pbc$year

> splitID <- split(pbc[c("start", "years")], pbc$id)

> pbc$stop <- unlist(lapply(splitID,
    function (d) c(d$start[-1], d$years[1]) ))

> pbc$event <- with(pbc, ave(status2, id,
    FUN = function (x) c(rep(0, length(x)-1), x[1]) ))
```

In particular, remember that in the counting process formulation we construct the interval (start, stop], with the important mathematical constraint that computations done at $t = $ stop utilize covariate data known before this stop time. This formalizes the fact that exogenous covariates are assumed predictable processes (see Section 3.4). For example, for Patient 3 we obtain the result:

```
> pbc[pbc$id == "3", ]
   id serBilir      drug      year    years status2 spiders
12  3     1.4 D-penicil 0.0000000 2.770781       1      No
13  3     1.1 D-penicil 0.4818749 2.770781       1     Yes
14  3     1.5 D-penicil 0.9966050 2.770781       1      No
15  3     1.8 D-penicil 2.0342788 2.770781       1     Yes
        start       stop event
12 0.0000000 0.4818749     0
13 0.4818749 0.9966050     0
14 0.9966050 2.0342788     0
15 2.0342788 2.7707809     1
```

To fit the joint model with spiders as an exogenous time-dependent covariate, we first need to fit the corresponding extended Cox model using the counting process notation and data in the long format constructed above. In addition, because jointModel() requires to distinguish between the measurements of the patients in the survival data in the long format, the patient id variable should be included as a cluster() component in the right-hand side of the formula argument of coxph(), and, moreover, argument model should be set to TRUE.

```
> tdCox.pbc <-
      coxph(Surv(start, stop, event) ~ drug * spiders + cluster(id),
          data = pbc, x = TRUE, model = TRUE)
```

Then the call to jointModel() is the same as in the example we have seen before, with the fitted extended Cox model provided as the survObject argument. We should mention that joint models with both exogenous and endogenous time-dependent covariates are only available under the spline-approximated baseline risk function, that is, for the method argument of jointModel() only option "spline-PH-aGH" is available, e.g.,

```
> jointFit8.pbc <- jointModel(lmeFit.pbc, tdCox.pbc, timeVar = "year",
      method = "spline-PH-aGH")

> summary(jointFit8.pbc)
```

. . .

Event Process
```
                          Value Std.Err z-value p-value
drugD-penicil           -0.2268  0.3164 -0.7169  0.4735
spidersYes               0.4731  0.2763  1.7122  0.0869
drugD-penicil:spidersYes 0.2544  0.4043  0.6292  0.5292
Assoct                   1.2223  0.1113 10.9839 <0.0001
```
. . .

The analysis shows that serum bilirubin remains the most important predictor, whereas there is not enough evidence to support that existence of spiders is associated with the risk for the composite event. The comparison of the joint model with the extended Cox model that treats both serum bilirubin and spiders as exogenous covariates reveals that the strength of the association between log serum bilirubin and the risk for an event is underestimated from the Cox model.

```
> tdCox2.pbc <- coxph(Surv(start, stop, event) ~ drug * spiders +
      log(serBilir), data = pbc)

> tdCox2.pbc


Call:
coxph(formula = Surv(start, stop, event) ~ drug * spiders + log(serBilir),
    data = pbc)


                           coef exp(coef) se(coef)      z    p
drugD-penicil            -0.310     0.734   0.3029 -1.023 0.31
spidersYes                0.419     1.521   0.2681  1.563 0.12
log(serBilir)             1.073     2.924   0.0932 11.514 0.00
drugD-penicil:spidersYes  0.294     1.341   0.3890  0.755 0.45
 . . .
```

In particular, the 95% confidence intervals for the hazard ratio for the logarithm of serum bilirubin under the two models show that the upper bound from the Cox model is only slightly larger than the point estimate from the joint model.

```
> exp(confint(jointFit8.pbc, parm = "Event"))
                              2.5 %       est.    97.5 %
drugD-penicil             0.4286782 0.7970458 1.481956
spidersYes                0.9338199 1.6050347 2.758708
drugD-penicil:spidersYes  0.5839259 1.2896589 2.848341
Assoct                    2.7297554 3.3950626 4.222521


> exp(confint(tdCox2.pbc))
                              2.5 %   97.5 %
drugD-penicil             0.4051017 1.328313
spidersYes                0.8990105 2.571901
log(serBilir)             2.4362185 3.510596
drugD-penicil:spidersYes  0.6257112 2.874938
```

5.3   Stratified Relative Risk Models

In many real examples it is not realistic to assume that the sample at hand comes from a homogeneous population. For instance, in multicenter clinical trials the different centers are expected to have different baseline survival functions due to varying patient populations and referral patterns. A standard extension of relative risk models that handles such settings is to allow for multiple strata. In particular, patients are assumed to be divided in different strata, with each stratum having its own baseline hazard function, but common values for the regressions coefficients γ and α. Under a stratified model, the risk for patient i belonging to stratum k is given by

$$h_{ik}(t) = h_{0k}(t) \exp\{\gamma^\top w_i + \alpha m_i(t)\}, \tag{5.9}$$

with $h_{0k}(t)$ denoting the baseline hazard function for stratum k. Joint models with a stratified relative risk submodel are available in package **JM** under the B-spline-approximated baseline risk function (4.4). A joint model for the PBC dataset, with a stratified survival submodel according to the presence or absence of hepatomegaly, is fitted by

```
> lmeFit.pbc <- lme(log(serBilir) ~ drug * (year + I(year^2)),
      random = ~ year + I(year^2) | id, data = pbc2)

> coxFit2.pbc <- coxph(Surv(years, status2) ~ drug + strata(hepatomegaly),
      data = pbc2.id, x = TRUE)

> jointFit9.pbc <- jointModel(lmeFit.pbc, coxFit2.pbc, timeVar = "year",
      method = "spline-PH-aGH")

> summary(jointFit9.pbc)
```

```
. . .
Event Process
                       Value  Std.Err  z-value  p-value
drugD-penicil         0.0430   0.1676   0.2564   0.7977
Assoct                1.2944   0.0941  13.7569  <0.0001
bs1(hepatomegaly=No) -3.6329   0.7995  -4.5441  <0.0001
bs2(hepatomegaly=No) -5.7295   1.1899  -4.8152  <0.0001
bs3(hepatomegaly=No) -4.2104   1.0735  -3.9220   0.0001
bs4(hepatomegaly=No) -5.4117   0.8184  -6.6129  <0.0001
bs5(hepatomegaly=No) -4.4717   0.7222  -6.1917  <0.0001
bs6(hepatomegaly=No) -4.1540   0.7493  -5.5439  <0.0001
bs7(hepatomegaly=No) -3.5401   1.5440  -2.2929   0.0219
bs8(hepatomegaly=No) -9.5100   3.2027  -2.9694   0.0030
bs9(hepatomegaly=No) -0.7835   1.8491  -0.4237   0.6718
bs1(hepatomegaly=Yes)-4.3688   0.5872  -7.4397  <0.0001
bs2(hepatomegaly=Yes)-4.7974   0.6758  -7.0990  <0.0001
```

```
bs3(hepatomegaly=Yes) -3.6573  0.6603 -5.5388 <0.0001
bs4(hepatomegaly=Yes) -4.1759  0.5591 -7.4686 <0.0001
bs5(hepatomegaly=Yes) -3.1475  0.6051 -5.2013 <0.0001
bs6(hepatomegaly=Yes) -5.3199  0.9146 -5.8164 <0.0001
bs7(hepatomegaly=Yes) -1.1899  1.6687 -0.7131  0.4758
bs8(hepatomegaly=Yes) -6.0432  3.3647 -1.7961  0.0725
bs9(hepatomegaly=Yes) -7.2148  6.9496 -1.0382  0.2992
. . .
```

As can been seen from the output for the event process, different spline coefficients are assumed for patients with and without hepatomegaly. If we would like to fit a model with multiple stratification factors, these should be included as extra arguments in the `strata()` function, e.g., to stratify with respect to both presence/absence of hepatomegaly and sex, the code would have been `strata(hepatomegaly, sex)`.

Contrary to the stratified Cox model in which no direct estimate of the importance of the strata is produced, in the stratified relative risk model with a spline-approximated baseline risk function it is possible to utilize a formal statistical inferential procedure to test whether stratification improves the fit of the model. This is because in the spline approach we use a flexible yet parametric model to estimate the baseline hazard, whereas in the Cox model it is left completely unspecified. The only requirement for such a statistical test to be valid is that the knots for the B-spline approximation of the log baseline risk function should be the same across strata, which is the default in package **JM**. A likelihood ratio test can be performed by fitting the unstratified joint model, and comparing it with the stratified one using function `anova()`. To perform the corresponding Wald test, function `wald.strata()` can be used that directly constructs the appropriate contrasts matrix:

```
> wald.strata(jointFit9.pbc)
        Wald Test for Stratification Factors

X^2 = 24.1423, df = 9, p-value = 0.0041
alternative hypothesis: spline coefficients for the baseline risk
        function are not equal among strata
```

For the stratified joint model fitted to the PBC data, this test suggests that there is strong evidence of a difference between the underlying survival curves of the sub-populations of patients with and without hepatomegaly.

The standard formulation of stratified relative risk models assumes that the effect of every covariate is constant across strata. However, this is not always reasonable, because in many cases some covariates may have a different effect per strata. For instance, in a multicenter randomized trial with similar patient populations in each center, it may be reasonable to assume that the effect of age is the same across centers, but assuming that the treatment effect to be uniform across center may be less defendable. To accommodate such possibilities we extend model (5.9) by allowing for strata by covariate interactions, i.e.,

$$h_i(t) = h_{0k}(t) \exp\{\gamma_k^\top w_i + \alpha_k m_i(t)\}, \tag{5.10}$$

where not only the baseline risk function $h_{0k}(t)$ but also the regression co-efficients γ_k and α_k now depend on the stratum k. In the following example we extend the stratified joint model fitted to the PBC data, by also including in the linear predictor the interaction terms of drug and serum bilirubin with hepatomegaly. As was illustrated in Section 5.1.1, such terms can be added in the survival submodel using the `interFact` argument,

```
> coxFit3.pbc <- coxph(Surv(years, status2) ~ drug * hepatomegaly +
      strata(hepatomegaly), data = pbc2.id, x = TRUE)

> jointFit10.pbc <- update(jointFit9.pbc, survObject = coxFit3.pbc,
      interFact = list(value = ~ hepatomegaly, data = pbc2.id))

> summary(jointFit10.pbc)
```

. . .

Event Process

	Value	Std.Err	z-value	p-value
drugD-penicil	-0.0896	0.2869	-0.3123	0.7548
drugD-penicil:hepatomegalyYes	0.2289	0.3529	0.6486	0.5166
Assoct	1.1974	0.1329	9.0099	<0.0001
Assoct:hepatomegalyYes	0.1854	0.1871	0.9910	0.3217

. . .

We observe that the strength of the association between the risk of the composite event and log serum bilirubin is not statistically different between patients with and without hepatomegaly. The marginal survival functions for the two hepatomegaly groups can be calculated according to the approximate formula

$$\mathcal{S}(t) = \int \mathcal{S}_i(t \mid b_i; \hat{\theta}) \, p(b_i; \hat{\theta}) \, db_i \approx n^{-1} \sum_i \mathcal{S}_i(t \mid \hat{b}_i; \hat{\theta}),$$

where $\hat{b}_i$ denotes the empirical Bayes estimates for the random effects (see Section 4.5), and are depicted for the stratified joint model `jointFit9.pbc` in Figure 5.5. The corresponding syntax to produce the figure entails just a simple call to the `plot()` method, i.e.,

```
> plot(jointFit9.pbc, which = 3)
```

Function `plot()` can be used to produce diagnostic plots of the fitted joint model. From the available options, argument `which` specifies that we want the third one that corresponds to the marginal survival function. Other options of the `plot()` function are illustrated in Chapter 6.

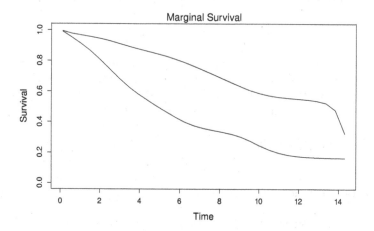

FIGURE 5.5: Marginal survival functions for patients with (dashed line) and without (solid line) hepatomegaly for the PBC dataset.

5.4   Latent Class Joint Models

Another class of joint models related to the stratified joint model presented in Section 5.3, is the latent class joint model (Proust-Lima et al., 2009; Lin et al., 2004, 2002). The motivation behind this type of joint models is also to account for possible heterogeneity in the population. However, and contrary to the stratified joint model, latent class joint models assume that the subpopulations that constitute the population are *latent*, in the sense that heterogeneity is not captured by any of the observed covariates.

To define latent class joint models, we assume that there are G subpopulations that constitute our original population and we introduce the unobserved class indicator $c_i = 1, \ldots, G$ that denotes the class membership of the ith subject. These models work under the following set of conditional independence assumptions:

$$
\begin{aligned}
p(T_i, \delta_i, y_i \mid c_i = g, b_i; \theta) &= p(T_i, \delta_i \mid c_i = g; \theta)\, p(y_i \mid c_i = g, b_i; \theta), \quad \text{and} \\
p(y_i \mid c_i = g, b_i; \theta) &= \prod_j p\{y_i(t_{ij}) \mid c_i = g, b_i; \theta\}.
\end{aligned}
$$

In particular, these models assume that the correlations between the repeated measurements in the longitudinal outcome are captured by the random effects b_i, whereas the association between the event time and longitudinal processes is explained by the shared latent class indicator c_i. The use of two latent components is advantageous from the point of view that it allows for more flexible association structures compared to the classical joint model that assumes the same set of random effects b_i to account for both types of association (see Section 4.3.2). Under the above conditional independence assumptions, a general definition of the latent class joint model involves the following submodels:

$$
\begin{cases}
h_i(t \mid c_i = g) &= h_{0g}(t) \exp(\gamma_g^\top w_i), \\[2mm]
\{y_i(t) \mid c_i = g\} &= x_i^\top(t)\beta_g + z_i^\top(t)b_{ig} + \varepsilon_i(t), \quad \varepsilon_i(t) \sim \mathcal{N}(0, \sigma^2), \\[2mm]
\Pr(c_i = g) &= \exp(\lambda_g^\top u_i) \big/ \sum_{l=1}^G \exp(\lambda_l^\top u_i),
\end{cases}
\tag{5.11}
$$

where we postulate that patients in different latent groups have both different longitudinal evolutions and different risks for an event. The last equation specifies a multinomial submodel for the latent class membership probabilities, with u_i denoting the vector of covariates associated with these probabilities with a corresponding vector of regression coefficients vector $\lambda^\top = (\lambda_1^\top, \ldots, \lambda_G^\top)$, with $\lambda_G = 0$ for identifiability. The random effects $b_{ig} \sim \mathcal{N}(\mu_g, \sigma_g^2 D)$ are also assumed to be latent-class specific, though for computational stability, their covariance matrix is typically assumed to depend on c_i only via the scalar variance parameter σ_g^2.

An advantageous byproduct of the above specification of the latent class joint model is that the log-likelihood under this model takes the following form:

$$
\begin{aligned}
\ell(\theta) &= \sum_{i=1}^n \log \left\{ \sum_{g=1}^G \Pr(c_i = g; \theta)\, h_i(T_i \mid c_i = g; \theta)^{\delta_i}\, S_i(T_i \mid c_i = g; \theta) \right. \\
&\qquad\qquad \left. \times \int \left[\prod_j p\{y_i(t_{ij}) \mid c_i = g, b_i; \theta\} \right] p(b_i \mid c_i = g; \theta)\, db_i \right\} \\
&= \sum_{i=1}^n \log \left\{ \sum_{g=1}^G \Pr(c_i = g; \theta)\, h_i(T_i \mid c_i = g; \theta)^{\delta_i}\, S_i(T_i \mid c_i = g; \theta) \right. \\
&\qquad\qquad \left. \times\, p(y_i \mid c_i = g; \theta) \right\},
\end{aligned}
$$

which is much more tractable to compute compared to the classical joint model because it does not require numerical integration neither for the calculation of the survival function as in (4.2) nor for the calculation of the likelihood as in (4.9). In particular, the former integral in the definition of the survival function has a closed-form (depending, however, also on the model for the baseline risk function) because it does not involve any time-dependent components of the longitudinal process, and the latter integral with respect to the random effects also has a closed-form solution because it only entails the conditional longitudinal model $p(y_i \mid c_i = g, b_i)$ and the random effects density $p(b_i \mid c_i = g)$, which, as we have seen in Section 2.2.1, under the normality assumption for both components leads to a multivariate Gaussian distribution. However, an issue with latent class joint models is that the log-likelihood may have multiple local maxima, and it is therefore recommended to refit the model a number of times using different sets of initial values and investigate convergence. It is evident that this problem in fact almost nullifies the computational advantage of not having to numerically approximate integrals because refitting the model, even though simpler than fitting the classical joint model, still remains a computationally demanding task. This problem is also enhanced by the fact that the appropriate number of latent classes is not known a priori. Thus, it is required to fit several models with an increasing number of classes, and statistically choose the number that provides the best fit to the data. This choice is typically based on information criteria.

An additional issue with latent class joint models is that the interpretability regarding the association structure is not straightforward. In particular, under the latent class formulation there is no set of parameters that directly quantifies the strength of the association between the longitudinal outcome and the risk of an event, which in many cases is of primary subject-matter interest. Thus, this type of joint models are primarily useful when interest is in recovering latent heterogeneity in the target population, but not when direct interest is in providing an easy interpretation behind the association mechanism of the two processes.

In R latent class joint models are fitted using function `Jointlcmm()` from package **lcmm** (Proust-Lima et al., 2011). Contrary to function `jointModel()` that requires to first separately fit the linear mixed-effects and survival models, function `Jointlcmm()` requires providing separate formula arguments that specify the different parts of the model. In particular, arguments `fixed` and `random` accept the formulas that define the fixed- and random-effects parts of the longitudinal submodel, and argument `survival` accepts the formula that specifies the survival submodel. The model for the baseline risk function is specified in argument `hazard` and its dependence on the latent classes by argument `hazardtype`. The last two formula arguments are `classmb` that specifies the linear predictor of the multinomial model in (5.11), and `mixture` that specifies which components of the fixed effects in the longitudinal model are assumed to be depended on c_i. Finally, using argument `ng` we specify that we want to fit a joint model with two latent classes. As an illustration we perform a latent class joint model analysis of the AIDS dataset. For the longitudinal part we include in the fixed part the main effect of time and treatment and in the random part random intercepts and random slopes:

$$\{y_i(t) \mid c_i = g\} = \beta_{0g} + \beta_{1g}t + \beta_{2g}\mathtt{ddI}_i + b_{0i} + b_{1i}t + \varepsilon_i(t).$$

We assume that both covariates in the fixed part are class dependent. For the survival submodel we assume latent class specific baseline risk function and treatment effect,

$$h_i(t \mid c_i = g) = h_{0g}(t)\exp(\gamma_g\mathtt{ddI}_i).$$

The class-specific baseline risk functions are assumed piecewise-constant with six knots placed at the corresponding percentiles of event times distribution.

TABLE 5.2: Log-likelihood and information criteria values for four latent class joint models fitted to the AIDS dataset with an increasing number of latent classes

# Classes	logLik	AIC	BIC
2	−4258.74	8565.48	8665.00
3	−4223.03	8516.06	8661.18
4	−4198.63	8489.26	8679.99
5	−4192.98	8499.96	8736.30

Finally, in the latent membership multinomial model we assume that the prior probability of each patient belonging to a certain class depends on treatment,

$$\Pr(c_i = g) = \frac{\exp(\lambda_{0g} + \lambda_{1g}\mathtt{ddI}_i)}{\sum_{l=1}^{G} \exp(\lambda_{0l} + \lambda_{1l}\mathtt{ddI}_i)}.$$

We fitted four joint models with two, three, four and five latent classes, respectively. The AIC and BIC values are given in Table 5.2. We observe a quite strong disagreement between the two information criteria. Namely, the AIC decreases steadily as the number of classes increases and favors the four class model, while the optimal model according to BIC is the three class model. Empirical studies in the literature have illustrated that the BIC more often suggests the model with the correct number of latent subgroups (Proust-Lima et al., 2009; Lin et al., 2004). Following this recommendation we choose here the model with three latent classes. The corresponding syntax to fit this model is

```
> aidsLC <- aids[c("patient", "CD4", "obstime", "drug", "Time", "death")]

> aidsLC$drug <- c(aidsLC$drug) - 1

> aidsLC <- aidsLC[complete.cases(aidsLC), ]

> lcjmFit.aids <- Jointlcmm(fixed = CD4 ~ obstime + drug,
      mixture = ~ obstime + drug, random = ~ obstime,
      classmb = ~ drug, subject = "patient", ng = 3, data = aids,
      survival = Surv(Time, death) ~ mixture(drug),
      hazard = "6-quant-piecewise", hazardtype = "Specific")

> summary(lcjmFit.aids)
```

· · ·

Maximum Likelihood Estimates:

*** Fixed effects in the class-membership model:

	coef	Se	Wald	p-value
intercept class1	1.89106	0.23570	8.023	0.00000
intercept class2	0.37732	0.31209	1.209	0.22665
drug class1	-0.61612	0.30357	-2.030	0.04240
drug class2	-0.83398	0.43408	-1.921	0.05470

*** Parameters in the proportional hazard model:

	coef	Se	Wald	p-value
+/-sqrt(piecewise1) class1	0.16281	0.01534	10.613	0.00000
+/-sqrt(piecewise2) class1	0.17828	0.01677	10.628	0.00000
+/-sqrt(piecewise3) class1	0.20624	0.01960	10.523	0.00000
+/-sqrt(piecewise4) class1	0.28446	0.02605	10.919	0.00000
+/-sqrt(piecewise5) class1	0.21988	0.02175	10.108	0.00000
+/-sqrt(piecewise1) class2	-0.07036	0.03972	-1.771	0.07649
+/-sqrt(piecewise2) class2	-0.00005	0.13878	0.000	0.99973
+/-sqrt(piecewise3) class2	-0.00006	0.06075	-0.001	0.99925
+/-sqrt(piecewise4) class2	-0.00001	0.06136	0.000	0.99988
+/-sqrt(piecewise5) class2	0.17793	0.05338	3.333	0.00086
+/-sqrt(piecewise1) class3	0.01161	0.02731	0.425	0.67074
+/-sqrt(piecewise2) class3	0.01104	0.02626	0.420	0.67425
+/-sqrt(piecewise3) class3	0.02034	0.04690	0.434	0.66457
+/-sqrt(piecewise4) class3	0.00000	0.01179	0.000	0.99982
+/-sqrt(piecewise5) class3	0.00000	0.01223	0.000	0.99997
drug class1	0.28098	0.15892	1.768	0.07704
drug class2	-0.38993	0.94958	-0.411	0.68134
drug class3	3.78385	4.62508	0.818	0.41329

*** Fixed effects in the longitudinal model:

	coef	Se	Wald	p-value
intercept class1	4.55138	0.20977	21.697	0.00000
intercept class2	11.97218	0.61159	19.575	0.00000
intercept class3	15.38392	0.50256	30.611	0.00000
obstime class1	-0.13510	0.01743	-7.750	0.00000
obstime class2	-0.33377	0.04416	-7.558	0.00000
obstime class3	0.00773	0.03110	0.249	0.80364
drug class1	0.19309	0.27229	0.709	0.47824
drug class2	-0.35690	0.90091	-0.396	0.69199
drug class3	-1.03255	0.57001	-1.811	0.07007

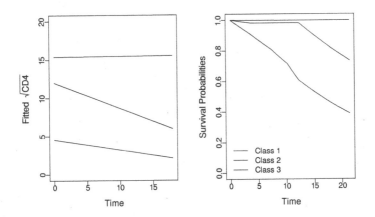

FIGURE 5.6: Fitted average longitudinal evolutions and event-free survival probabilities for the three class joint model fitted to the AIDS dataset.

```
*** Variance-covariance matrix of the random-effects:
           intercept      obstime
intercept  4.9973730
obstime    -0.2399735 0.01740456

                          coef         se
*** Residual standard error: 1.733884 0.04702784
```

The current version of the package (1.4-3) does not automatically exclude missing data, and does not create dummy variables for factors; the user is required to do these operations manually. We observe that for some parameters, such as the slope in the longitudinal part, there seem to be significant differences between classes. Though a more useful summary of the fitted latent class joint model is given in Figure 5.6 that illustrates the average longitudinal evolutions of the square root CD4 cells count for the three latent classes and the corresponding survival probabilities. It is evident that the model has identified three distinct subpopulations. In particular, one group with relatively high and stable CD4 cell count levels that also enjoys high event-free survival rates, a second group that starts with moderate CD4 cell count levels at baseline and deteriorates rather fast and shows high survival rates up to month 12 and then deteriorates, and a third group that starts with low CD4 cell counts levels also deteriorates in time, though slower than group 2, and exhibits the lowest survival probabilities.

Using the fitted model we can also derive the posterior classification for the patients in the sample. This is achieved by taking the maximum of the posterior probabilities,

$$\Pr(c_i = g \mid T_i, \delta_i, y_i; \hat{\theta}) =$$

$$\frac{\Pr(c_i = g; \hat{\theta})\, h_i(T_i \mid c_i = g; \hat{\theta})^{\delta_i} S_i(T_i \mid c_i = g; \hat{\theta})\, p(y_i \mid c_i = g; \hat{\theta})}{\sum_{l=1}^{G} \Pr(c_i = l; \hat{\theta})\, h_i(T_i \mid c_i = l; \hat{\theta})^{\delta_i} S_i(T_i \mid c_i = l; \hat{\theta})\, p(y_i \mid c_i = l; \hat{\theta})},$$

that is subject i is classified to group g, using

$$\hat{c}_i = \arg\max_{g}\{\Pr(c_i = g \mid T_i, \delta_i, y_i; \hat{\theta})\}$$

which is similar in spirit to the empirical Bayes estimates for the random effects described in Section 4.5. A summary of these probabilities and of the posterior classification is provided by function `postprob()`,

```
> postprob(lcjmFit.aids)
Posterior classification based on longitudinal and time-to-event data:
   class1 class2 class3
N 335.00  62.00  70.00
% 71.73  13.28  14.99

Posterior classification table:
     --> mean of posterior probabilities in each class
          prob1  prob2  prob3
class1 0.9686 0.0299 0.0015
class2 0.0961 0.8304 0.0734
class3 0.0048 0.0642 0.9309


Posterior classification based only on longitudinal data:
   class1 class2 class3
N 338.00  61.00  68.00
% 72.38  13.06  14.56
```

Class 1 contains the largest percentage of subjects, with classes 2 and 3 evenly matched. Moreover, the high means of posterior probabilities for each class suggests that for the majority of the patients the class allocation was evident.

5.5   Multiple Failure Times

5.5.1   Competing Risks

As we have also mentioned in Section 1.3, in longitudinal studies we often collect a wealth of follow-up information for the patients under study. This could include several biomarkers but also multiple failure times. Here we focus on studying the association between a single endogenous time-dependent covariate and time to different types of failure (the consideration of multiple biomarkers is deferred to Section 5.8). For example, in all our previous analyses of the PBC dataset, we have considered the association between serum bilirubin and the risk for the composite event, death or transplantation, whatever comes first. However, it could also be of interest to distinguish between the events, and investigate how covariates affect the risk for transplantation separately from how they affect the risk for death. One of the traditional types of analysis in such settings is the cause-specific hazard regression, which postulates separate relative risk models for each of the competing events (Putter et al., 2007). When only baseline and exogenous time-dependent covariates need to be considered in an analysis, we can fit separate Cox models for each cause, treating failure from the other cause as censored observations. Nevertheless, when there is interest in the association between endogenous time-dependent covariates and the risk for either of the causes, a joint modeling approach should be utilized instead. In particular, joint models of this type have been studied by Elashoff et al. (2008), Williamson et al. (2008), Hu et al. (2009), and Huang et al. (2011).

To handle different failure types we need to extend the notation for the survival process. In particular, assuming K different causes of failure, we let $T_{i1}^*, \ldots, T_{iK}^*$ denote the true failure times for each one of those. The observed data for the ith subject comprise of the observed event time $T_i = \min(T_{i1}^*, \ldots, T_{iK}^*, C_i)$, with C_i denoting the censoring time, and the event indicator takes values $\delta_i \in \{0, 1, \ldots, K\}$, with 0 corresponding to censoring, and $1, \ldots, K$ to the competing events. For each of the K causes, and as mentioned above, we postulate the standard relative risk model

$$h_{ik}(t) = h_{0k}(t) \exp\{\gamma_k^\top w_i + \alpha_k m_i(t)\}, \tag{5.12}$$

which includes the effects of the baseline covariates w_i and of the current value of the longitudinal marker $m_i(t)$. The specification of the joint model is completed by positing a suitable mixed-effects model for the observed longitudinal responses $y_i(t)$. Estimation of such joint models is based on exactly the same principles as for joint models with a single failure type. The only difference is in the construction of the likelihood part for the event process. This in particular takes the form:

$$p(T_i, \delta_i \mid b_i; \theta_t, \beta) = \prod_{k=1}^{K} \left[h_{0k}(T_i) \exp\{\gamma_k^\top w_i + \alpha_k m_i(T_i)\} \right]^{I(\delta_i = k)}$$

$$\times \exp\left(-\sum_{k=1}^{K} \int_0^{T_i} h_{0k}(s) \exp\{\gamma_k^\top w_i + \alpha_k m_i(s)\} \, ds \right). \tag{5.13}$$

From a computational point of view, this part of the likelihood can be more easily calculated by transforming the data in the competing risk long format (which is different from the counting process long format of Section 3.5). In particular, if there are K competing events, then each subject has K rows, one for each possible cause. The observed event time T_i of each subject is repeated K times, and there are two indicator variables, namely one identifying the cause, and one indicating whether the corresponding event type is the one that occurred. Standard survival datasets that included a single row per patient, e.g.,

```
> head(pbc2.id[c("id", "years", "status")], 5)
  id     years      status
1  1  1.095170        dead
2  2 14.152338       alive
3  3  2.770781        dead
4  4  5.270507        dead
5  5  4.120578 transplanted
```

can be easily transformed to the competing risks long format using function crLong(). This accepts as main arguments the survival data in the standard format that has a single row per patient, the name of the status variable, and the level in this status variable that corresponds to censoring. For the first five patients from the PBC dataset presented above we obtain:

```
> pbc2.idCR <- crLong(pbc2.id, statusVar = "status",
      censLevel = "alive", nameStrata = "CR")
```

```
> head(pbc2.idCR[c("id", "years", "status", "CR", "status2")], 10)
     id     years        status           CR status2
1     1  1.095170          dead         dead       1
1.1   1  1.095170          dead transplanted       0
2     2 14.152338         alive         dead       0
2.1   2 14.152338         alive transplanted       0
3     3  2.770781          dead         dead       1
3.1   3  2.770781          dead transplanted       0
4     4  5.270507          dead         dead       1
4.1   4  5.270507          dead transplanted       0
5     5  4.120578  transplanted         dead       0
5.1   5  4.120578  transplanted transplanted       1
```

Note that each patient is now represented by two rows (we have two possible causes of discontinuation from the study, death and transplantation), the time variable years is identical in both rows of each patient, variable CR denotes the cause for the specific line of the long dataset, and variable status2 equals 1 if the corresponding event occurred. Using the data in the long format, we can easily compute the logarithm of $p(T_i, \delta_i \mid b_i; \theta_t, \beta)$, as presented above, by simply treating variable CR as a stratification factor, taking interaction terms of this variable with all other variables we wish to include in the linear predictor of the cause-specific relative risk models, using `status2` as the event variable, and calculating the sum of the rows corresponding to the ith subject.

As an illustration, we fit a joint model to the PBC dataset, treating transplantation and death as separate competing events. For the longitudinal bilirubin responses we assume the linear mixed-effects model of Section 5.1.1 with quadratic evolutions in time for each patient with different average effects per treatment group:

$$y_i(t) = \beta_0 + \beta_1 \texttt{D-pnc}_i + \beta_2 t + \beta_3 t^2 + \beta_4 \{\texttt{D-pnc}_i \times t\} + \beta_5 \{\texttt{D-pnc}_i \times t^2\}$$
$$+ b_{i0} + b_{i1} t + b_{i2} t^2 + \varepsilon_i(t).$$

The call to function `lme()` to fit this model is

```
> lmeFit.pbc <- lme(log(serBilir) ~ drug * (year + I(year^2)),
      random = ~ year + I(year^2) | id, data = pbc2)
```

For the event process we assume the cause-specific relative risks models:

$$\begin{cases} h_{i1}(t) = h_{01}(t) \exp\{\gamma_{11}\texttt{D-pnc}_i + \gamma_{12}\texttt{Age}_i + \alpha_1 m_i(t)\}, \\[2mm] h_{i2}(t) = h_{02}(t) \exp\{(\gamma_{11} + \gamma_{21})\texttt{D-pnc}_i + (\gamma_{12} + \gamma_{22})\texttt{Age}_i \\[2mm] \qquad\qquad\qquad\qquad + (\alpha_1 + \alpha_2) m_i(t)\}. \end{cases}$$

Under this formulation parameters γ_{11}, γ_{12} and α_1 denote the effects of treatment, age, and log serum bilirubin, respectively, on the risk for transplantation, and γ_{21}, γ_{22} and α_2 denote the additional effects of treatment, age and log serum bilirubin, respectively on the risk for death. For example, $\gamma_{21} = 0$ means that the hazard ratio for treatment is the same for both transplantation and death. Using dataset `pbc2.idCR` we fit the corresponding cause-specific Cox regressions by including the interaction terms of age and treatment with variable `CR`, and further including it as a stratification variable using `strata()`:

```
> coxFit4.pbc <-
      coxph(Surv(years, status2) ~ (drug + age) * CR + strata(CR),
          data = pbc2.idCR, x = TRUE)
```

The warning message regarding the singularity of the design matrix that appears when fitting this model is due to the fact that we both include the main effect of `CR` and we treat it as a stratification factor. Since we assume different and completely unspecified baseline risk functions for the two causes, the main effect of `CR` on the hazard cannot be identified. As before, the joint model is fitted by providing the mixed-effects and Cox models as main argument to `jointModel()`. Since a `strata()` term has been included in `coxph()`, only option `"spline-PH-aGH"` (or `"spline-PH-GH"`) is available for the `method` argument of `jointModel()`. In addition, to specify that the survival part of the likelihood of the joint model needs to be computed according to (5.13), we also need to set argument `CompRisk` to `TRUE`, i.e.,

```
> jointFit11.pbc <- jointModel(lmeFit.pbc, coxFit4.pbc,
    timeVar = "year", method = "spline-PH-aGH", CompRisk = TRUE,
    interFact = list(value = ~ CR, data = pbc2.idCR))

> summary(jointFit11.pbc)
```

. . .

```
Event Process
                          Value  Std.Err  z-value  p-value
drugD-penicil            -0.3968  0.3874  -1.0243  0.3057
age                      -0.0860  0.0245  -3.5105  0.0004
drugD-penicil:CRdead      0.3756  0.4240   0.8860  0.3756
age:CRdead                0.1523  0.0259   5.8795 <0.0001
Assoct                    1.0223  0.1920   5.3246 <0.0001
Assoct:CRdead             0.4490  0.2185   2.0554  0.0398
```

. . .

The `interFact` is used to additionally include in the linear predictor of the survival submodel the main effect of log serum bilirubin $m_i(t)$, and its interaction with the failure type indicator `CR`. The results indicate that each one unit increase of the current value of log serum bilirubin is associated with a 2.8-fold increase (95% CI: 1.9; 4) in a patient's risk for transplantation, and a 4.4-fold increase (95% CI: 3.5; 5.4) in a patient's risk for death. In addition, we observe that younger patients have a higher risk of getting a transplant (hazard ratio for one year decrease in age equals 1.09), whereas older patients have a higher risk of dying (hazard ratio for one year increase in age equals 1.07).

Furthermore, the different parameterizations we have introduced in Section 5.1 can also be utilized in the specification of the cause-specific hazard regression models (5.12). As an example, we extend the competing risks joint model fitted to the PBC dataset above by allowing the risk for death and transplantation to additionally depend on the slope of the true trajectory of the log serum bilirubin $m_i'(t) = dm_i(t)/dt$. In particular, the cause-specific hazard models take the form:

$$\begin{cases} h_{i1}(t) &= h_{01}(t)\exp\{\gamma_{11}\text{D-pnc}_i + \gamma_{12}\text{Age}_i + \alpha_{11}m_i(t) + \alpha_{12}m_i'(t)\}, \\ h_{i2}(t) &= h_{02}(t)\exp\{(\gamma_{11}+\gamma_{21})\text{D-pnc}_i + (\gamma_{12}+\gamma_{22})\text{Age}_i \\ &\quad + (\alpha_{11}+\alpha_{21})m_i(t) + (\alpha_{12}+\alpha_{22})m_i'(t)\}. \end{cases}$$

where, as in Section 5.1.3, $m_i'(t)$ is given by

$$m_i'(t) = \beta_2 + 2\beta_3 t + \beta_4\text{D-pnc}_i + 2\beta_5\{\text{D-pnc}_i \times t\} + b_{i1} + 2b_{i2}t.$$

To incorporate these terms in our analysis, we take advantage of the functionality provided by the `derivForm` and `interFact` arguments of `jointModel()`. More specifically, to include term $m_i'(t)$ in the linear predictors of the cause-specific hazards models, we use option `"both"` for the `parameterization` argument, and provide the list that specifies the fixed- and random-effects parts of $m_i'(t)$ in the `derivForm` argument. This list takes the form:

```
> dform <- list(fixed = ~ I(2*year) * drug, indFixed = 3:6,
      random = ~ I(2*year), indRandom = 2:3)
```

To additionally specify that the effect of the slope of the true trajectory is different for the two failure types we add the component `slope` in the list provided in the `interFact` argument. Similar to the `value` component the `slope` component is a formula that specifies the interaction factors for the time-dependent slope $m_i'(t)$. In particular, the call to `jointModel()` is

```
> jointFit12.pbc <- update(jointFit11.pbc,
      parameterization = "both", derivForm = dform,
      interFact = list(value = ~ CR, slope = ~ CR, data = pbc2.idCR))
```

The `summary()` method provides the detailed output:

```
> summary(jointFit12.pbc)
```

. . .

```
Event Process
                        Value  Std.Err  z-value  p-value
drugD-penicil          -0.3208  0.3914  -0.8196   0.4125
age                    -0.0808  0.0241  -3.3516   0.0008
drugD-penicil:CRdead    0.2569  0.4263   0.6026   0.5468
age:CRdead              0.1307  0.0255   5.1252  <0.0001
Assoct                  0.9905  0.2109   4.6976  <0.0001
Assoct:CRdead           0.2787  0.2346   1.1878   0.2349
Assoct.s                1.4072  1.6032   0.8777   0.3801
Assoct.s:CRdead         0.7498  1.7097   0.4386   0.6610
```

. . .

We observe that a unit increase in the value of the slope of the true trajectory of log serum bilirubin results in a log hazard ratio of 1.4 (95% CI: -1.7; 4.5) for transplantation, and 2.2 (95% CI: 1; 3.3) for death. To statistically test whether the extension to include the time-dependent slopes component $m_i'(t)$ improves the fit of the competing risks joint model, we perform a likelihood ratio test between models `jointFit11.pbc` and `jointFit12.pbc` using function `anova()`:

```
> anova(jointFit11.pbc, jointFit12.pbc)

                  AIC      BIC   log.Lik    LRT df p.value
jointFit11.pbc 3866.90 4005.39 -1896.45
jointFit12.pbc 3858.07 4004.05 -1890.04 12.83  2  0.0016
```

The level of the p-value suggests that there is strong enough evidence to reject the null hypothesis which posits that $\alpha_{12} = \alpha_{22} = 0$.

5.5.2 Recurrent Events

In the previous section we focused on the association between a longitudinal marker and different failure types. A similar setting emerges however when we are interested in a single event that may occur several times for each subject. For example, in the AIDS study, introduced in Section 1.2.2, patients provided CD4 cell count measurements, but they were also checked for the occurrence of opportunistic diseases. In this setting we may conjecture that higher CD4 cell counts are associated with a lower risk for opportunistic diseases, and in turn, that higher CD4 cell counts and a lower risk of opportunistic disease are associated with a lower risk for death. To statistically validate this hypothesis it is required to postulate a model that relates the three outcomes, namely, the occurrence of opportunistic diseases, death, and the CD4 cell count. Another situation where it may be required to account for recurrent events in our analysis is encountered when the visiting process is informative. In particular, as we have noted in Section 4.3.2, the joint modeling analyses we have performed were based on the assumption that the time elapsed between the visits of the patients may only depend on the observed longitudinal history. Nevertheless, this assumption may be violated in practice, when, for instance, patients in a severe disease stage visit the hospital more often than patients in a mild stage. In this case, and even though we may be primarily interested in the terminating event, it would be required to model the visiting process in order to obtain valid results. Detailed descriptions of the different modeling approaches available for the analysis of recurrent event time can be found in Hougaard (2000) and Therneau and Grambsch (2000), whereas joint models that combine recurrent and terminating events with longitudinal endogenous covariates have been proposed by Liu et al. (2008) and Liu and Huang (2009).

To introduce joint models that can handle this type of survival data, we let U_{ik}, $k = 1, \ldots, K_i$ denote the recurrent event times from the study onset, and d_{ik} the indicator for the kth recurrent event of subject i. For the terminal event we use the same notation as in the previous sections, with T_i denoting the observed terminal event time, taken as the minimum of the true terminal event time T_i^* and of the censoring time C_i. The terminal event indicator is analogously defined as $\delta_i = I(T_i^* \leq C_i)$. We assume that true value of the longitudinal marker $m_i(t)$ is associated with both the risk for the recurrent events and for the terminal event. In particular, we postulate two separate relative risk models for the two processes:

$$\begin{cases} r_i(t) &= r_0(t)\exp\{\gamma_r^\top w_{ri} + \alpha_r m_i(t) + \mathrm{v}_i\}, \\ h_i(t) &= h_0(t)\exp\{\gamma_h^\top w_{hi} + \alpha_h m_i(t) + \zeta\mathrm{v}_i\}, \end{cases} \tag{5.14}$$

where w_{ri} denotes the baseline covariates affecting the risk for a recurrent event, and w_{hi} the ones affecting the risk for the terminating event, with corresponding regression coefficients γ_r and γ_h, respectively. Analogously, parameters α_r and α_h measure the strength of the association between the current value of the longitudinal marker and the risk for a recurrent and terminal event, respectively. Term v_i is a random effect (also known as a frailty term in the survival analysis context) that accounts for the correlation in the recurrent events. Subjects with a higher value for v_i will have a higher risk for a recurrent event. Parameter ζ in the terminating event relative risk model measures how strongly associated is the risk of a terminating event with the risk for a recurrent event.

The definition of the likelihood of this type of joint model is based on extended set of conditional independence assumptions. In particular, the three processes, namely the recurrent event process, the terminating event process and the longitudinal process, are assumed independent given both sets of random effects $\{b_i, \mathrm{v}_i\}$. Moreover, the recurrent event times for subject i are assumed independent given her frailty term v_i, and, as before, the longitudinal responses $y_i(t_{ij})$ are assumed independent given b_i. Formally, these statements are given by the following set of equations:

$$\begin{aligned} p(T_i, \delta_i, U_i, d_i, y_i \mid b_i, \mathrm{v}_i; \theta) &= p(T_i, \delta_i \mid b_i, \mathrm{v}_i; \theta) \\ &\quad \times p(U_{ik}, d_{ik} \mid b_i, \mathrm{v}_i; \theta)\, p(y_i \mid b_i; \theta), \end{aligned}$$

$$p(U_i, d_i \mid b_i \mathrm{v}_i; \theta) = \prod_k p(U_{ik}, d_{ik} \mid b_i, \mathrm{v}_i; \theta), \quad \text{and}$$

$$p(y_i \mid b_i; \theta) = \prod_j p\{y_i(t_{ij}) \mid b_i; \theta\},$$

where $U_i^\top = (U_{i1}, \dots, U_{ik})$ and similarly, $d_i^\top = (d_{i1}, \dots, d_{ik})$. Under these assumptions, the likelihood contribution for the ith subject is

$$p(T_i, \delta_i, y_i; \theta) = \int p(T_i, \delta_i \mid b_i, \mathrm{v}_i; \theta)\, p(U_{ik}, d_{ik} \mid; \theta)\, p(y_i \mid b_i; \theta)\, p(b_i; \theta)\, db_i,$$

where $p(T_i, \delta_i \mid b_i, \mathrm{v}_i; \theta)$ and $p(y_i \mid b_i; \theta)p(b_i; \theta)$ are formulated similarly to (4.10) and (4.11), respectively, and

$$p(U_{ik}, d_{ik} \mid; \theta) = \int p(U_{ik}, d_{ik} \mid \mathrm{v}_i; \theta)\, p(\mathrm{v}_i; \theta)\, d\mathrm{v}_i,$$

with

$$p(U_{ik}, d_{ik} \mid v_i; \theta) = \prod_{k=1}^{K_i} \left[r_0(U_{ik}) \exp\{\gamma_r^\top w_{ri} + \alpha_r m_i(U_{ik}) + v_i\} \right]^{\delta_{ik}}$$

$$\times \exp\left(-\int_0^{U_{ik}} r_0(s) \exp\{\gamma_r^\top w_{ri} + \alpha_r m_i(s) + v_i\} \, ds \right).$$

The specification of the model is completed by assuming an appropriate distribution for the frailty terms v_i. A standard choice in the frailty models context is to assume that $\log(v_i)$ has a Gamma distribution with mean one and variance σ_V, because it leads to a closed-form expression for the marginal distribution of the event times (Duchateau and Janssen, 2008). However, under the joint model formulation presented above, and because the integral with respect to time

$$\int_0^{U_{ik}} r_0(s) \exp\{\gamma_r^\top w_{ri} + \alpha_r m_i(s) + v_i\} \, ds$$

also involves the term $m_i(s)$, the integral with respect to the frailty term v_i in the definition of $p(U_{ik}, d_{ik} \mid v_i; \theta)$ no longer has an analytical solution, and therefore a numerical integration approach is required for its evaluation. This requirement is, however, alleviated if we opt for a random-effects parameterization, similar to the one presented in Section 5.1.5, i.e.,

$$r_i(t) = r_0(t) \exp(\gamma_r^\top w_{ri} + \alpha_r^\top b_i + v_i).$$

Then the integral with respect to time takes the form

$$\int_0^{U_{ik}} r_0(s) \exp\{\gamma_r^\top w_{ri} + \alpha_r^\top b_i + v_i\} \, ds = R_0(U_{ik}) \exp(\gamma_r^\top w_{ri} + \alpha_r^\top b_i + v_i),$$

with $R_0(\cdot)$ denoting the cumulative hazard function corresponding to $r_0(\cdot)$, and this in turn leads to the following expression for the marginal distribution of the recurrent events process:

$$p(U_{ik}, d_{ik} \mid v_i; \theta)$$

$$= \frac{\Gamma(d_i + \vartheta) \prod_k \{r_0(U_{ik}) \exp(\gamma_r^\top w_{ri} + \alpha_r^\top b_i + v_i)\}^{d_{ik}}}{\{\vartheta + \sum_k R_0(U_{ik}) \exp(\gamma_r^\top w_{ri} + \alpha_r^\top b_i + v_i)\}^{d_i + \vartheta} \, \sigma_V^\vartheta \Gamma(\vartheta)},$$

where $\Gamma(\cdot)$ denotes the Gamma function, $d_i = \sum_k d_{ik}$, and $\vartheta = 1/\sigma_V$. Nevertheless, this property is lost when v_i is assumed to follow another distribution, such as the normal.

5.6 Accelerated Failure Time Models

An alternative modeling framework for event time data when the proportionality assumption in (4.1) fails is the accelerated failure time (AFT) models. These model specify that predictors act multiplicatively on the failure time or additively on the log failure time. The idea is that predictors alter the rate at which a subject proceeds along the time axis, i.e., accelerate or decelerate the time of failure (Kalbfleisch and Prentice, 2002). AFT models are typically defined as

$$\log T_i^* = \gamma^\top w_i + \sigma_t \varepsilon_{ti}, \tag{5.15}$$

where parameter σ_t is a scale parameter and ε_{ti} is assumed to follow a specific distribution. Parameter γ_j denotes the change in the expected log failure time for a unit change in the corresponding covariate w_{ij}. Equivalently, a unit change in w_{ij} increases the failure time by a factor of $\exp(\gamma_j)$. Standard options for the distribution of the error terms ε_{ti} are the normal, Student's-t, and the extreme value distribution. The last option corresponds to a Weibull distribution for T_i^*, which is the only distribution (together with its special case, the exponential) that accepts both a relative risk and an AFT model formulation.

In order to incorporate time-dependent covariates within this framework, we let $\mathcal{S}_0$ denote an absolutely continuous baseline survival function, and we follow the formulation of Cox and Oakes (1984, Section 5.2) that postulates

$$\left\{ \int_0^{T^*} \exp\{\gamma^\top w + \alpha m(s)\} \, ds \right\} \sim \mathcal{S}_0.$$

This can be reexpressed in terms of the risk rate function for subject i as

$$h_i(t \mid \mathcal{M}_i(t), w_i) = h_0(V_i(t)) \exp\{\gamma^\top w_i + \alpha m_i(t)\}, \tag{5.16}$$

with

$$V_i(t) = \int_0^t \exp\{\gamma^\top w_i + \alpha m_i(s)\} \, ds.$$

Similar to (4.1), the baseline risk function $h_0(\cdot)$ can be assumed of a specific parametric form or modeled flexibly. An important difference of (5.16) compared to (4.1) is that in the former the entire covariate history $\mathcal{M}_i(t)$ is assumed to influence the subject-specific risk $h_i(t)$ because $h_0(\cdot)$ is evaluated at $V_i(t)$. An issue when introducing time-varying covariates in AFT models is that interpretation becomes more complicated because parameter α is involved in both terms in the right-hand side of (5.16). In particular, the survival function for a subject with covariate history $\mathcal{M}_i(t)$ is $\mathcal{S}_i(t \mid \mathcal{M}_i(t)) = \mathcal{S}_0(V_i(t))$, which means that this subject ages on an accelerated schedule $V_i(t)$ compared to $\mathcal{S}_0$; for more information we refer to Cox and Oakes (1984, Section 5.2). Within the joint modeling framework, accelerated failure time models have been discussed by Tseng et al. (2005).

Currently, the only AFT model available in package **JM** is the Weibull model, i.e., model (5.16) with $h_0(t) = \sigma_t t^{\sigma_t - 1}$ using the option `"weibull-AFT-aGH"` for the `method` argument. We should note that when time-dependent covariates are considered the unique property of the Weibull model that can be expressed under both the relative risk and AFT formulations is lost. That is, the default option `"weibull-PH-aGH"` for argument `method` that fits a joint model with a Weibull relative risk submodel is not equivalent to `"weibull-AFT-aGH"`. We compare the two formulations for the AIDS dataset. For the longitudinal outcome we postulate a linear mixed model with fixed effects time and its interaction with treatment, and as random effects the intercept term and time. In the survival submodel we include the effects of treatment, gender, and AZT (i.e., whether the patient has AZT intolerance or failure):

```
> lmeFit.aids <- lme(CD4 ~ obstime + obstime:drug,
      random = ~ obstime | patient, data = aids)

> coxFit.aids <- coxph(Surv(Time, death) ~ drug + gender + AZT,
      data = aids.id, x = TRUE)

> jointFit3.aids <- jointModel(lmeFit.aids, coxFit.aids,
      timeVar = "obstime")

> jointFit4.aids <- update(jointFit3.aids, method = "weibull-AFT-aGH")
```

Since these models are not nested, we can only compare them using information criteria, and therefore we specify in the call to `anova()` that we do not wish to perform the likelihood ratio test:

```
> anova(jointFit3.aids, jointFit4.aids, test = FALSE)

                   AIC      BIC   log.Lik df
jointFit3.aids 8674.95 8728.86 -4324.48
jointFit4.aids 8675.79 8729.69 -4324.90  0
```

We observe that both models practically provide the same fit to the data, with almost indistinguishable log-likelihood values. The parameter estimates and standard errors for the event process under the two formulations are presented in Table 5.3. As expected, the estimated regression coefficients for the same covariates have different values and opposite signs under the two formulations since they, in fact, have different interpretations.

TABLE 5.3: Parameter estimates and standard errors for the Weibull model fitted to the AIDS dataset under the relative risk and accelerated failure time formulations

	Rel. Risk		AFT	
	Value	Std. Err.	Value	Std. Err.
(Intercept)	-2.988	0.388	2.342	0.225
drugddI	0.359	0.156	-0.277	0.122
gendermale	-0.362	0.259	0.280	0.201
AZTfailure	0.329	0.156	-0.257	0.122
Assoct	-0.265	0.036	0.204	0.034
log(shape)	0.234	0.073	0.247	0.078

5.7 Joint Models for Categorical Longitudinal Outcomes

5.7.1 The Generalized Linear Mixed Model (GLMM)

So far we have primarily focused on continuous longitudinal responses. However, in many cases interest may lie in the association between a categorical longitudinal outcome and a time-to-event. In this context it is evident that the linear mixed model (4.5) cannot be used anymore, since it is only applicable for normally distributed biomarkers. An alternative framework which is nowadays routinely used for the analysis of discrete repeated measures data is the generalized linear mixed model (Breslow and Clayton, 1993). The two main reasons for its widespread applicability are that it is a straightforward extension of the generalized linear models (McCullagh and Nelder, 1989) to multivariate data, and that it is currently possible to fit this type of models in a wide range of software packages.

To define GLMMs, let $y_i(t)$ denote the outcome measure at time t for subject i, $i = 1, \dots, n$. We also denote by $y_i = \{y_{ij}, j = 1, \dots, n_i\}$ the n_i-dimensional vector of observed longitudinal responses for the ith subject. Conditionally on a q_b-dimensional random-effects vector b_i, assumed to be independently drawn from $\mathcal{N}(0, D)$, the outcomes y_{ij} are independent with densities from the exponential family of distributions

$$p(y_i \mid b_i; \beta, \varphi) = \exp\left\{ \sum_{j=1}^{n_i} \left[y_{ij}\psi_{ij}(b_i) - c\{\psi_{ij}(b_i)\} \right] \Big/ a(\varphi) - d(y_{ij}, \varphi) \right\}, \quad (5.17)$$

where $\psi_{ij}(b_i)$ and φ denote the natural and dispersion parameters in the exponential family, respectively, and $c(\cdot)$, $d(\cdot)$ and $a(\cdot)$ are known functions specifying the member of the exponential family. Different choices for these functions cover the Binomial, Poisson, Gamma, and normal distributions among others. We complete the specification of the model by defining the mean of $y_i(t)$

conditional on the random effects

$$E(y_i(t) \mid b_i) = \frac{\partial c\{\psi_i(t \mid b_i)\}}{\partial \psi_i(t \mid b_i)} = g^{-1}\{x_i^\top(t)\beta + z_i^\top(t)b_i\}, \qquad (5.18)$$

where $g(\cdot)$ denotes a known monotonic link function, and $x_i(t)$ and $z_i(t)$ denote the design vectors for the fixed effects β and the random effects b_i, respectively. Since the normal distribution is a member of the exponential family of distributions, the linear mixed model of Section 4.1.2 is a special case of a generalized linear mixed model, with $p(y_i \mid b_i; \beta, \varphi)$ denoting the normal density with variance parameter φ, and $g(\cdot)$ is the identity link function.

One of the traditional estimation approaches for the parameters of GLMMs is the marginal maximum likelihood method. This proceeds in a very similar manner as for linear mixed models, presented in Section 2.2.1. In particular, the marginal log-likelihood function for GLMMs takes the form

$$
\begin{aligned}
\ell(\beta, \varphi, D) &= \sum_{i=1}^{n} p(y_i; \beta, \varphi, D) \\
&= \sum_{i=1}^{n} \int \prod_{j=1}^{n_i} p(y_{ij} \mid b_i; \beta, \varphi)\, p(b_i; D)\, db_i, \qquad (5.19)
\end{aligned}
$$

where we exploit the fact that y_{ij} are assumed independent conditionally on the random effects b_i. In general, no analytic expressions are available for the n integrals in the definition of (5.19). The well-known exception where these integrals can be solved analytically is the linear mixed model under which, and as we have seen in Section 2.2.1, the marginal density $p(y_i; \beta, \varphi, D)$ is the n_i-dimensional normal density with mean $X_i\beta$ and variance-covariance matrix $V_i = Z_i D Z_i^\top + \varphi I_{n_i}$. Another example where an analytic solution can be fashioned is the probit-normal model (Molenberghs and Verbeke, 2005, Chapter 13); however, in this case integral approximations are still required but instead for the calculation of the multivariate normal cumulative distribution function. When an analytic solution is not possible, then the numerical integration techniques discussed in Section 4.3.5 for joint models are also directly applicable to GLMMs. In fact, it should be noted that there is a lengthy literature on methods to approximate such integrals, and many of the numerical integration techniques used in joint models have been originally applied to GLMMs. The performance of (adaptive) Gaussian quadrature integration rules has been studied by Pinheiro and Chao (2006), Pinheiro and Bates (1995), and Lesaffre and Spiessens (2001), Monte Carlo integration specifically designed for GLMMs has been developed by Booth and Hobert (1999) and McCulloch (1997), and Laplace approximations have been discussed by Raudenbush et al. (2000). After the numerical integration technique has been chosen, the maximum likelihood estimates are obtained using either the EM algorithm (treating the random effects as 'missing data') or Newton-type algorithms. For a more detailed presentation of the GLMMs framework, along with a discussion of alternative estimation procedures and inference, we refer to Molenberghs and Verbeke (2005, Chapters 14 and 16), Fitzmaurice et al. (2004, Chapters 12 and 13), and Diggle et al. (2002, Chapter 9).

5.7.2 Combining Discrete Repeated Measures with Survival

Working under the GLMMs framework presented in Section 5.7.1, it is rather straightforward to define a joint model for a categorical longitudinal outcome. In particular, utilizing the same conditional independence assumptions (4.7) and (4.8), as in the case of continuous responses, we can define separate sub-models for the longitudinal and event time processes, conditional on the random effects b_i. In principle, all extensions that we have seen so far are directly applicable for categorical markers as well. Following the model formulation of Section 5.1 that allows for different parameterizations, a general definition of a joint model for a longitudinal and a survival outcome is

$$
\begin{cases}
p(y_i(t) \mid b_i) &= \exp\left\{ \sum_{j=1}^{n_i} \left[y_{ij}\psi_{ij}(b_i) - c\{\psi_{ij}(b_i)\} \right] \Big/ a(\varphi) - d(y_{ij}, \varphi) \right\}, \\[2mm]
m_i(t) &= E(y_i(t) \mid b_i) = g^{-1}\{x_i^\top(t)\beta + z_i^\top(t)b_i\}, \\[2mm]
b_i &\sim \mathcal{N}(0, D), \\[2mm]
h_i(t) &= h_0(t)\exp\left[\gamma^\top w_{i1} + f\{m_i(t-c), b_i, w_{i2}; \alpha\}\right],
\end{cases}
$$

where, as in Section 4.1.1, $h_0(\cdot)$ can be assumed to be the hazard function of a known distribution (e.g., Weibull), it can be modeled flexibly using step-functions or splines, or it can be left completely unspecified. Note that since the normal distribution is a member of the exponential family, this definition also includes the standard joint model for continuous longitudinal responses presented in Chapter 4. The interpretation for the vector of association parameters α under the different parameterizations remains the same as it was explained in Sections 5.1.1 – 5.1.5. For instance, for the standard current-value parameterization,

$$
f\{m_i(t-c), b_i, w_{i2}; \alpha\} = \alpha m_i(t),
$$

parameter α measures the strength of the association between the risk for an event at time t and the expected value of the longitudinal outcome at the same time point. Moreover, the other extensions presented in the previous sections, that is, including stratification factors in the relative risk model or replacing the relative risk model with an accelerated failure time model, are also easily incorporated under the conditional independence assumption (4.7).

Maximum likelihood estimation proceeds in a similar manner as described for the joint model for continuous longitudinal responses. In particular, the log-likelihood takes the form,

$$
\begin{aligned}
\ell(\theta) \ &= \ \sum_{i=1}^{n} \int p(T_i, \delta_i \mid b_i; \theta) \Big\{ \prod_{j=1}^{n_i} p(y_{ij} \mid b_i; \theta) \Big\} p(b_i; \theta) \, db_i \\
&= \ \sum_{i=1}^{n} \int \Big\{ h_0(T_i) \exp\big[\gamma^\top w_{i1} + f\{m_i(T_i - c), b_i, w_{i2}; \alpha\}\big] \Big\}^{\delta_i} \\
&\quad \times \exp\Big(-\int_0^{T_i} h_0(s) \exp\big[\gamma^\top w_{i1} + f\{m_i(s - c), b_i, w_{i2}; \alpha\}\big] \, ds \Big) \\
&\quad \times \exp\Big\{ \sum_{j=1}^{n_i} \big[y_{ij}\psi_{ij}(b_i) - c\{\psi_{ij}(b_i)\} \big] \Big/ a(\varphi) - d(y_{ij}, \varphi) \Big\} \\
&\quad \times (2\pi)^{-q_b/2} \det(D)^{-1/2} \exp(-b_i^\top D^{-1} b_i / 2) \, db_i.
\end{aligned}
$$

The maximization of $\ell(\theta)$ with respect to θ requires a combination of numerical integration and optimization routines. In particular, numerical integration is required for both the integral with respect to the random effects in the definition of the log-likelihood as well as for the integral with respect to time in the survival function

$$
\mathcal{S}_i(t \mid \mathcal{M}_i(t), w_i) = \exp\Big(-\int_0^t h_0(s) \exp\big[\gamma^\top w_{i1} + f\{m_i(s - c), b_i, w_{i2}; \alpha\}\big] \, ds \Big).
$$

In the literature joint models for categorical longitudinal responses have received relatively little attention compared to joint models for continuous outcomes. The focus has been on either handling nonrandom dropout in discrete longitudinal responses (Pulkstenis et al., 1998; Albert and Follmann, 2000; Albert et al., 2002) or investigating the association structure between the categorical longitudinal process and the censored event time data (Faucett et al., 1998; Rizopoulos et al., 2008; Yao, 2008; Li et al., 2010).

5.8   Joint Models for Multiple Longitudinal Outcomes

The extension of joint models to handle more than one longitudinal outcome (either continuous or categorical) is mathematically straightforward under the GLMMs framework of Section 5.7.1. In particular, to accommodate for different types of longitudinal responses in a unified framework, we postulate a multivariate generalized linear mixed-effects model, with the conditional distribution of qth outcome given a vector of random effects vector b_{iq} being a member of the exponential family (5.17), with linear predictor given by

$$
g_q\{E(y_{iq}(t) \mid b_{iq})\} = x_{iq}^\top(t)\beta + z_{iq}^\top(t)b_{iq},
$$

where $g_q(\cdot)$, as in Section 5.7.1, denotes a known one-to-one monotonic link function, and $y_{iq}(t)$ denotes the value of the qth longitudinal outcome for the ith subject at time point t. Moreover, we extend the set of conditional independence assumptions of Section 4.3.2, and in addition assume that the random effects also account for the associations between the Q longitudinal outcomes. In particular, we assume that

$$p(T_i, \delta_i, y_i \mid b_i; \theta) \quad = \quad p(T_i, \delta_i \mid b_i; \theta)\, p(y_i \mid b_i; \theta),$$

$$p(y_i \mid b_i; \theta) \quad = \quad \prod_q p(y_{iq} \mid b_{iq}; \theta_q), \quad \text{and}$$

$$p(y_{iq} \mid b_{iq}; \theta_q) \quad = \quad \prod_j p\{y_{iq}(t_{ij}) \mid b_{iq}; \theta_q\},$$

where $y_i^\top = (y_{i1}^\top, \ldots, y_{iQ}^\top)$, $y_{iq}^\top = (y_{iq}(t_{i1}), \ldots, y_{iq}(t_{in_i}))$, and $b_i^\top = (b_{i1}^\top, \ldots, b_{iQ}^\top)$. The complete vector of random effects b_i is assumed to follow a multivariate normal distribution with mean zero and general covariance matrix D. The linear predictor of the relative risk model for the survival process is similarly expanded to accommodate for all longitudinal outcomes, i.e.,

$$h_i(t) = h_0(t) \exp\left[\gamma^\top w_{i1} + \sum_q f_q\{m_{iq}(t - c), b_{iq}, w_{i2q}; \alpha_q\}\right],$$

where again the general formulation of Section 5.1 is used in order to explicitly note that all extensions we have seen before are also, in principle, applicable for multivariate joint models.

Estimation of the multivariate joint model proceeds by maximizing the corresponding log-likelihood function, which is very similar in form to the one presented in Section 5.7.2 for categorical longitudinal responses. In fact, the only difference is the density for the longitudinal part that under the multivariate model takes the form:

$$p(y_i \mid b_i; \theta) \quad = \quad \exp\left\{\sum_{q=1}^{Q} \sum_{j=1}^{n_{iq}} \left[y_{ij,q}\psi_{ij,q}(b_{iq}) - c_q\{\psi_{ij,q}(b_{iq})\}\right] \middle/ a_q(\varphi_q) \right.$$
$$\left. - d_q(y_{ij,q}, \varphi_q) \right\},$$

where we explicitly denote that functions $c_q(\cdot)$, $d_q(\cdot)$, and $a_Q(\cdot)$ that define the respective member of the exponential family depend on q, implying that we can simultaneously handle both continuous and categorical longitudinal responses.

Even though the extension from a univariate to a multivariate joint model is relatively straightforward, the main practical problem in fitting multivariate joint models is their computational complexity due to the requirement for numerical integration with respect to the random effects. In particular, since we assume a different set of random effects per outcome, it is evident that the dimensionality of the random effects vector is considerably increased when the number of longitudinal outcomes Q is moderate to large. The problem is even further exaggerated when, in some of the outcomes, the subject-specific longitudinal profiles are nonlinear requiring thus even higher-dimensional random effects vectors. Multivariate joint models of this type have been considered by Rizopoulos and Ghosh (2011), Chi and Ibrahim (2006), Brown et al. (2005), and Lin et al. (2002) among others.

An alternative approach that reduces the computational burden has been proposed by Proust-Lima et al. (2009). These authors postulated a multivariate joint model in which the longitudinal outcomes are considered as realizations of a single latent process $\Lambda_i(t)$, which is defined in continuous time and represents the common unobserved factor that drives the observed longitudinal trajectories. More specifically, the model takes the form

$$
\begin{cases}
\Lambda_i(t) & = & x_i^\top(t)\beta + z_i^\top(t)b_i \\[2ex]
g_q\{E(y_{iq}(t) \mid b_i)\} & = & \Lambda_i(t) + u_{iq},
\end{cases}
$$

with $y_{it}(t)$ belonging to the exponential family and $b_i \sim \mathcal{N}(0, D)$, as before. The extra random effects u_{iq} are assumed normally distributed with mean zero and variance σ_u^2, independent of b_i, i.e., $\text{cov}(b_i, u_{iq}) = 0$, and independent of each other, i.e., $\text{cov}(u_{iq}, u_{iq'}) = 0$ for $q, q' = 1, \ldots, Q$ with $q \neq q'$. These subject-and-marker specific random-intercept terms represent interindividual variability not accounted for by the common latent structure $\Lambda_i(t)$. Another way to view these two sets of random effects is that b_i's account for both the association between the outcomes and the correlation in the repeated measurements of each outcome, and u_{iq}'s for the extra correlation in the repeated measurements of outcome q not captured by b_i. The advantage of the latent process approach is that only a single extra random effect u_{iq} is added for each of the Q outcomes, thus keeping the dimensionality of the random effects vectors relatively low, and making this model computationally feasible. On the other hand, the disadvantage is that the postulated association structure between the outcomes is more restrictive because only a single set of random effects b_i is used to explain the interrelationships between them.

Chapter 6

Joint Model Diagnostics

The previous chapters have focused on different formulations and several extensions of joint models. However, when it comes to using these models in practice, a prerequisite step is to validate the model's assumptions. The standard tools to assess these assumptions are residual plots. Properties and features of residuals, when longitudinal and survival outcomes are separately modeled, have been extensively studied in the literature. However, this topic has not received much attention in the joint modeling literature, with the only exception being the conditional residuals of Dobson and Henderson (2003) and the multiple imputation residuals of Rizopoulos et al. (2010). In this chapter we present different types of residuals for the longitudinal and event time outcomes, and we provide a thorough discussion of the implications of the nonrandom dropout caused by the occurrence of events.

6.1 Residuals for Joint Models

6.1.1 Residuals for the Longitudinal Part

In the standard linear mixed-effects model, two types of residuals are often used, namely the subject-specific (conditional) residuals, and the marginal (population averaged) residuals (see e.g., Nobre and Singer, 2007; Verbeke and Molenberghs, 2000). The subject-specific residuals aim to validate the assumptions of the hierarchical version of the model, i.e.,

$$
\begin{cases}
y_i &= X_i\beta + Z_ib_i + \varepsilon_i, \\
b_i &\sim \mathcal{N}(0, D), \quad \varepsilon_i \sim \mathcal{N}(0, \sigma^2),
\end{cases}
\tag{6.1}
$$

and are defined as:

$$
r_i^{ys}(t) = \{y_i(t) - x_i^\top(t)\hat{\beta} - z_i^\top(t)\hat{b}_i\},
\tag{6.2}
$$

with corresponding standardized version

$$
r_i^{yss}(t) = \{y_i(t) - x_i^\top(t)\hat{\beta} - z_i^\top(t)\hat{b}_i\}/\hat{\sigma},
$$

where, as before, $\hat{\beta}$ and $\hat{\sigma}$ denote the MLEs, and $\hat{b}_i$ the empirical Bayes estimates for the random effects. These residuals predict the conditional errors $\varepsilon_i(t)$, and can be used for checking the homoscedasticity and normality assumptions. On the other hand, the marginal residuals focus on the marginal model for y_i implied by the hierarchical representation, that is,

$$
\begin{cases}
y_i &= X_i\beta + \varepsilon_i^*, \\
\varepsilon_i^* &\sim \mathcal{N}(0, Z_iDZ_i^\top + \sigma^2 \mathrm{I}_{n_i}),
\end{cases}
\tag{6.3}
$$

and are defined as:

$$
r_i^{ym} = y_i - X_i\hat{\beta},
\tag{6.4}
$$

with corresponding standardized version

$$
r_i^{ysm} = \hat{V}_i^{-1/2}(y_i - X_i\hat{\beta}),
$$

where $\hat{V}_i = Z_i\hat{D}Z_i^\top + \hat{\sigma}^2 \mathrm{I}_{n_i}$ denotes the estimated marginal covariance matrix of y_i. These marginal residuals r_i^{ym} predict the marginal errors $y_i - X_i\beta = Z_ib_i + \varepsilon_i$, and can be used to investigate misspecification of the mean structure $X_i\beta$ as well as to validate the assumptions for the within-subjects covariance structure V_i.

Both types of residuals can be used to check the assumptions of the longitudinal part of a joint model as well. As an illustration, we produce residuals plots for the simple joint model fitted to the AIDS dataset in Section 4.2. In particular, in the longitudinal part we assume linear subject-specific evolutions in time for the square root of the CD4 cell count, whereas in the survival part we control for treatment and the effect of the *true* CD4 cell count, and we assume a piecewise-constant baseline risk function. The corresponding R code to fit the model is

```
> lmeFit.aids <- lme(CD4 ~ obstime + obstime:drug,
        random = ~ obstime | patient, data = aids)
```

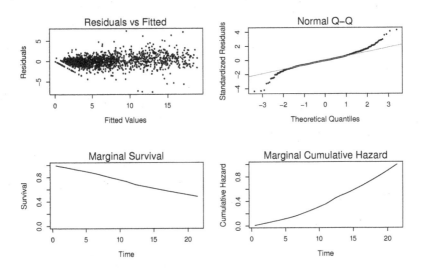

FIGURE 6.1: Default diagnostic plots for the joint model fitted to the AIDS dataset.

```
> coxFit.aids <- coxph(Surv(Time, death) ~ drug, data = aids.id,
    x = TRUE)

> jointFit.aids <- jointModel(lmeFit.aids, coxFit.aids,
    timeVar = "obstime", method = "piecewise-PH-aGH")
```

Some basic residuals diagnostic plots are directly available by calling the `plot()` method for `jointModel` objects; for our fitted joint model these are illustrated in Figure 6.1, and include the plots of the subject-specific residuals versus the corresponding fitted values, the Q-Q plot of the subject-specific residuals, and the marginal survival and cumulative risk functions for the event process.

```
> par(mfrow = c(2, 2))

> plot(jointFit.aids)
```

The marginal survival function presented is estimated using the approximate formula:

$$\mathcal{S}(t) = \int \mathcal{S}_i(t \mid b_i; \hat{\theta}) \, p(b_i; \hat{\theta}) \, db_i \approx n^{-1} \sum_i \mathcal{S}_i(t \mid \hat{b}_i; \hat{\theta}),$$

and the marginal cumulative risk function is simply calculated as $H(t) =$

$-\log \mathcal{S}(t)$. Additional residual plots can be easily produced by first calculating the specific type of residuals of interest, and then plotting them against the corresponding fitted values or covariates. As it is standard in R, the residuals and fitted values can be extracted from a fitted model using the generic functions `residuals()` and `fitted()`, respectively. The extra arguments `process` and `type` specify the submodel for which we want to calculate residuals (i.e., longitudinal or survival), and the type of residuals (i.e., subject-specific, marginal or the standardized versions). For example, the following piece of code calculates the standardized marginal residuals r_i^{ysm} and the marginal fitted values $X_i\widehat{\beta}$.

```
> resMargY.aids <- residuals(jointFit.aids, process = "Longitudinal",
    type = "Marginal")
```

```
> fitMargY.aids <- fitted(jointFit.aids, process = "Longitudinal",
    type = "Marginal")
```

The corresponding scatterplot can be produced by a call to the standard `plot()` function of R; however, here we use the following wrapper function:

```
> plotResid <- function (x, y, col.loess = "black", ...) {
    plot(x, y, ...)
    lines(lowess(x, y), col = col.loess, lwd = 2)
    abline(h = 0, lty = 3, col = "grey", lwd = 2)
}
```

which also includes the loess smooth of the scatterplot, and help us to easily locate potential problems.

```
> plotResid(fitMargY.aids, resMargY.aids, xlab = "Fitted Values",
    ylab = "Marginal Residuals")
```

The resulting plot is shown in Figure 6.2. We observe that the fitted loess curve in the plot of the standardized marginal residuals versus the fitted values shows a systematic trend with more positive residuals for small fitted values. This may be an indication that the form of the design matrix of the fixed effects X is not the appropriate one. We will return to this issue in Section 6.2.

6.1.2   Residuals for the Survival Part

A standard type of residuals for the relative risk submodel of the joint model is the martingale residuals. These are based on the counting process notation of time-to-event data, briefly introduced in Section 3.5, and in particular on the subject-specific counting process martingale, which is defined for the ith

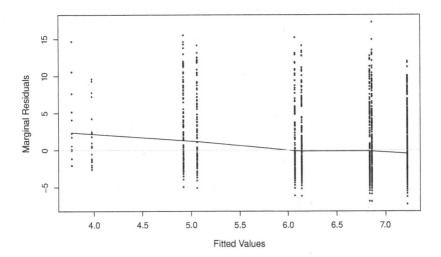

FIGURE 6.2: Marginal standardized residuals versus fitted values for the longitudinal outcome for the AIDS dataset.

subject as

$$r_i^{tm}(t) = N_i(t) - \int_0^t R_i(s) h_i(s \mid \hat{\mathcal{M}}_i(s); \hat{\theta}) \, ds$$

$$= N_i(t) - \int_0^t R_i(s) \hat{h}_0(s) \exp\{\hat{\gamma}^\top w_i + \hat{\alpha} \hat{m}_i(s)\} \, ds, \qquad (6.5)$$

where $N_i(t)$ is the counting process denoting the number of events for subject i by time t, $R_i(t)$ is the left continuous at risk process with $R_i(t) = 1$ if subject i is at risk at time t, and $R_i(t) = 0$ otherwise, $\hat{m}_i(t) = x_i^\top(t)\hat{\beta} + z_i^\top(t)\hat{b}_i$, and $\hat{h}_0(\cdot)$ denotes the estimated baseline risk function. The idea behind these residuals is based on the Doob-Meyer decomposition of a counting process to a compensator plus a martingale process, which can be seen analogous, in a broad sense, to the classical statistical decomposition in which the data are described by a model plus noise. Thus, the martingale process can been seen as the equivalent of the residual term in the standard statistical decomposition. In plain terms, the residual $r_i^{tm}(t)$ can be viewed as the difference between the observed number of events for the ith subject by time t, and the expected number of events by the same time based on the fitted model. The theoretical framework behind the use of martingales to investigate the fit of relative risk models has been provided by Barlow and Prentice (1988) and Therneau et al. (1990). The main use of these residuals is for a direct identification of excess events (i.e., to reveal subjects that are poorly fit by the model) and for evaluating whether the appropriate functional form for a covariate interest has been used in the model.

An alternative type of residuals for survival models, related to the martingale residuals, is the Cox-Snell residuals (Cox and Snell, 1968). For each subject, these are calculated as the value of the estimated cumulative risk function evaluated at the observed event time T_i, that is,

$$r_i^{tcs} = \int_0^{T_i} h_i(s \mid \hat{\mathcal{M}}_i(s); \hat{\theta}) \, ds$$

$$= \int_0^{T_i} \hat{h}_0(s) \exp\{\hat{\gamma}^\top w_i + \hat{\alpha}\hat{m}_i(s)\} \, ds, \tag{6.6}$$

and thus, $r_i^{tcs} = N_i(T_i) - r_i^{tm}(T_i)$. According to the probability integral transform, when the assumed model fits the data well we expect that the probability of failure after time t, i.e., $\mathcal{S}(t) = \Pr(T_i^* > t)$ will have a uniform distribution in $[0, 1]$, and therefore the cumulative hazard, defined as $\mathcal{H}(t) = -\log \mathcal{S}(t)$ will have a unit exponential distribution. This identity implies that we can check the overall goodness-of-fit of our relative risk submodel by checking whether the Cox-Snell residuals r_i^{tcs} are unit exponentially distributed. However, a complexity in the practical use of these residuals is that they are evaluated at the observed event time T_i, and thus when T_i is censored, r_i^{tcs} will be censored as well. Hence, in order to check the fit of the model, while accounting for the fact that r_i^{tcs} is actually a censored sample from a unit exponential distribution, we compare the survival function of the unit exponential distribution, $\mathcal{S}_{exp}(t) = \exp(-t)$, with the Kaplan-Meier estimate of the survival function of r_i^{tcs}.

We illustrate the use of the martingale and Cox-Snell residuals in R by continuing the residuals analysis for the joint model fitted to the AIDS dataset, presented in Section 6.1.1, and validate the fit of the survival part. Similar to the calculation of residuals for the longitudinal process, both types of residuals for the survival submodel are extracted using the `residuals()` generic function. We start by examining the chosen functional form for the time-dependent marker. Namely, in the relative risk submodel defined in the previous section, we have assumed that the current value of the marker is associated with the risk for death, that is

$$h_i(t) = h_0(t) \exp\{\gamma \texttt{ddI}_i + \alpha m_i(t)\}.$$

However, as we have seen in Section 5.1, there are several alternative parameterizations that can be used to describe the relationship between the risk for an event and the marker, which may be more appropriate. As we have seen in that section, these parameterizations can be, in general, formulated as

$$h_i(t) = h_0(t) \exp[\gamma \texttt{ddI}_i + \alpha f\{m_i(t)\}],$$

where $f(\cdot)$ denotes an unknown function, and our aim is to explore whether the default choice of $f(x) = x$ is an appropriate one. Therneau et al. (1990) have shown that, under certain conditions, the scatterplot of martingale residuals from a null model versus a predictor of interest can reveal the true form of the $f(\cdot)$ function. In our example, where we have already fitted the relative risk model assuming the current value term $m_i(t)$, we can instead inspect the scatterplot of the martingale residuals $r_i^{tm}(t)$ versus $m_i(t)$ for systematic trends. These residuals are calculated from a fitted joint model using the option `process = "Event"` in the call to `residuals()`,

```
> martRes <- residuals(jointFit.aids, process = "Event")

> mi.t <- fitted(jointFit.aids, process = "Longitudinal",
      type = "EventTime")
```

Function `residuals()` calculates the martingale residuals for all the time points where we have available information for the failure status of the patient. These include the times $\{t_{ij}, j = 1, \ldots, n_i\}$ at which longitudinal responses were recorded,[1] and the observed event time T_i. To calculate the current value term $m_i(t)$ at the same time points, we use option `type = "EventTime"` in the call to the `fitted()` generic function. Figure 6.3 shows the corresponding scatterplot with a superimposed loess curve, produced using function `plotResid()` defined in Section 6.1.1:

```
> plotResid(mi.t, martRes, col.loess = "grey62",
      ylab = "Martingale Residuals",
      xlab = "Subject-Specific Fitted Values Longitudinal Outcome")
```

We can observe that for small fitted values there is a slight deviation of the loess smoother from zero. To further investigate the appropriateness of the chosen functional form for the CD4 cell count, it is advisable to additionally check for systematic trends in the martingale residuals when we condition on other baseline covariates. As an illustration, we produce an updated version of Figure 6.3 by conditioning on the randomized treatment. The scatterplots for the ddI and ddC groups can be produced using function `xyplot()` from package **lattice**:

```
> xyplot(martRes ~ mi.t | drug, data = aids, type = c("p", "smooth"),
      col = "black", lwd = 3, ylab = "Martingale Residuals",
      xlab = "Subject-Specific Fitted Values Longitudinal Outcome")
```

The option `type = c("p", "smooth")` in the call to `xyplot()` specifies that we want to plot both the points and the fit of the loess smoother. The resulting

---

[1] Baseline measurements at $t = 0$ are excluded from the calculation of $r_i^{tm}(t)$ because these always have a zero martingale residual.

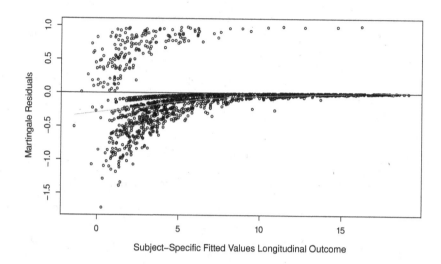

FIGURE 6.3: Martingale residuals versus the subject-specific fitted values of the longitudinal outcome for the AIDS dataset. The grey solid line denotes the fit of the loess smoother.

plot is shown in Figure 6.4. We again observe some small deviations from the null horizontal line for both treatments, but to a lesser degree for the ddI group.

We proceed in our residuals analysis for the survival outcome by assessing the overall fit of the survival submodel using the Cox-Snell residuals. These are again calculated in R using the **residuals()** function but now using option **type = "CoxSnell"**:

```
> resCST <- residuals(jointFit.aids, process = "Event",
    type = "CoxSnell")
```

To calculate the Kaplan-Meier estimate of the survival function of the Cox-Snell residuals we use function **survfit()** from package **survival**. The syntax of this function is very similar to the syntax of **coxph()** used so far to fit Cox models. In particular, it accepts as a main argument an R formula, which in the left-hand side uses function **Surv()** to provide the censored responses and the corresponding event indicator, and on the right-hand side it may include potential stratification factors. Note that in our case the censored responses are not the observed failure times of the patients, but rather the Cox-Snell residuals. The corresponding event indicator is extracted from the **aids.id** data frame supplied in the **data** argument. The graph of the Kaplan-Meier

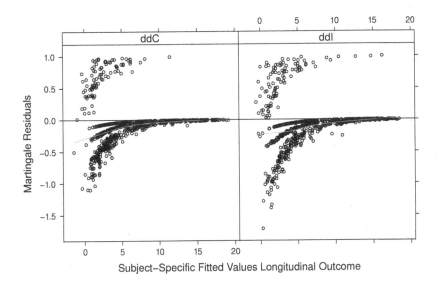

FIGURE 6.4: Martingale residuals versus the subject-specific fitted values of the longitudinal outcome per treatment group for the AIDS dataset. The grey solid lines denote the fit of the loess smoother.

estimate is produced with a call to the `plot()` function, and is depicted in Figure 6.5:

```
> sfit <- survfit(Surv(resCST, death) ~ 1, data = aids.id)

> plot(sfit, mark.time = FALSE, conf.int = TRUE,
      xlab = "Cox-Snell Residuals", ylab = "Survival Probability",
      main = "Survival Function of Cox-Snell Residuals")

> curve(exp(-x), from = 0, to = max(aids.id$Time), add = TRUE,
      col = "grey62", lwd = 2)
```

The `curve()` function is used to superimpose the survival function of the unit exponential distribution, i.e., $\mathcal{S}_{exp}(t) = \exp(-t)$. Comparing the fit of the Kaplan-Meier estimate to the expected asymptotic distribution, we observe some discrepancies, especially for residuals greater than 0.8 (even though, strictly speaking, the survival function of the unit exponential distribution lies within the 95% pointwise confidence intervals of the Kaplan-Meier estimate, except around one). To further scrutinize the fit of the model, we stratify the residuals by treatment, and we plot separate survival function estimates; the corresponding R code is

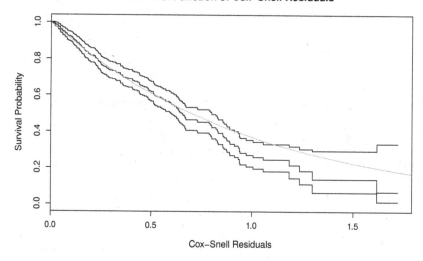

FIGURE 6.5: Cox-Snell residuals for the AIDS dataset. The black solid line denotes the Kaplan-Meier estimate of the survival function of the residuals (with the dashed lines corresponding the 95% pointwise confidence intervals), and the grey solid line, the survival function of the unit exponential distribution.

```
> sfit <- survfit(Surv(resCST, death) ~ drug, data = aids.id)

> plot(sfit, mark.time = FALSE, xlab = "Cox-Snell Residuals",
    ylab = "Survival Probability",
    main = "Survival Function of Cox-Snell Residuals")

> curve(exp(-x), from = 0, to = max(aids.id$Time), add = TRUE,
    col = "grey62", lwd = 2)
```

When the model fits the data well, we expect the survival function estimates for each strata to hover around the unit exponential distribution. Figure 6.6 shows the Kaplan-Meier estimates of the Cox-Snell residuals for the two treatment groups, from which we can again observe some lack of fit for residual values greater than one, though to a lesser degree than in Figure 6.5.

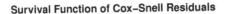

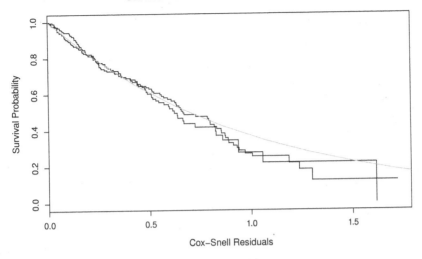

FIGURE 6.6: Cox-Snell residuals for the AIDS dataset. The black solid lines denote the Kaplan-Meier estimates of the survival functions of the Cox-Snell residuals for the two treatment groups, and the grey solid line, the survival function of the unit exponential distribution.

6.2 Dropout and Residuals

The previous section introduced the basic types of residuals plots that are routinely used to validate the assumptions behind mixed models and relative risk models when these are separately fitted. Even though the same type of diagnostic plots can be easily constructed to inspect the fit of joint models, a problem is that the reference distribution of the residuals for the longitudinal process is affected by the dropout caused by the occurrence of events. In particular, as we have discussed in Section 4.6, when a patient experiences the event of interest this corresponds to a discontinuation of the collection of longitudinal information because either follow-up measurements can no longer be collected or their distribution changes after the event occurred and therefore are considered irrelevant. As we have seen in Section 4.6, the dropout mechanism implied by joint models is of a nonrandom nature, that is, it corresponds to a missing not at random mechanism (see Section 2.3.1). The implication of the nonrandom nature of the dropout mechanism is that the observed data, upon which the residuals are calculated, do not constitute a random sample of the target population (Verbeke et al., 2008; Fitzmaurice et al., 2004, Section 14.2). This in turn implies that residual plots based on the observed data alone can be misleading because these residuals should not be expected to exhibit standard properties, such as zero mean and independence. For example, in Figure 6.2 we observed that for small fitted values we have more positive than negative residuals. However, small fitted values correspond to lower levels of square root CD4 cell count, which in turn corresponds to a worsening of the patient's condition and therefore to higher chance of dropout. Thus, the residuals corresponding to small fitted values are only based on patients with a 'good' health condition. Therefore, due to the dropout we cannot discern that the systematic trend seen in Figure 6.2 is truly attributed to a misspecification of the design matrix X of the fixed effects.

To further illustrate how the nonrandom dropout affects the use of residuals based on the observed data alone, we show in Figure 6.7 plots of the standardized marginal and standardized subject-specific residuals versus the corresponding fitted values for the PBC dataset. These are based on a joint model that assumes linear subject-specific evolutions for log serum bilirubin, and a relative risk model for the time-to-event (death or transplantation), which controls for treatment and hepatomegaly, and assumes a piecewise-constant baseline risk function. The R syntax to fit the model is

```
> lmeFit2.pbc <- lme(log(serBilir) ~ year * drug,
      random = ~ year | id, data = pbc2)

> coxFit.pbc <- coxph(Surv(years, status2) ~ drug + hepatomegaly,
      data = pbc2.id, x = TRUE)

> jointFit2.pbc <- jointModel(lmeFit2.pbc, coxFit.pbc, timeVar = "year",
      method = "piecewise-PH-aGH")
```

As for the AIDS dataset in Section 6.1, we compute the residuals and fitted values using suitable calls to the generic functions `residuals()` and `fitted()`, respectively.

```
> resSubY.pbc <- residuals(jointFit2.pbc, process = "Longitudinal",
      type = "stand-Subject")

> fitSubY.pbc <- fitted(jointFit2.pbc, process = "Longitudinal",
      type = "Subject")

> resMargY.pbc <- residuals(jointFit2.pbc, process = "Longitudinal",
      type = "stand-Marginal")

> fitMargY.pbc <- fitted(jointFit2.pbc, process = "Longitudinal",
      type = "Marginal")
```

Figure 6.7 is then produced with the code:

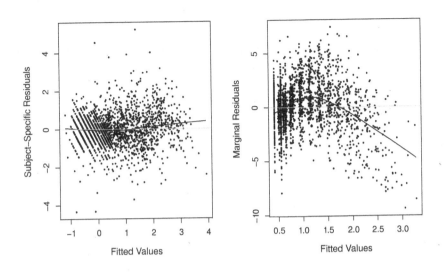

FIGURE 6.7: Scatterplots of observed residuals versus fitted values for the longitudinal process for the PBC dataset.

```
> par(mfrow = c(1,2))

> plotResid(fitSubY.pbc, resSubY.pbc, xlab = "Fitted Values",
      ylab = "Subject-Specific Residuals")

> plotResid(fitMargY.pbc, resMargY.pbc, xlab = "Fitted Values",
      ylab = "Marginal Residuals")
```

We again observe that the fitted loess curve in the plot of the standardized marginal residuals versus the fitted values shows a systematic trend. Note, however, that high levels of serum bilirubin indicate a worsening of a patient's condition resulting in higher death rates (i.e., dropout). Similar to Figure 6.2, we cannot definitely conclude from this figure that the lack-of-fit is attributed to a misspecification of X. Thus, both the AIDS and PBC data examples illustrate that residual plots based on the observed data alone can be proven misleading when it comes to validating the joint model's assumptions.

6.3   Multiple Imputation Residuals

6.3.1   Fixed Visit Times

To overcome the problems caused by the nonrandom dropout and produce residuals for the longitudinal process that can be readily used in diagnostic plots, Rizopoulos et al. (2010) proposed to augment the observed data with randomly imputed longitudinal responses under the complete data model, corresponding to the longitudinal outcomes that would have been observed had the patients not dropped out. Using these augmented longitudinal responses, residuals are then calculated for the complete data, and a multiple imputation approach is used to properly account for the uncertainty in the imputed values due to missingness (Gelman et al., 2005).

To present this idea, we will borrow the notation of Section 4.6, and denote by $y_i^o = \{y_i(t_{ij}) : t_{ij} < T_i, j = 1, \ldots, n_i\}$ the observed part of the longitudinal response vector that contains all observed longitudinal measurements of the ith subject before the observed event time, and by $y_i^m = \{y_i(t_{ij}) : t_{ij} \geq T_i, j = 1, \ldots, n_i'\}$ the missing part that contains the longitudinal measurements that would have been taken until the end of the study, had the event not occurred. We also assume that the joint model has been fitted to the dataset at hand, and that we have obtained the maximum likelihood estimates $\hat{\theta}$ and an estimate of their asymptotic covariance matrix $\hat{\text{var}}(\hat{\theta})$. Moreover, we assume that longitudinal measurements are planned to be taken at a set of prespecified time points $t_0, t_1, \ldots, t_{max}$, and that, for the ith subject, measurements are available up to the last prespecified visit time earlier than T_i. To put ideas forward, we adopt a Bayesian formulation of the joint model, since multiple imputation has Bayesian grounds (Little and Rubin, 2002, Chapter 10). In particular, the multiple imputation approach is based on repeated sampling from the posterior distribution of y_i^m given the observed data, averaged over the posterior distribution of the parameters. Under the joint model (4.9), and the dropout mechanism (4.20), the density for this distribution can be expressed as

$$p(y_i^m \mid y_i^o, T_i, \delta_i) = \int p(y_i^m \mid y_i^o, T_i, \delta_i; \theta)\, p(\theta \mid y_i^o, T_i, \delta_i)\, d\theta. \qquad (6.7)$$

The first part of the integrand in (6.7) can be derived from (4.20) taking also into account the conditional independence assumptions (4.7) and (4.8), i.e.,

$$p(y_i^m \mid y_i^o, T_i, \delta_i; \theta) = \int p(y_i^m \mid b_i, y_i^o, T_i, \delta_i; \theta)\, p(b_i \mid y_i^o, T_i, \delta_i; \theta)\, db_i$$

$$= \int p(y_i^m \mid b_i; \theta)\, p(b_i \mid y_i^o, T_i, \delta_i; \theta)\, db_i. \qquad (6.8)$$

For the second part, which is the posterior distribution of the parameters given the observed data, we use arguments of standard asymptotic Bayesian theory (Cox and Hinkley, 1974, Section 10.6), and assume that the sample size n is sufficiently large, such that $\{\theta \mid y_i^o, T_i, \delta_i\}$ can be well approximated by $\mathcal{N}\{\hat{\theta}, \text{vâr}(\hat{\theta})\}$. This assumption, combined with (6.7) and (6.8), suggests the following simulation scheme:

S1: Draw $\theta^{(l)} \sim \mathcal{N}\{\hat{\theta}, \text{vâr}(\hat{\theta})\}$.

S2: Draw $b_i^{(l)} \sim \{b_i \mid y_i^o, T_i, \delta_i, \theta^{(l)}\}$.

S3: Draw $y_i^{m(l)}(t_{ij}) \sim \mathcal{N}\left\{\hat{m}_i^{(l)}(t_{ij}), \hat{\sigma}^{2,(l)}\right\}$, for the prespecified visit times $t_{ij} \geq T_i$, $j = 1, \ldots, n_i'$ that were not observed for the ith subject, where $\hat{m}_i^{(l)}(t_{ij}) = x_i^{\top}(t_{ij})\hat{\beta}^{(l)} + z_i^{\top}(t_{ij})\hat{b}_i^{(l)}$.

Steps 1–3 are repeated for each subject, $l = 1, \ldots, L$ times, where L denotes the number of imputations. Steps 1 and 2 account for the uncertainties in the parameter and empirical Bayes estimates, respectively, whereas Step 3 imputes the missing longitudinal responses. Steps 1 and 3 are straightforward to perform since they require sampling from a multivariate normal distribution; on the contrary, the posterior distribution for the random effects given the observed data in Step 2 is of a non-standard form, and thus a more sophisticated approach is required to sample from it. Rizopoulos et al. (2010) proposed to use a Metropolis-Hastings algorithm with independent proposals from a multivariate t distribution centered at the empirical Bayes estimates $\hat{b}_i$, with scale matrix $\text{vâr}(\hat{b}_i)$, and four degrees of freedom. A similar approach has been used by Booth and Hobert (1999) to simulate from the posterior distribution of the random effects in the generalized linear mixed models context. In the joint modeling framework, the justification for a multivariate t proposal is two fold. First, Rizopoulos et al. (2008) have shown that, as n_i increases, the leading term of the log posterior distribution of the random effects is the logarithm of the density of the linear mixed model $\log p(y_i \mid b_i; \theta^{(l)}) = \sum_j \log p\{y_i(t_{ij}) \mid b_i; \theta^{(l)}\}$, which is quadratic in b_i and will resemble the shape of a multivariate normal distribution, and second, for small n_i, the heavier tails of the t distribution will ensure sufficient coverage. The simulated $y_i^{m(l)}(t_{ij})$ values together with y_i^o can now be used to calculate residuals according to (6.2) or (6.4). A key advantage of the multiply-imputed residuals is that they inherit the properties of the complete data model. This facilitates common graphical model checks without requiring formal derivation of the reference distribution of the observed data residuals. We should note, however, that in some clinical studies in which the terminating event is death, such as in the AIDS and PBC datasets, it may not be conceptually reasonable to consider potential values of the longitudinal outcome after the event time; for instance, see Kurland and Heagerty (2005). Nonetheless, the multiply-imputed residuals are merely used as a mechanism to help us investigate the fit of the model, and we are not actually interested in inferences after the event time.

The simulation scheme described above is available in the `residuals()` method, and can be invoked using the logical argument MI. As an illustration, we calculate the multiply-imputed standardized marginal residuals for the AIDS dataset:

```
> set.seed(123) # we set the seed for reproducibility

> resMI.aids <- residuals(jointFit.aids, process = "Longitudinal",
      type = "Marginal", MI = TRUE)

> fitMargYmiss.aids <- resMI.aids$fitted.valsM

> resMargYmiss.aids <- resMI.aids$resid.valsM
```

Contrary to the standard call to `residuals()` that returns a numeric vector of residuals (as illustrated above), setting MI to TRUE returns a list with several components useful in the further processing of the multiply-imputed residuals. The two components that we extract here are the fitted values and the multiply-imputed standardized marginal residuals that correspond to y_i^m, as defined in Section 6.1.1. Object `fitMargY.miss` is a numeric vector, whereas `resMargY.miss` is a numeric matrix with columns representing the realizations of the residuals based on the multiple-imputations for y_i^m (default is 50 multiple-imputations; this is controlled by argument M of function `residuals()`). The following code produces Figure 6.8 that depicts the multiply-imputed residuals together with the observed residuals versus their corresponding fitted values:

```
> M <- ncol(resMargYmiss.aids) # number of imputations
> resMargYmi.aids <- c(resMargY.aids, resMargYmiss.aids)
> fitMargYmi.aids <- c(fitMargY.aids, rep(fitMargYmiss.aids, M))
> plot(range(fitMargYmi.aids), range(resMargYmi.aids), type = "n",
      xlab = "Fitted Values",
      ylab = "MI Standardized Marginal Residuals")
> abline(h = 0, lty = 2)
> points(rep(fitMargYmiss.aids, M), resMargYmiss.aids, cex = 0.5,
      col = "grey")
> points(fitMargY.aids, resMargY.aids)
```

The black loess curve in Figure 6.8 is, in fact, the same curve as in Figure 6.2, and is produced by

```
> lines(lowess(fitMargY.aids, resMargY.aids), lwd = 2)
```

However, to produce the grey loess curve, which describes the relationship

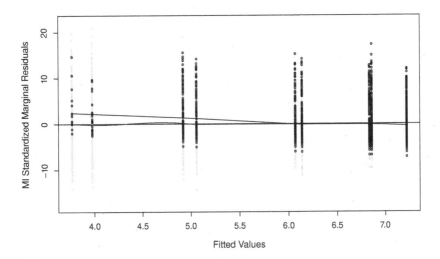

FIGURE 6.8: Observed standardized marginal residuals (black points), augmented with all the multiply imputed residuals produced by the $L = 50$ imputations (grey points) for the AIDS dataset. The superimposed solid lines represent a loess fit based only on the observed residuals (black line), and a weighted loess fit based on all residuals (black dashed line).

between the complete residuals (i.e., the multiply-imputed residuals together with the observed residuals) versus their corresponding fitted values, some extra steps are required. In particular, we need to take into account that, for each of the time points the ith subject did not appear in the study center, we have M = 50 multiply-imputed residuals, whereas for the times that she did appear we only have one. Thus, in the calculation of the loess curve we will use case weights with the value 1 for the observed residuals and $1/M = 1/50 = 0.02$ for the multiply-imputed ones, i.e.,

```
> datResid <- data.frame(
    resid = resMargYmi.aids,
    fitted = fitMargYmi.aids,
    weight = c(rep(1, length(resMargY.aids)),
        rep(1/M, length(resMargYmiss.aids)))
)

> fitLoess.aids <- loess(resid ~ fitted, data = datResid,
    weights = weight)

> nd.aids <- data.frame(fitted = seq(min(fitMargYmi.aids),
```

```
        max(fitMargYmi.aids), length.out = 100))

> prdLoess.aids <- predict(fitLoess.aids, nd.aids)

> lines(nd.aids$fit, prdLoess.aids, lwd = 2, lty = 2)
```

A comparison between the two loess smoothers reveals that indeed the systematic trends that were present in the residual plots based on the observed data alone are mainly attributed to the nonrandom dropout and not to a model lack-of-fit.

6.3.2   Random Visit Times

The multiple imputation scheme presented in Section 6.3.1 assumes that visit times were prespecified by the protocol and all patients adhere to them. However, in observational studies the time points at which the longitudinal measurements are taken are not fixed by design but rather determined by the physician or even the patients themselves. This may even occur in randomized studies that, by the protocol, have prespecified visit times. For instance, for the PBC dataset and during the first two years of follow-up, measurements of serum bilirubin were taken at baseline, 0.5, 1, and 2 years, with little variability, however, in the latter years the variability in the visit times increased considerably. Under the noninformativeness assumption mentioned in Section 4.3.2, and provided that the joint model is correctly specified, the visiting process can be ignored without influencing the asymptotic properties of the maximum likelihood estimators.

However, the possibility of random visit times complicates the computation of multiple imputation residuals, presented in Section 6.3.1. In particular, the time points at which the ith subject was supposed to provide measurements after the observed event time T_i are not available, and thus the corresponding rows $x_i^\top(t_{ij})$ and $z_i^\top(t_{ij})$, for $t_{ij} \geq T_i$, of the design matrices X_i and Z_i, respectively, cannot be specified. This issue cannot be overcome by a naive approach of imputing y_i^m at arbitrary specified fixed time points because it may contaminate the residuals plots by producing either too many or too few positive residuals in specific ranges of the data where there are few observations. An alternative approach is to fit a suitable model for the visiting process and use it to simulate future visit times for each individual. Formally, we assume, without loss of generality, that all subjects have at least one measurement and we let u_{ik} ($k = 2, \ldots, n_i$) denote the time elapsed between visit $k-1$ and visit k for the ith subject. Let also Y_i^* denote the complete longitudinal response vector, that is all longitudinal responses that would have been observed for subject i by time t, if she had not dropped out. Under these definitions, the noninformativeness assumption for the visiting process can be formulated as

$$p(u_{ik} \mid u_{i2}, \ldots, u_{i,k-1}, Y_i^*; \theta_v)$$

$$= \quad p\{u_{ik} \mid u_{i2}, \ldots, u_{i,k-1}, y_i(t_1), \ldots, y_i(t_{k-1}); \theta_v\}, \qquad (6.9)$$

where θ_v is the vector parameterizing the visiting process density, and $\{\theta, \theta_v\}$ have disjoint parameter spaces. To formulate a model for the visiting process, we need to account for the fact that the visit times $u_i^\top = (u_{i2}, \ldots, u_{in_i})$ of each subject are correlated. For multivariate survival data there are mainly two families of models, namely, marginal models and conditional/frailty models (Hougaard, 2000; Therneau and Grambsch, 2000). Marginal models are based on a similar idea as the generalized estimating equations approach of Liang and Zeger (1986), which entails fitting an ordinary Cox model to the multivariate data treating them as independent (i.e., ignoring the correlation), and then adjust the estimated standard errors using a sandwich-type of estimator. On the other hand, conditional models explicitly model the correlation using latent variables. Similar to mixed models, we make a conditional independence assumption that states that the multivariate survival responses are independent given the frailty term. Therefore, frailty models require the specification of both a model for the multivariate survival responses conditional on the frailty term, and appropriate distributional assumptions for the frailty term itself (Duchateau and Janssen, 2008).

For our purposes, and because we want to simulate visit times for each subject, we need to provide a full specification of the conditional distribution $p\{u_{ik} \mid u_{i2}, \ldots, u_{i,k-1}, y_i(t_1), \ldots, y_i(t_{k-1}); \theta_v\}$, and therefore a conditional model is more appropriate. In particular, we use a Weibull model with a multiplicative Gamma frailty, defined as:

$$\lambda(u_{ik} \mid x_{vi}, \omega_i) = \lambda_0(u_{ik}) \omega_i \exp(x_{vi}^\top \gamma_v), \quad \omega_i \sim \text{Gamma}(\sigma_\omega, \sigma_\omega), \qquad (6.10)$$

where $\lambda(\cdot)$ is the risk function conditional on the frailty term ω_i, x_{vi} denotes the covariate vector that may contain a functional form of the observed longitudinal responses $y_i(t_{i1}), \ldots, y_i(t_{i,k-1})$, γ_v is the vector of regression coefficients, and σ_ω^{-1} is the unknown variance of ω_i's. The Weibull baseline risk function is given by $\lambda_0(u_{ik}) = \phi\psi u_{ik}^{\psi-1}$, with $\psi, \phi > 0$. Our choice for this model is motivated, not only by its flexibility and simplicity, but also by the fact that the posterior distribution of the frailty term, given the observed data, is of standard form (Sahu et al., 1997), which as will be shown below, facilitates simulation.

Similarly to Section 6.3.1, we assume that both the joint model and the visiting process model (6.10) have been fitted to the data at hand, and that the maximum likelihood estimates $\hat\theta$ and $\hat\theta_v$, and their corresponding asymptotic covariance matrices, $\text{vâr}(\hat\theta)$ and $\text{vâr}(\hat\theta_v)$, respectively, have been obtained. Let also t_{max} denote the end of the study, and $\delta_{v,ik}$ the event indicator corresponding to u_{ik}. Furthermore, taking into consideration the noninformativeness assumption (6.9), the future elapsed visit time u_{i,n_i+1} can be simulated independently from $y_i^m(t_{i,n_i+1})$. Thus, the simulation scheme under the random visit times setting takes the following form:

S1: Parameter Values

    a. Draw $\theta_v^{(l)} \sim \mathcal{N}\{\hat{\theta}_v, \hat{\mathrm{var}}(\hat{\theta}_v)\}$.

    b. Draw $\theta^{(l)} \sim \mathcal{N}\{\hat{\theta}, \hat{\mathrm{var}}(\hat{\theta})\}$.

S2: Frailties and Random Effects

    a. Draw

$$\omega_i^{(l)} \sim \mathrm{Gamma}(A, B),$$

with $A = \sigma_\omega^{(l)} + \sum_{k=2}^{n_i} \delta_{v,ik}$, and $B = \sigma_\omega^{(l)} + \phi^{(l)} \sum_{k=2}^{n_i} u_{ik}^{\psi^{(l)}} \exp(x_{vi}^\top \gamma_v^{(l)})$ for subjects with two or more visits, and

$$\omega_i^{(l)} \sim \mathrm{Gamma}(\sigma_\omega^{(l)}, \sigma_\omega^{(l)}),$$

for subjects with one visit.

    b. Draw $b_i^{(l)} \sim \{b_i \mid y_i^o, T_i, \delta_i, \theta^{(l)}\}$.

S3: Outcomes

    a. Draw $u_i^{(l)} \sim \mathrm{Weibull}\left\{\psi^{(l)}, \phi^{(l)}\omega_i^{(l)} \exp(x_{vi}^\top \gamma_v^{(l)})\right\}$.

    b. Set $\tilde{t}_i = u_i^{(l)} + t_{in_i}$, where t_{in_i} denotes the last observed visit time for the ith subject. If $\tilde{t}_i > t_{max}$, no y_i^m need to be imputed for this subject; otherwise draw $y_i^{m(l)}(\tilde{t}_i) \sim \mathcal{N}\left\{\hat{m}_i^{(l)}(\tilde{t}_i), \hat{\sigma}^{2,(l)}\right\}$, where $\hat{m}_i^{(l)}(\tilde{t}_i) = x_i^\top(\tilde{t}_i)\hat{\beta}^{(l)} + z_i^\top(\tilde{t}_i)\hat{b}_i^{(l)}$.

    c. Set $t_{in_i} = \tilde{t}_i$, and repeat a–b until $t_{in_i} > t_{max}$ for all i.

Steps 1–3 are repeated $l = 1, \ldots, L$ times. As in Section 6.3.1, Steps 1–3 simultaneously account for uncertainties in both the joint and visiting process models. Furthermore, note that subjects who have only one longitudinal measurement provide no information to the visiting process model. For these cases, in Step 3a, we can only simulate future elapsed visit times using a simulated frailty value from the Gamma prior distribution (Step 2a).

An important aspect in applying the above simulation scheme is the form of the linear predictor of the visiting process model. More specifically, we should note that assumption (6.9) is the weakest assumption under which the joint model provides valid inferences even if the visiting process is ignored, but a model satisfying (6.9) involves many parameters, and thus it may be unstable. A set of stronger but perhaps more plausible assumptions is

$$p(u_{ik} \mid u_{i2}, \ldots, u_{i,k-1}, Y_i^*; \theta_v)$$

$$= p\{u_{ik} \mid u_{i2}, \ldots, u_{i,k-1}, y_i(t_{k-1}); \theta_v\}, \qquad (6.11)$$

and

$$p(u_{ik} \mid u_{i2}, \ldots, u_{i,k-1}, Y_i^*; \theta_v) = p\{u_{ik} \mid y_i(t_{k-1}); \theta_v\}. \qquad (6.12)$$

Equation (6.11) posits that the time elapsed between visit $k-1$ and visit k depends on the previous elapsed times and the last observed longitudinal measurement, whereas under (6.12) it depends only on the last observed longitudinal measurement. These assumptions describe the situation in which physicians base their decision for a future visit for a patient on the last observed outcome and possibly the past visiting pattern.

We illustrate the practical use of the multiple imputation approach to augment the standardized residuals for the longitudinal process for the joint model fitted to the PBC dataset in Section 6.2. As a first step, we need to specify the visiting process model. For the sake of illustration, we assume here a simple model that postulates that the elapsed time u_{ik} between visits $k-1$ and k depends on the previous visit times, and the current value of serum bilirubin. This model corresponds to assumption (6.11), and it takes the following form:

$$\lambda(u_{ik} \mid y_i^*(t), \omega_i) = \lambda_0(u_{ik})\omega_i \exp\{\gamma_v y_i(t_{k-1})\}, \quad \omega_i \sim \text{Gamma}(\sigma_\omega, \sigma_\omega).$$

To fit this model, we need first to extract the time elapsed between visits $\{u_{ik}, k = 2, \ldots, n_i\}$, and the lagged response vector $\{y_i(t_{k-1}), k = 2, \ldots, n_i\}$ for each subject from the pbc2 data frame. This is achieved with the following piece of code:

```
> diff.time <- with(pbc2, tapply(year, id, diff))

> prev.y <- with(pbc2, tapply(log(serBilir), id, head, -1))

> one.visit <- sapply(diff.time, length) == 0

> diff.time[one.visit] <- prev.y[one.visit] <- NA
```

In particular, object diff.time is a list with the elapsed between visits for each patient, and object prev.y is a list with the level of log serum bilirubin at the previous visit time $y_i(t_{k-1})$ for each patient. The last two lines of the code set to NA the elements of diff.time and prev.y that correspond to patients with a single serum bilirubin measurement. Next, we construct the data frame that contains all patient information for the visiting process:

```
> dataVT <- data.frame(
      "id" = rep(names(prev.y), sapply(prev.y, length)),
      "diff.Times" = unlist(diff.time),
      "prev.y" = unlist(prev.y),
      "event" = 1)
```

Model (6.10) can be fitted in R using function `weibull.frailty()` from package **JM**. This function has very similar syntax as `coxph()` from package **survival**, and in particular, its main arguments are argument `formula` specifying the survival information and the linear predictor of the model, argument `data` providing the data frame with all the variables, and argument `id` specifying the name of the variable in the `data` that corresponds to the patient identifier variable.

```
> WeibFrl <- weibull.frailty(Surv(diff.Times, event) ~ prev.y,
      id = "id", data = dataVT)

> summary(WeibFrl)
        Weibull Relative Risk Model with Gamma Frailty

Call:
weibull.frailty(formula = Surv(diff.Times, event) ~ prev.y, data = dataVT,
    id = "id")

Data Descriptives:
Number of groups: 285
Number of observations: 1633
Total Number of Events:  1633

Model Summary:
   log.Lik       AIC       BIC
  -665.254 1338.508 1353.118

Coefficients:
          value std.err z-value p-value
prev.y -0.5084  0.0616  -8.249 <0.0001

Shape: 3.7618
Scale: 7.2209
Frailty variance: 2.7283
```

The detailed output provided by the **summary()** method shows that the timing of the next visit is strongly associated with the current value of serum bilirubin, and also that there is considerable heterogeneity (i.e., large frailty variance) in the visiting patterns of the patients.

The next steps are very similar to those in Section 6.3.1. In particular, setting argument MI to TRUE in the call to residuals() implements the multiple-imputation simulation scheme for random visit times described above. In order for residuals() to simulate future visit time for the patients who dropped out, we need to provide the fitted Weibull frailty model as the argument time.points. Moreover, for some internal computations, it is required to add as an extra attribute to WeibFrl the name of the variable that corresponds to $y_i(t_{k-1})$, which in our case is prev.y; this is achieved with the code

```
> attr(WeibFrl, "prev.y") <- "prev.y"
```

Then, the call to residuals() is

```
> set.seed(123) # we set the seed for reproducibility
```

```
> resMI.pbc <- residuals(jointFit2.pbc, type = "stand-Marginal",
    MI = TRUE, M = 10, time.points = WeibFrl)
```

As in Section 6.3.1, we first extract the standardized marginal residuals and the corresponding fitted values for the multiply-imputed responses, and then construct the data frame that contains the complete data, i.e., the multiply-imputed and observed residuals and fitted values, respectively.

```
> fitMargYmiss.pbc <- unlist(resMI.pbc$fitted.valsM)
```

```
> resMargYmiss.pbc <- unlist(resMI.pbc$resid.valsM)
```

```
> M <- length(resMI.pbc$fitted.valsM)
```

```
> datResid <- data.frame(
    resid = c(resMargY.pbc, resMargYmiss.pbc),
    fitted = c(fitMargY.pbc, fitMargYmiss.pbc),
    weight = c(rep(1, length(resMargY.pbc)),
        rep(1/M, length(resMargYmiss.pbc))))
```

```
> datResid <- datResid[complete.cases(datResid), ]
```

To help us spot any systematic trends in the residuals versus fitted values scatterplot, we calculate the loess smoother. Again the loess smoother for the completed data needs to account for the fact that residuals after the dropout time are over-represented. As in Section 6.3.1, we achieve that using the weighted loess smoother, with weights $1/L = 1/10 = 0.1$ for the residuals after dropout. The corresponding code is

```
> fitLoess.pbc <- loess(resid ~ fitted, data = datResid,
    weights = weight)
```

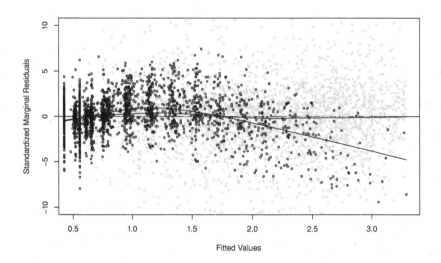

FIGURE 6.9: Observed standardized marginal residuals (black points), augmented with all the multiply-imputed residuals produced by the $L = 10$ imputations (grey points) for the PBC dataset. The superimposed solid lines represent a loess fit based only on the observed residuals (black solid line), and a weighted loess fit based on all residuals (black dashed line).

```
> nd.pbc <- data.frame(fitted = seq(min(datResid$fitted, na.rm = TRUE),
      max(datResid$fitted, na.rm = TRUE), len = 100))

> prdLoess.pbc <- predict(fitLoess.pbc, nd.pbc)
```

Finally, the scatterplot of the residuals versus the fitted values, including the two loess smoothers (i.e., the one based on the observed data alone, and the one based on the completed data) is produced with the code

```
> plot(range(fitMargYmiss.pbc, na.rm = TRUE),
      range(resMargYmiss.pbc, na.rm = TRUE),
      type = "n", xlab = "Fitted Values",
      ylab = "Standardized Marginal Residuals")
> abline(h = 0, lty = 2)
> points(fitMargY.pbc, resMargY.pbc)
> points(fitMargYmiss.pbc, resMargYmiss.pbc, col = "grey")
> lines(lowess(fitMargY.pbc, resMargY.pbc), lwd = 2)
> lines(nd.pbc$fit, prdLoess.pbc, lwd = 2, lty = 2)
```

As it was also the case for the AIDS dataset, we observe from Figure 6.9 that the weighted loess that is based on the completed data does not exhibit the systematic trend that was clearly seen in the loess curve based on the observed data alone. This is a strong indication that this systematic trend was primarily due to dropout and not model misfit.

＊

6.4   Random-Effects Distribution

The last component of the joint model for which we have made distributional assumptions is the random effects. As we have already seen, in mixed models, in general, the standard choice is to assume that the random effects are normally distributed with mean zero and covariance matrix D, even though, many times, this choice is not actually made on computational grounds. The main problem in checking the appropriateness of the normal distribution is that the random effects are latent quantities that do not lend themselves to a straightforward construction of residuals, i.e., observed quantity minus expected/fitted quantity. Nonetheless, in the standard mixed models literature, it has been shown that linear mixed-effects models are relatively robust to misspecification of this distribution (Verbeke and Lesaffre, 1997). However, in generalized linear mixed models there is more ambiguity regarding this topic, with some authors reporting sensitivity of the derived inferences to the distribution of the random effects (Heagerty and Kurland, 2001; Agresti et al., 2004; Litière et al., 2007, 2008), and some others reporting robustness (Neuhaus et al., 1992, 1994, 2011).

In joint models and for mainly two reasons, there has been even more concern regarding how much a potential misspecification of the random-effects distribution may influence the derived inferences. First, random effects have a more prominent role in joint models because they are used to capture both the correlations between the repeated measurements in the longitudinal outcome and to build the association between the longitudinal and event time processes. Second, as we have already explained in Section 6.2, the nonrandom dropout caused by the occurrence of events complicates matters because in the missing data literature it is known that inferences in nonrandom dropout settings can be highly sensitive to modeling assumptions (Copas and Li, 1997; Molenberghs et al., 2008).

These features motivated Song et al. (2002) to propose a flexible model for this distribution based on the class of smooth densities studied by Gallant and Nychka (1987) and Tsiatis and Davidian (2001) to propose a semiparametric estimating equations approach that provides valid inferences without requiring to specify the random-effects distribution. However, simulation findings of these authors suggested that parameter estimates and standard errors were rather robust to misspecification. This feature has been later theoretically corroborated by Rizopoulos et al. (2008) and Huang et al. (2009), who showed that, as the number of repeated measurements per subject n_i increases, misspecification of the random-effects distribution has a minimal effect in parameter estimators and standard errors.

Chapter 7

Prediction and Accuracy in Joint Models

Often the motivation behind building a statistical model is to provide predictions for an outcome of interest. In this chapter we illustrate how fitted joint models can be used to provide individualized predictions for the survival and longitudinal outcomes. An important characteristic of the setting we consider here is that these predictions have a dynamic nature, that is, as time progresses additional information is recorded for the patient, and therefore her predictions can be updated utilizing the new information. To assess the quality of these predictions we present discrimination measures based on Receiver Operating Characteristic (ROC) methodology.

7.1 Dynamic Predictions of Survival Probabilities

7.1.1 Definition

We first turn our attention to predictions of survival probabilities. In particular, for a specific patient and at a specific time point during follow-up, we would like to utilize all available information we have at hand (including both baseline information and accumulated biomarker levels) to produce predictions of survival probabilities. Access to this information will enable physicians to gain a better understanding of the disease dynamics, and ultimately take the most optimal decision at that specific time point. Due to current trends in

171

medical practice towards personalized medicine, and the prominent role such individualized predictions can play in that respect, there has recently been a lot of interest within the joint modeling framework on this front (Rizopoulos, 2011; Proust-Lima and Taylor, 2009; Yu et al., 2008; Garre et al., 2008).

To put it more formally, based on a joint model fitted in a random sample $\mathcal{D}_n = \{T_i, \delta_i, y_i; i = 1, \ldots, n\}$, we are interested in predicting survival probabilities for a new subject i that has provided a set of longitudinal measurements $\mathcal{Y}_i(t) = \{y_i(s); 0 \leq s < t\}$, and has a vector of baseline covariates w_i. As we have seen in Section 3.4, an important characteristic of the endogenous nature of $y_i(t)$ is that it is directly related to the failure mechanism, that is, providing longitudinal measurements up to t, in fact, implies survival up to this time point. Hence, it is more relevant to focus on the conditional probability of surviving time $u > t$ given survival up to t, i.e.,

$$\pi_i(u \mid t) = \Pr(T_i^* \geq u \mid T_i^* > t, \mathcal{Y}_i(t), w_i, \mathcal{D}_n; \theta^*), \quad t > 0, \tag{7.1}$$

where θ^* denotes the true parameter values. From its definition note that $\pi_i(u \mid t)$ has a dynamic nature. That is, when new information will be recorded for the patient at time $t' > t$, we can update these predictions and obtain $\pi_i(u \mid t')$, with $u > t'$, and therefore proceed in a *time dynamic* manner.

7.1.2   Estimation

The estimation of the subject-specific conditional survival probabilities takes full advantage of the conditional independence assumptions used to define the joint model. Namely, under condition (4.7) we observe that (7.1) can be rewritten as (conditioning on the covariates w_i is assumed but omitted from the notation):

$$\Pr(T_i^* \geq u \mid T_i^* > t, \mathcal{Y}_i(t); \theta)$$
$$= \int \Pr(T_i^* \geq u \mid T_i^* > t, \mathcal{Y}_i(t), b_i; \theta)$$
$$\times p(b_i \mid T_i^* > t, \mathcal{Y}_i(t); \theta) \, db_i$$
$$= \int \Pr(T_i^* \geq u \mid T_i^* > t, b_i; \theta) \, p(b_i \mid T_i^* > t, \mathcal{Y}_i(t); \theta) \, db_i$$
$$= \int \frac{\mathcal{S}_i\{u \mid \mathcal{M}_i(u, b_i, \theta); \theta\}}{\mathcal{S}_i\{t \mid \mathcal{M}_i(t, b_i, \theta); \theta\}} \, p(b_i \mid T_i^* > t, \mathcal{Y}_i(t); \theta) \, db_i, \tag{7.2}$$

where $\mathcal{S}_i(\cdot)$, as before, denotes the survival function, and furthermore we explicitly note that the longitudinal history $\mathcal{M}_i(\cdot)$, as approximated by the linear mixed-effects model, is a function of both the random effects and the parameters.

Based on (7.2) we can derive a first-order estimate of $\pi_i(u \mid t)$ using the empirical Bayes estimate for b_i, that is,

$$\tilde{\pi}_i(u \mid t)$$
$$= \mathcal{S}_i\{u \mid \mathcal{M}_i(u, \hat{b}_i^{(t)}, \hat{\theta}); \hat{\theta}\} \Big/ \mathcal{S}_i\{t \mid \mathcal{M}_i(t, \hat{b}_i^{(t)}, \hat{\theta}); \hat{\theta}\} + O([n_i(t)]^{-1}), \quad (7.3)$$

where $\hat{\theta}$ denotes the maximum likelihood estimates, $\hat{b}_i^{(t)}$ denotes the mode of the conditional distribution $\log p(b_i \mid T_i^* > t, \mathcal{Y}_i(t); \hat{\theta})$, and $n_i(t)$ denotes the number of longitudinal responses for subject i by time t. Simulation studies in Rizopoulos (2011) have shown that this estimator works relatively well in practice; however, deriving its standard error and confidence intervals for $\pi_i(u \mid t)$ is a rather difficult task due to the fact that we need to account for the variability of both the maximum likelihood and empirical Bayes estimates. To resolve this issue and produce valid standard errors, Rizopoulos (2011) and Proust-Lima and Taylor (2009) have alternatively proposed to use Monte Carlo simulation schemes. These are in fact very similar in spirit to the simulation schemes presented in Section 6.3 for the multiple imputation residuals, and they can be motivated by an asymptotic Bayesian formulation of the joint model. In particular, the posterior expectation of (7.1) can be derived as

$$\Pr(T_i^* \geq u \mid T_i^* > t, \mathcal{Y}_i(t), \mathcal{D}_n)$$
$$= \int \Pr(T_i^* \geq u \mid T_i^* > t, \mathcal{Y}_i(t); \theta) \, p(\theta \mid \mathcal{D}_n) \, d\theta. \quad (7.4)$$

The first part of the integrand, and as shown above, is given by (7.2). For the second part, which is the posterior distribution of the parameters given the observed data, we use similar arguments as in Section 6.3, and assume that the sample size n is sufficiently large such that $\{\theta \mid \mathcal{D}_n\}$ can be well approximated by $\mathcal{N}\{\hat{\theta}, \hat{\text{var}}(\hat{\theta})\}$. Combining (7.4) with (7.2) and $\{\theta \mid \mathcal{D}_n\} \sim \mathcal{N}\{\hat{\theta}, \hat{\text{var}}(\hat{\theta})\}$, we can derive a Monte Carlo estimate of $\pi_i(u \mid t)$ using the following simulation scheme:

S1: Draw $\theta^{(l)} \sim \mathcal{N}\{\hat{\theta}, \hat{\text{var}}(\hat{\theta})\}$.

S2: Draw $b_i^{(l)} \sim \{b_i \mid T_i^* > t, \mathcal{Y}_i(t), \theta^{(l)}\}$.

S3: Compute

$$\pi_i^{(l)}(u \mid t) = \mathcal{S}_i\{u \mid \mathcal{M}_i(u, b_i^{(l)}, \theta^{(l)}); \theta^{(l)}\} \Big/ \mathcal{S}_i\{t \mid \mathcal{M}_i(t, b_i^{(l)}, \theta^{(l)}); \theta^{(l)}\}.$$

Steps 1–3 are repeated $l = 1, \ldots, L$ times, where L denotes the number of

Monte Carlo samples. Note that, in fact, the above simulation scheme entails calculating the first-order estimator (7.3), but using $\theta^{(l)}$ and $b_i^{(l)}$ instead of $\hat{\theta}$ and $\hat{b}_i^{(t)}$, in order to propagate the uncertainty in the maximum likelihood and empirical Bayes estimates, respectively. Moreover, similarly to Section 6.3, Step 2 is based on a Metropolis-Hastings algorithm with independent proposals from a multivariate t distribution with four degrees of freedom, centered at the empirical Bayes estimates $\hat{b}_i^{(t)}$, and with scale matrix $\mathrm{v\hat{a}r}(\hat{b}_i^{(t)}) = \left\{ -\partial^2 \log p(T_i^* > t, \mathcal{Y}_i(t), b; \hat{\theta}) / \partial b^\top \partial b \big|_{b=\hat{b}_i^{(t)}} \right\}^{-1}$.

The realizations $\{\pi_i^{(l)}(u \mid t), l = 1, \ldots, L\}$ can be used to derive point estimates of $\pi_i(u \mid t)$, such as

$$\hat{\pi}_i(u \mid t) = \mathrm{median}\{\pi_i^{(l)}(u \mid t), l = 1, \ldots, L\} \tag{7.5}$$

or

$$\hat{\pi}_i(u \mid t) = L^{-1} \sum_{l=1}^{L} \pi_i^{(l)}(u \mid t), \tag{7.6}$$

and compute standard errors using the sample standard deviation over the Monte Carlo samples, and confidence intervals using the Monte Carlo sample percentiles. Compared to (7.3), estimators (7.5) and (7.6) not only provide a straightforward manner to calculate standard errors, but they are also expected to yield more accurate results because they properly approximate the integrals in the definition of $\pi_i(u \mid t)$.

7.1.3   Implementation in R

The dynamic survival probabilities are calculated in package **JM** using function `survfitJM()`. This function accepts as main arguments a fitted joint model and a data frame that contains the longitudinal and covariate information for the subjects for which we wish to calculate the predicted survival probabilities. To illustrate its use, we compute survival probabilities for Patients 2 and 25 from the PBC dataset. The observed longitudinal trajectories of log serum bilirubin for these two patients are depicted in Figure 7.1. We observe that Patient 2 shows an increasing profile in her log serum bilirubin levels, which is indicative of a worsening in her condition. On the other hand, Patient 25 shows a much more stable profile of lower serum bilirubin levels, and therefore we expect her to enjoy higher survival probabilities.

We base the estimation of the conditional survival probabilities $\pi_i(u \mid t)$ for these two patients on a joint model that uses B-splines to approximate the subject-specific longitudinal trajectories $m_i(t)$. More specifically, for the

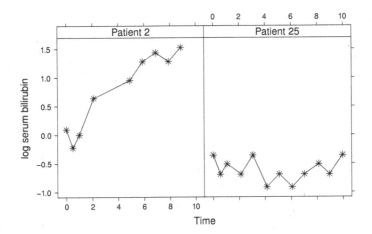

FIGURE 7.1: Observed longitudinal trajectories for Patients 2 and 25 from the PBC dataset.

longitudinal log serum bilirubin measurements, we assume the model

$$y_i(t) = m_i(t) + \varepsilon_i(t)$$

$$= (\beta_0 + b_{i0}) + (\beta_k + b_{ik})^\top B(t, 4, 4) + \varepsilon_i(t),$$

where $B(t, df, q)$ denotes a B-spline basis matrix for $q - 1$ degree splines with $df - q + 1$ internal knots placed at the corresponding percentiles of the follow-up times, and β_k and b_{ik} denote the vectors of fixed and random effects corresponding to the B-spines matrix. For the survival process we assume that the risk for the composite event (death or transplantation) depends on treatment, abnormal prothrombin time and the true level of log serum bilirubin, i.e.,

$$h_i(t) = h_0(t) \exp\{\gamma_1 \texttt{D-pnc}_i + \gamma_2 \texttt{ProtTime}_i + \alpha m_i(t)\},$$

where `ProtTime` denotes a dummy variable taking the value 1 when the prothrombin time at baseline was outside the normal range of [10 sec, 13 sec]. The baseline hazard is assumed piecewise-constant. We start by fitting the corresponding joint model using the same syntax:

```
> pbc2.id$Pro <- with(pbc2.id, factor(pro >= 10 & pro <= 13,
      labels = c("Abnormal", "Normal")))

> pbc2$Pro <- rep(pbc2.id$Pro, tapply(pbc2$id, pbc2$id, length))
```

```
> lmeFitBsp.pbc <- lme(
      fixed = log(serBilir) ~ bs(year, 4, Boundary.knots = c(0, 15)),
      random = list(
          id = pdDiag(form = ~ bs(year, 4, Boundary.knots = c(0, 15)))),
      data = pbc2)

> coxFit.pbc <- coxph(Surv(years, status2) ~ drug + Pro,
      data = pbc2.id, x = TRUE)

> jointFitBsp.pbc <- jointModel(lmeFitBsp.pbc, coxFit.pbc,
      timeVar = "year", method = "piecewise-PH-aGH")
```

The first part of the code constructs the factor variable denoting whether the prothrombin time at baseline was within the normal range. Function bs() from package **splines** automatically constructs the required B-spline basis matrix. Its second argument corresponds to the degrees of freedom, and argument Boundary.knots is used to ensure that the boundary knots of the B-spline basis extend to the combined range of the follow-up times $\{t_{ij}, i = 1, \ldots, n; j = 1, \ldots, n_i\}$ and the observed event times $\{T_i, i = 1, \ldots, n\}$.

We will first focus on Patient 2 and calculate her conditional survival probabilities $\pi_i(u \mid t)$. In particular, we provide as first argument to survfitJM() the fitted joint model, and in the newdata argument, the data we have for this patient. The function assumes that the patient has survived up to the last time point t in newdata for which a serum bilirubin measurement was recorded, and will produce survival probabilities for a set of predefined $u > t$ values.[1]

```
> set.seed(123) # we set the seed for reproducibility

> survPrbs <- survfitJM(jointFitBsp.pbc, newdata = pbc2[pbc2$id == 2, ])

> survPrbs


Prediction of Conditional Probabilities for Event
          based on 200 Monte Carlo samples

$2
      times   Mean Median  Lower  Upper
1    8.8325 1.0000 1.0000 1.0000 1.0000
1    8.9405 0.9835 0.9845 0.9666 0.9926
2    9.3609 0.9197 0.9252 0.8379 0.9655
3    9.7813 0.8567 0.8695 0.7022 0.9403
```

---

[1]By default survfitJM() constructs a regular sequence of 35 equidistant points from the minimum to the maximum observed event time, and computes $\pi_i(u \mid t)$ for the $u > t$ in this sequence.

```
 4  10.2017 0.7944 0.8140 0.5633 0.9138
 5  10.6221 0.7524 0.7769 0.4848 0.9014
 6  11.0425 0.7162 0.7462 0.4026 0.8933
 7  11.4629 0.6791 0.7101 0.3405 0.8837
 8  11.8833 0.6412 0.6773 0.2516 0.8718
 9  12.3037 0.6027 0.6501 0.1561 0.8559
10  12.7241 0.5641 0.6182 0.0728 0.8466
11  13.1445 0.5265 0.5847 0.0131 0.8405
12  13.5649 0.4906 0.5509 0.0003 0.8335
13  13.9853 0.4566 0.5216 0.0000 0.8326
14  14.4057 0.4251 0.4853 0.0000 0.8193
```

The output is rather self-explanatory. In particular, for each different subject in newdata and for a series of time points u, we obtain the median (7.5) and average (7.6) Monte Carlo estimates of $\pi_i(u \mid t)$, along with the corresponding 95% confidence intervals, calculated from the percentiles of the Monte Carlo samples. By default, 200 Monte Carlo samples are used, but this number can be suitably adjusted by specifying the M argument of survfitJM(). The first row in the output corresponds to the last time point for which we know the subject was still event free, and therefore the corresponding estimates and limits of the confidence interval are set to one. Alternatively, when interest is only in point estimates of $\pi_i(u \mid t)$, then we could also utilize the faster approximate first order estimator (7.3). This can be invoked by setting the simulate argument to FALSE, e.g.,

```
> survPrbsEB <- survfitJM(jointFitBsp.pbc,
      newdata = pbc2[pbc2$id == 2, ], simulate = FALSE)

> survPrbsEB


Prediction of Conditional Probabilities for Events

$2
      times predSurv
 1   8.8325   1.0000
 1   8.9405   0.9859
 2   9.3609   0.9314
 3   9.7813   0.8780
 4  10.2017   0.8255
 5  10.6221   0.7917
 6  11.0425   0.7636
 7  11.4629   0.7349
 8  11.8833   0.7053
 9  12.3037   0.6746
10  12.7241   0.6427
11  13.1445   0.6090
12  13.5649   0.5734
```

```
13 13.9853    0.5354
14 14.4057    0.4946
```

Comparing the estimates of $\pi_i(u \mid t)$ from the approximate and Monte Carlo estimators, we observe rather minor differences. This corroborates the statement of Section 7.1.2 that, in practice, estimator (7.3) performs very well in relation to estimators (7.5) and (7.6), which are expected to yield more accurate results because they properly approximate the integrals in the definition of $\pi_i(u \mid t)$.

Moreover, in some occasions, we may also have additional information regarding the failure status of a patient at a specific time point after the last available longitudinal measurement. For instance, according to the data of Patient 2:

```
> pbc2[pbc2$id == 2, c("id", "years", "status", "serBilir", "year")]
   id    years status serBilir      year
3   2 14.15234  alive      1.1 0.0000000
4   2 14.15234  alive      0.8 0.4983025
5   2 14.15234  alive      1.0 0.9993429
6   2 14.15234  alive      1.9 2.1027270
7   2 14.15234  alive      2.6 4.9008871
8   2 14.15234  alive      3.6 5.8892783
9   2 14.15234  alive      4.2 6.8858833
10  2 14.15234  alive      3.6 7.8907020
11  2 14.15234  alive      4.6 8.8325485
```

we know that she was still in the study and alive up to year 14.2, whereas the last serum bilirubin measurement was collected at year 8.8. This information can be provided in survfitJM() by specifying the last.time argument, which should be either a character string with the name of the variable in newdata holding this information or the last time point(s) itself as a numeric vector.

```
> set.seed(123)

> survPrbs2 <- survfitJM(jointFitBsp.pbc,
      newdata = pbc2[pbc2$id == 2, ], last.time = "years")

> survPrbs2


Prediction of Conditional Probabilities for Event
        based on 200 Monte Carlo samples

$2
    times   Mean Median  Lower  Upper
1 14.1523 1.0000 1.0000 1.0000 1.0000
1 14.4057 0.9414 0.9842 0.5686 0.9998
```

Note that due to the default approach to compute the sequence of time points u, when we specify that Patient 2 was alive up to year 14.2, $\pi_i(u \mid t)$ is estimated for a single time point. If we alternatively wish to estimate $\pi_i(u \mid t)$ for specific us, this can be achieved by argument `survTimes`. For instance, the 14.5 and 15 years Monte Carlo estimates of $\pi_i(u \mid t)$ are produced by the call

```
> set.seed(123)

> survfitJM(jointFitBsp.pbc, newdata = pbc2[pbc2$id == 2, ],
      survTimes = c(14.5, 15), last.time = "years")


Prediction of Conditional Probabilities for Event
          based on 200 Monte Carlo samples

$2
    times    Mean Median  Lower   Upper
1 14.1523 1.0000 1.0000 1.0000 1.0000
1 14.5000 0.9225 0.9783 0.4382 0.9997
2 15.0000 0.8385 0.9486 0.0549 0.9995
```

The estimates of $\pi_i(u \mid t)$ can also be graphically illustrated using the `plot()` method for objects of class `survfitJM`. In particular, the following simple call to `plot()` produces Figure 7.2:

```
> plot(survPrbs, lty = c(1:2,3,3), conf.int = TRUE)
```

The dashed and solid lines represent the median (7.5) and mean (7.6) estimators, respectively, whereas the `conf.int` argument specifies that we also want to plot the corresponding 95% pointwise confidence intervals, which are denoted by the dotted lines. This plot is based on object `survPrbs` produced by the first call to `survfitJM()`, and which assumed that the last time point the patient was still alive was at year 8.8 when she provided her last serum bilirubin measurement. Therefore, for all the previous time points $u < t$, $\pi_i(u \mid t) = 1$.

In the following we focus on the dynamic predictions of the conditional survival probabilities. In particular, we will dynamically update $\pi_i(u \mid t)$ for Patient 2 after each extra longitudinal measurement has been recorded. To program this we use a standard `for`-loop

```
> ND <- pbc2[pbc2$id == 2, ]
> survPreds <- vector("list", nrow(ND))
> for (i in 1:nrow(ND)) {
    set.seed(123)
    survPreds[[i]] <- survfitJM(jointFitBsp.pbc, newdata = ND[1:i, ])
  }
```

Subject 2

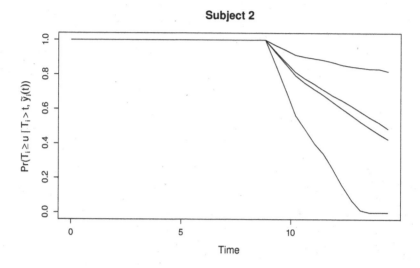

FIGURE 7.2: Survival probabilities for Patient 2 from the PBC dataset. The dashed and solid lines correspond to the median (7.5) and mean (7.6) estimators (7.5), respectively, and the dotted lines to the corresponding 95% pointwise confidence intervals.

The idea behind the loop is to simply provide in each iteration the updated data frame that contains one extra measurement in the **newdata** argument of **survfitJM()**. The results are saved in the list **survPreds**. We plot the updated survival curves after the baseline, third, fifth, and seventh measurements, respectively, with the code

```
> par(mfrow = c(2, 2), oma = c(0, 2, 0, 2))
> for (i in c(1,3,5,7)) {
      plot(survPreds[[i]], estimator = "median", conf.int = TRUE,
          include.y = TRUE, main = paste("Follow-up time:",
              round(survPreds[[i]]$last.time, 1)))
  }
> mtext("log serum bilirubin", side = 2, line = -1, outer = TRUE)
> mtext("Survival Probability", side = 4, line = -1, outer = TRUE)
```

Again, a **for**-loop is used to produce the plots. The **include.y** argument is used to simultaneously include in the plot the fitted longitudinal profile for Patient 2 up to the time point of the last available serum bilirubin measurements, and the estimated survival probabilities after this point. Moreover, the option **"median"** for argument **estimator** specifies that we only want the median estimator (7.5) to be plotted. The four plots are included in Figure 7.3. We observe that after the third measurement, where a clear increase in the

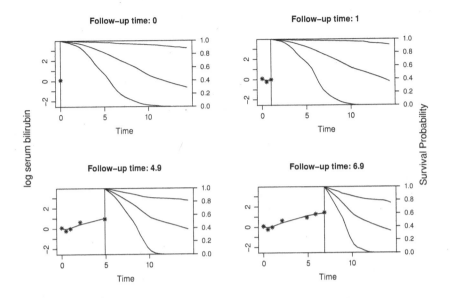

FIGURE 7.3: Dynamic survival probabilities for Patient 2 from the PBC dataset during follow-up. The vertical dotted lines represent the time point of the last serum bilirubin measurement. Left of this vertical line, the fitted longitudinal trajectory is depicted. Right of the vertical line, the solid line represents the median estimator (7.5) for $\pi_i(u \mid t)$, and the dashed lines the corresponding 95% pointwise confidence intervals.

true level of serum bilirubin is observed, the rate of decrease of the conditional survival function $\pi_i(u \mid t)$ becomes considerably more steep.

To illustrate how changes in the serum bilirubin profiles are reflected in changes in the dynamic updates of the survival probabilities, we make a comparison of the estimates $\pi_i(u \mid t)$ between Patients 2 and 25. These are presented in Figure 7.4. In each panel of this figure we have four estimates of $\pi_i(u \mid t)$ (along with the corresponding 95% confidence intervals) for $t = 0$, 0.5, 2 and 5 years, and $u = t + \Delta t$, with a different value of Δt for each panel. In particular, the left panels correspond to $\Delta t = 1$ year, the middle panels to $\Delta t = 2$ years, and the right panels to $\Delta t = 4$ years. In general, we observe that Patient 25 who showed a much more stable serum bilirubin profile has a higher survival chance of not experiencing the composite event (death or transplantation) compared to Patient 2. In addition, if we take a closer look to Figure 7.1, which depicts the observed longitudinal trajectories for the two patients, we see that for both patients the level of serum bilirubin decreased from the baseline to the first measurement, indicating an improvement in their condition. This improvement is also noted in the corresponding

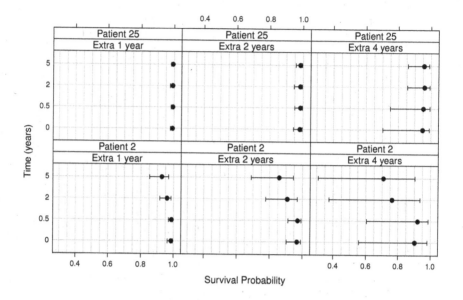

FIGURE 7.4: A comparison of dynamic survival probabilities for Patients 2 and 25 from the PBC dataset. In each panel four estimates (with associated 95% confidence intervals) of $\pi_i(u \mid t)$ are presented for t set to the time point the most recent serum bilirubin measurement was collected. The top panels correspond to Patient 25, the bottom panels to Patient 2, and in the left-hand side panels $u = t + 1$, in the middle panels $u = t + 2$, and in the right-hand side panels $u = t + 4$.

point estimates of survival probabilities in Figure 7.4 that at $t = 0.5$ are higher than the same probabilities at baseline ($t = 0$), albeit the confidence intervals of the two estimates overlap.

7.2 Dynamic Predictions for the Longitudinal Outcome

In many occasions interest may also lie in predictions for the longitudinal outcome. For example, in HIV-infected patients the CD4 cell count and the viral load are often used to determine when treatment should be initiated. In these settings it would be helpful to the treating physician to gain an insight into the projected longitudinal profile of the two markers in order to initiate treatment sooner than later. Such predictions can be defined and estimated in an analogous manner as it has been done for the survival process. In particular, for a specific subject i who is still alive by follow-up time t, we are interested in the expected value of her longitudinal outcome at time $u > t$ given her observed responses up to that time point $\mathcal{Y}_i(t) \doteq \{y_i(s), 0 \leq s < t\}$, that is,

$$\omega_i(u \mid t) = E\{y_i(u) \mid T_i^* > t, \mathcal{Y}_i(t), \mathcal{D}_n; \theta^*\}, \quad u > t. \tag{7.7}$$

Similar to the conditional survival probabilities (7.1), these predictions are also dynamically updated in time as extra information is recorded for that subject. That is, the prediction $\omega_i(u \mid t)$ for $y_i(u)$ that is based on the information that we have available up to time t, can be updated at time t' with $t < t' < u$, to produce the new prediction $\omega_i(u \mid t')$ that uses the additional longitudinal information up to the latter time point.

For the estimation of $\omega_i(u \mid t)$ we can utilize an analogous procedure to the one followed for the estimation of $\pi_i(u \mid t)$ in Section 7.1.2. More specifically, in order to account for the fact that we do not know the true parameter values θ^*, we proceed again under an asymptotic Bayesian formulation of the joint model, and calculate the expectation of $\omega_i(u \mid t)$ with respect to the posterior distribution of the parameters $\{\theta \mid \mathcal{D}_n\}$ as

$$
\begin{aligned}
&E\{y_i(u) \mid T_i^* > t, \mathcal{Y}_i(t), \mathcal{D}_n\} \\
&= \int E\{y_i(u) \mid T_i^* > t, \mathcal{Y}_i(t); \theta\} \, p(\theta \mid \mathcal{D}_n) \, d\theta.
\end{aligned} \tag{7.8}
$$

The first part of the integrand can be simplified by exploiting the conditional independence assumptions (4.7) and (4.8) as follows:

$$
\begin{aligned}
&E\{y_i(u) \mid T_i^* > t, \mathcal{Y}_i(t); \theta\} \\
&= \int E\{y_i(u) \mid T_i^* > t, \mathcal{Y}_i(t), b_i; \theta\} \, p(b_i \mid T_i^* > t, \mathcal{Y}_i(t); \theta) \, db_i \\
&= \int E\{y_i(u) \mid b_i\} \, p(b_i \mid T_i^* > t, \mathcal{Y}_i(t); \theta) \, db_i \\
&= \int \{x_i^\top(u)\beta + z_i^\top(u)b_i\} \, p(b_i \mid T_i^* > t, \mathcal{Y}_i(t); \theta) \, db_i \\
&= x_i^\top(u)\beta + z_i^\top(u)\bar{b}_i^{(t)},
\end{aligned} \tag{7.9}
$$

where

$$\bar{b}_i^{(t)} = \int b_i \, p(b_i \mid T_i^* > t, \mathcal{Y}_i(t); \theta) \, db_i.$$

Under these derivations a straightforward estimator of $\omega_i(u \mid t)$ is obtained by simply replacing θ with $\hat{\theta}$, and calculating the mean of the posterior distribution $p(b_i \mid T_i^* > t, \mathcal{Y}_i(t); \hat{\theta})$. In the same spirit, a similar estimator is derived when instead of the mean $\bar{b}_i^{(t)}$ of the posterior distribution we use its mode $\hat{b}_i^{(t)} = \arg\max_b \log p(b \mid T_i^* > t, \mathcal{Y}_i(t); \hat{\theta})$, i.e.,

$$\tilde{\omega}_i(u \mid t) = x_i^\top(u)\hat{\beta} + z_i^\top(u)\hat{b}_i^{(t)} + O(n_i^{-1}). \tag{7.10}$$

This is justified from the standard relationship (Tierney and Kadane, 1986):

$$\bar{b}_i^{(t)} = \hat{b}_i^{(t)} + O\big([n_i(t)]^{-1}\big),$$

that holds under sufficient smoothness of $\log p(b \mid T_i^* > t, \mathcal{Y}_i(t); \hat{\theta})$, and in which $n_i(t)$ denotes the number of longitudinal responses for subject i by time t. As we have also noted in Section 4.5, the mean and the mode of the posterior distribution of the random effects are typically very close, and therefore we also expect negligible differences between the two aforementioned estimators of $\omega_i(u \mid t)$. For practical purposes, we prefer estimator (7.10), because the mode is usually a better location measure than the mean, especially when the posterior distribution is skewed. Nevertheless, obtaining the standard error of either of the two estimators is very difficult because both $\hat{b}_i^{(t)}$ and $\bar{b}_i^{(t)}$ are nonlinear functions of $\hat{\theta}$ that cannot be written in closed form. To overcome this and obtain confidence intervals for $\omega_i(u \mid t)$, we use a similar Monte Carlo approach as in Section 7.1.2. In particular, combining (7.8) with (7.9), and assuming again that the sample size is sufficiently large such that $\{\theta \mid \mathcal{D}_n\}$ can be well approximated by a normal distribution centered at the MLEs $\hat{\theta}$ and with variance-covariance matrix the inverse of the observed information matrix $\hat{\text{var}}(\hat{\theta}) = \{\mathcal{I}(\hat{\theta})\}^{-1}$, we obtain the following simulation scheme:

S1: Draw $\theta^{(l)} \sim \mathcal{N}\{\hat{\theta}, \hat{\text{var}}(\hat{\theta})\}$.

S2: Draw $b_i^{(l)} \sim \{b_i \mid T_i^* > t, \mathcal{Y}_i(t), \theta^{(l)}\}$.

S3: Compute $\omega_i^{(l)}(u \mid t) = x_i^\top(u)\beta^{(l)} + z_i^\top(u)b_i^{(l)}$.

Steps 1 and 2 are exactly the same as in the simulation scheme of Section 7.1.2, and are used to account for the variability in $\hat{\theta}$ and $\hat{b}_i^{(t)}$, respectively. Using the simulated values for the parameters and the random effects, Step 3 only entails the calculation of the predicted value for the unobserved longitudinal outcome $y_i(u)$. The corresponding 95% pointwise confidence intervals can be obtained from 2.5% and 97.5% percentiles of $\{\omega_i^{(l)}(u \mid t), l = 1, \ldots, L\}$. An advantageous feature of the above simulation scheme is that it can be easily modified to produce prediction intervals. More specifically, instead of setting $\omega_i^{(l)}(u \mid t)$ to the realization of the subject-specific mean, we simulate a value from the corresponding normal distribution, i.e., $\omega_i^{(l)}(u \mid t) \sim \mathcal{N}\{x_i^\top(u)\beta^{(l)} + z_i^\top(u)b_i^{(l)}, [\sigma^{(l)}]^2\}$.

Furthermore, note that, similar to Section 7.1.2, we can also alternatively estimate $\omega_i(u \mid t)$ using its Monte Carlo realizations, that is by

$$\hat{\omega}_i(u \mid t) = L^{-1} \sum_{l=1}^{L} \omega_i^{(l)}(u \mid t) \qquad (7.11)$$

or

$$\hat{\omega}_i(u \mid t) = \text{median}\{\omega_i^{(l)}(u \mid t), l = 1, \dots, L\}. \qquad (7.12)$$

However, numerical comparisons of (7.11)

and (7.12) versus (7.10) have shown that the resulting estimates from these estimators are almost indistinguishable. Therefore, for simplicity, we use $\tilde{\omega}_i(u \mid t)$ for point estimation, and the Monte Carlo approach to derive confidence or prediction intervals.

Subject-specific predictions for the longitudinal outcome are produced in R using function `predict()`. We have already seen this function in Section 4.4.2 where it was used to produce estimates of the average longitudinal evolutions $\mu = X\beta$, and their corresponding pointwise confidence intervals. The main arguments to this function are the fitted joint model of interest and the data frame `newdata`, providing the data on which to base predictions. For subject-specific predictions, this data frame should contain baseline covariates and the longitudinal responses up to time t, which will be used to estimate $\omega_i(u \mid t)$, $u > t$. By default `predict()` will produce predictions for the average longitudinal evolutions. When subject-specific are required instead, we set the option `type = "Subject"`. In the following we illustrate the use of this function to produce estimates of $\omega_i(u \mid t)$ along with the corresponding confidence intervals, for Patient 2 from the PBC study, and based on model `jointFitBsp.pbc`. In connection with the estimators for $\omega_i(u \mid t)$ presented above, function `predict()` returns as predictions the estimates according to (7.10), and when option `interval = "confidence"` is invoked it uses the Monte Carlo scheme to compute standard errors and confidence intervals.[2] To illustrate how the predictions for Patient 2 are updated when additional serum bilirubin measurements are recorded, we use a `for`-loop which at each iteration updates the `newdata` argument.

```
> ND <- pbc2[pbc2$id == 2, ]
> longPreds <- vector("list", nrow(ND))
> for (i in 1:nrow(ND)) {
      set.seed(123) # we set the seed for reproducibility
      longPreds[[i]] <- predict(jointFitBsp.pbc, newdata = ND[1:i, ],
          type = "Subject", interval = "confidence", returnData = TRUE)
      longPreds[[i]]$FollowUp <- round(max(ND[1:i, "year"]), 1)
}
```

The default output of `predict()` is a vector of predicted values for each one of the individuals included in `newdata`. The time points u at which these

---

[2]Prediction intervals can be computed using the option `interval = "prediction"`.

predictions are calculated are by default chosen as a regular sequence of length 25 from t (the last available measurement of the subject) to $t_{max} + \epsilon$ where t_{max} denotes the largest follow-up time in the sample at hand and ϵ is a small number.[3] However, by setting argument `returnData` to `TRUE`, the output of `predict()` is the data frame supplied in `newdata` augmented with extra lines for each subject with her predictions at time points u. The last line of the `for`-loop adds one extra column to data frame returned by `predict()`, denoting the last follow-up time t at which a longitudinal response has been recorded.

To visualize the resulting estimates we first collect all the results in a single data frame using the code

```
> longPreds.all <- do.call(rbind, longPreds)
> longPreds.all$FollowUp <- with(longPreds.all, factor(FollowUp,
    labels = paste("Follow-up time:", unique(FollowUp))))
```

The second line transforms column `FollowUp`, which holds the last available time point, to a factor with suitable levels. Using this data frame the following code produces the plot of the dynamic predictions of the longitudinal outcome:

```
> xyplot(pred + low + upp ~ year | FollowUp, data = longPreds.all,
    lty = c(1, 2, 2), type = "l", as.table = TRUE,
    xlab = "Time", ylab = "Predicted log serum bilirubin")
```

A more elaborate version of this plot is shown in Figure 7.5.[4] As expected, we observe that the width of the predictions intervals increases as time progresses, indicating that we have much stronger faith on predictions shortly after the last available longitudinal measurement. An important feature of these prediction intervals is that they are not restricted to be symmetric, since they are not based on an asymptotic normality of $\hat{\omega}_i(u \mid t)$. In particular, we expect the Monte Carlo approach to provide a relatively good approximation to the true sampling distribution of $\omega_i(u \mid t)$, and therefore obtain confidence intervals that have higher chance to satisfy the claimed coverage.

7.3   Effect of Parameterization on Predictions

In the previous sections we have seen how dynamic predictions for either the survival or the longitudinal outcome can be obtained under a fitted joint model. However, before deciding to utilize these predictions in practice, we should first investigate their stability and quality. The quality of these predictions will typically depend on two factors, first, on the capability of the longi-

---

[3]In particular, ϵ is set to `0.1 * mad(times)`, where `times` is the vector of the follow-up times $\{t_{ij}, i = 1, \ldots, n; j = 1, \ldots, n_i\}$, and `mad()` computes the median absolute deviation.

[4]The actual R code that reproduces Figure 7.5 is available from the web site of the book.

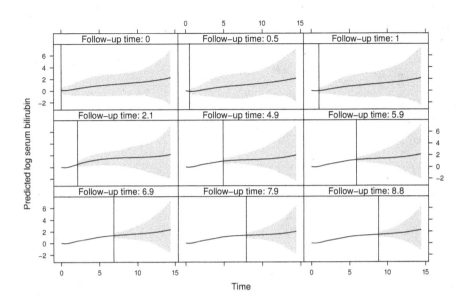

FIGURE 7.5: Dynamic predictions of longitudinal responses for Patient 2 from the PBC dataset. In each panel the dotted vertical line denotes the time point of the last observed longitudinal response. The solid line left to the dotted line denotes the fitted longitudinal trajectory prior to the last visit, and the dashed line right to the dotted line denotes the predicted longitudinal trajectory. The grey areas denote the 95% pointwise confidence intervals.

tudinal marker itself in predicting future events, and second, on the correct formulation of the joint model in order to reveal the true predictive performance of this marker. It is evident that the first factor has primarily to do with the biological mechanism that the marker attempts to describe, and how strongly this mechanism is related to the event outcome. Assuming that a marker has been chosen based on strong biological background, the purpose of the joint modeling exercise is then to reveal which features of the marker process are most strongly associated with the risk for an event. Due to the fact that we are dealing with time-dependent markers, the risk for an event may depend on an elaborate function of the longitudinal history $\mathcal{M}_i(t) = \{m_i(s), 0 \leq s < t\}$. In particular, as we have seen in Section 5.1, there are various parameterizations that can be used to link the two outcomes, and, as illustrated in Figure 5.3, they can considerably influence the shapes of the estimated subject-specific hazard functions.

To investigate how the posited association structure between the longitudinal and event time outcomes may affect the derived subject-specific predictions, we perform a sensitivity analysis under different parameterizations. For

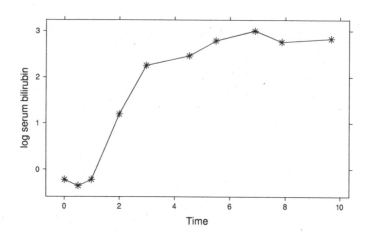

FIGURE 7.6: Observed longitudinal trajectory for Patient 51 from the PBC dataset.

our illustration we will use Patient 51 from the PBC study whose longitudinal trajectory of log serum bilirubin measurements is depicted in Figure 7.6. We can observe that this patient had stable bilirubin levels for the first three visits, but afterward she showed a steep increase in her longitudinal profile indicating a worsening of her condition. In our sensitivity analysis we will compare six joint models with different specifications for the relative risk submodel for the composite event (death or transplantation), namely:

$$
\begin{aligned}
\text{(I)} \quad h_i(t) &= h_0(t)\exp\{\gamma_1 \text{D-pnc}_i + \gamma_2 \text{ProtTime}_i + \alpha_1 m_i(t)\}, \\
\text{(II)} \quad h_i(t) &= h_0(t)\exp\{\gamma_1 \text{D-pnc}_i + \gamma_2 \text{ProtTime}_i + \alpha_2 m_i'(t)\}, \\
\text{(III)} \quad h_i(t) &= h_0(t)\exp\{\gamma_1 \text{D-pnc}_i + \gamma_2 \text{ProtTime}_i + \alpha_1 m_i(t) + \alpha_2 m_i'(t)\},
\end{aligned}
$$

$$
\begin{aligned}
\text{(IV)} \quad h_i(t) &= h_0(t)\exp\big[\gamma_1 \text{D-pnc}_i + \gamma_2 \text{ProtTime}_i + \alpha_1 m_i(t) \\
&\quad + \alpha_1^{int}\{\text{ProtTime}_i \times m_i(t)\}\big], \\
\text{(V)} \quad h_i(t) &= h_0(t)\exp\big[\gamma_1 \text{D-pnc}_i + \gamma_2 \text{ProtTime}_i + \alpha_2 m_i'(t) \\
&\quad + \alpha_2^{int}\{\text{ProtTime}_i \times m_i'(t)\}\big], \\
\text{(VI)} \quad h_i(t) &= h_0(t)\exp\big[\gamma_1 \text{D-pnc}_i + \gamma_2 \text{ProtTime}_i + \alpha_1 m_i(t) + \alpha_2 m_i'(t) \\
&\quad + \alpha_1^{int}\{\text{ProtTime}_i \times m_i(t)\} + \alpha_2^{int}\{\text{ProtTime}_i \times m_i'(t)\}\big],
\end{aligned}
$$

and the same longitudinal submodel, as presented in Section 7.1.3, which uses B-splines to flexibly capture the shapes of the subject-specific longitudinal trajectories:

$$y_i(t) \quad = \quad m_i(t) + \varepsilon_i(t)$$

$$= \quad (\beta_0 + b_{i0}) + (\beta_k + b_{ik})^\top B(t, 4, 4) + \varepsilon_i(t).$$

Relative risks models (I)–(III) assume that the risk for the composite event at time t depends on the true level of log serum bilirubin at the same time point, the slope of the true trajectory at t, or on both the true level and the slope at t, respectively. Similarly, models (IV)–(VI) assume the same type of relationships, but also include the interaction terms between the true level of the marker and/or the slope of the trajectory with the dummy variable of abnormal prothrombin time at baseline.

Before proceeding in fitting these models in R, we first need to derive the expression for the derivative $m_i'(t)$ under the B-splines representation for $m_i(t)$. From standard B-splines theory it is known that this derivative can be also written in terms of B-splines basis functions (Dierckx, 1993, Section 1.3.2). In particular, rewriting $m_i(t)$ in the form:

$$m_i(t) = (\beta_0 + b_{i0}) + \sum_k (\beta_k + b_{ik}) B_k(t, q),$$

with $B_k(t, q)$ denoting the B-spline basis of order q at knot λ_k, its derivative is given by the expression:

$$m_i'(t) = (q - 1) \sum_k \frac{c_{i,k+1} - c_{i,k}}{\lambda_{k+q+1} - \lambda_k} B_k(t, q - 1),$$

where $c_{i,k} = \beta_k + b_{ik}$. To specify the slope of the true trajectory using the `formula` interface of R, we rewrite $m_i'(t)$ using the mixed-effects model formulation, that is,

$$
\begin{aligned}
m_i'(t) \quad = \quad & [x_i^{sl}(t)]^\top \beta^{sl} + [z_i^{sl}(t)]^\top b_i^{sl} \\
= \quad & (q - 1) B(t, \lambda, q - 1)^\top (\beta_{k,-1}/D\lambda) - q B(t, \lambda, q - 1)^\top (\beta_{k,-c}/D\lambda) \\
& + q B(t, \lambda, q - 1)^\top (b_{ik,-1}/D\lambda) - q B(t, \lambda, q - 1)^\top (b_{ik,-c}/D\lambda),
\end{aligned}
$$

where λ denotes the knots of the B-spline basis in the specification of $m_i(t)$, $D\lambda$ denotes the $q + 1$ order differences of λ, and $\beta_{k,-l}$ and $b_{ik,-l}$ denote the vectors of fixed and random effects β_k and b_{ik}, respectively, excluding their lth element, with c denoting the last element. For our example, and due to the fact that we have only a single internal knot, the term $D\lambda_k = \lambda_{k+q+1} - \lambda_k$ in the denominator of $m_i'(t)$, always equals the range of the boundary knots, which we have manually set to the combined range of the follow-up times t_{ij} and observed event times T_i.

The code to fit the longitudinal and survival submodels is the same as in Section 7.1.3, that is

```
> lmeFitBsp.pbc <- lme(
      fixed = log(serBilir) ~ bs(year, 4, Boundary.knots = c(0, 15)),
      random = list(
          id = pdDiag(form = ~ bs(year, 4, Boundary.knots = c(0, 15)))),
      data = pbc2)

> coxFit.pbc <- coxph(Surv(years, status2) ~ drug + Pro,
      data = pbc2.id, x = TRUE)
```

To fit the joint models that include the slope term $m_i'(t)$, we will initially need to appropriately specify the `derivForm` argument of `jointModel()`, introduced in Section 5.1.3, using suitable R formulas that construct the fixed- and random-effects design matrices for this term. These take the form

```
> dform <- list(
      fixed = ~ -1
      + I(3 * bs(year, knots = 2.0534443,
          Boundary.knots = c(0, 15), degree = 2) / 15)
      + I(-3 * bs(year, knots = 2.0534443,
          Boundary.knots = c(0, 15), degree = 2) / 15),

      indFixed = c(3,4,5,2,3,4),

      random = ~ -1
      + I(3 * bs(year, knots = 2.0534443,
          Boundary.knots = c(0, 15), degree = 2) / 15)
      + I(-3 * bs(year, knots = 2.0534443,
          Boundary.knots = c(0, 15), degree = 2) / 15),

      indRandom = c(3,4,5,2,3,4))
```

The B-splines basis in the specification of $m_i'(t)$ should be calculated at exactly the same knots as the B-spline basis for $m_i(t)$. To do this we first extract the value of the internal knot with the code

```
> attr(lmeFitBsp.pbc$terms, "predvars")
list(log(serBilir), bs(year, degree = 3L, knots = 2.0534443105903,
    Boundary.knots = c(0, 15), intercept = FALSE))
```

and then we manually set the internal and boundary knots in the call to `bs()` using the `knots` and `Boundary.knots` arguments, respectively. In addition, the `degree` argument specifies the degree of the B-splines, and by default is set to three, meaning that the order q of the B-splines is four. Thus, in the above formulas and in order to construct the term $(q-1)B(t, \lambda, q-1)$, we multiply the B-splines basis with three, and set their `degree` to two. The `indFixed` component of the `dform` list corresponds to the indices that construct the vector $\beta^{sl} = (\beta_{k,-1}^{\top}, \beta_{k,-c}^{\top})^{\top}$, and `indRandom` is defined analogously. The six joint models with corresponding relative submodels given by (I)–(VI) above are fitted in R with the code:

```
> jointFitBsp.pbc <- jointModel(lmeFitBsp.pbc, coxFit.pbc,
    timeVar = "year", method = "piecewise-PH-aGH")

> jointFitBsp2.pbc <- update(jointFitBsp.pbc,
    parameterization = "slope", derivForm = dform)

> jointFitBsp3.pbc <- update(jointFitBsp.pbc,
    parameterization = "both", derivForm = dform)


> jointFitBsp4.pbc <- update(jointFitBsp.pbc,
    interFact = list(value = ~ Pro, data = pbc2.id))

> jointFitBsp5.pbc <- update(jointFitBsp2.pbc,
    interFact = list(slope = ~ Pro, data = pbc2.id))

> jointFitBsp6.pbc <- update(jointFitBsp3.pbc,
    interFact = list(value = ~ Pro, slope = ~ Pro, data = pbc2.id))
```

The estimated regression coefficients (with associated standard errors, and p-values) for the six relative risk submodels are presented in Table 7.1. To illustrate how predictions are affected under the different parameterizations, we show in Figures 7.7 and 7.8 estimates of the dynamically updated predictions for the longitudinal outcome $\omega_i(u \mid t)$, and the dynamically updated conditional survival probabilities $\pi_i(u \mid t)$ for the event outcome for Patient 51 from the PBC study. In each panel of these figures, t is set to the time point of the last available longitudinal response, and $u = t + 1$. From Figure 7.7 we clearly observe that the predictions for the longitudinal outcome, and their corresponding standard errors, are minimally affected by the chosen association structure. On the contrary, from Figure 7.8, and for some time points u the estimated conditional survival probabilities $\pi_i(u \mid t)$ show considerable variability between the six different parameterizations. For example, we observe that the predictions after each one of the first three visits, based on joint models (II) and (V) that only allow for the effect of the slope term $m_i'(t)$, show greater standard errors than the other models that also condition on the current value $m_i(t)$. However, for latter time points, and in particular after the sixth visit (i.e., $u = 5.5$), the opposite behavior emerges, with models (II) and (V) showing higher survival probabilities and smaller standard errors than the other models. This can be explained by the shape of the longitudinal profile of Patient 51 (see Figure 7.6), which is more nonlinear during the first five visits, but stabilizes afterwards.

The decision upon which of the six models we should base our predictions can be based on standard likelihood information approach. Table 7.2

TABLE 7.1: Parameter estimates and standard errors for the regression coefficients in relative risks models (I)–(VI) based on the corresponding joint models fitted to the PBC dataset

	Coefficient	Value	Std. Err.	z-value	p-value
`jointFitBsp.pbc`	γ_1	−0.02	0.16	−0.09	0.926
	γ_2	−0.08	0.22	−0.36	0.722
	α_1	1.30	0.09	14.15	< 0.001
`jointFitBsp2.pbc`	γ_1	−0.07	0.16	−0.45	0.649
	γ_2	0.31	0.21	1.50	0.135
	α_2	3.40	0.41	8.23	< 0.001
`jointFitBsp3.pbc`	γ_1	−0.02	0.17	−0.13	0.894
	γ_2	−0.05	0.22	−0.23	0.821
	α_1	1.29	0.10	13.51	< 0.001
	α_2	1.00	0.43	2.33	0.020
`jointFitBsp4.pbc`	γ_1	−0.00	0.17	−0.01	0.991
	γ_2	1.19	0.67	1.78	0.076
	α_1	1.89	0.31	6.08	< 0.001
	α_1^{int}	−0.69	0.33	−2.10	0.035
`jointFitBsp5.pbc`	γ_1	−0.07	0.16	−0.46	0.646
	γ_2	0.50	0.33	1.49	0.136
	α_2	3.86	0.75	5.17	< 0.001
	α_2^{int}	−0.59	0.82	−0.71	0.476
`jointFitBsp6.pbc`	γ_1	−0.01	0.17	−0.04	0.972
	γ_2	1.06	0.71	1.49	0.135
	α_1	1.89	0.32	5.88	< 0.001
	α_1^{int}	−0.68	0.34	−2.02	0.044
	α_2	0.41	0.89	0.47	0.642
	α_2^{int}	0.59	0.99	0.60	0.550

presents AIC and BIC values for all six models, as well as the results of the five likelihood ratio tests comparing the full model (VI) with the other five more parsimonious models. The AIC chooses the full model as the most appropriate, whereas the BIC model (IV) that assumes that only the current value of the marker is associated with the risk for the composite event, but the strength of this association differs between patients with normal and abnormal prothrombin time. The likelihood ratio tests also suggest model (IV),

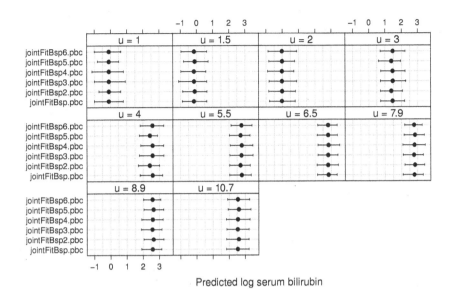

FIGURE 7.7: Dynamic predictions of the log serum bilirubin level for Patient 51 from the PBC dataset. Each panel depicts point estimates and the associated 95% confidence intervals of the log serum bilirubin one year after the last visit of the patient, based on the six joint models.

TABLE 7.2: Log-likelihood, AIC and BIC values for the six joint models fitted to the PBC data. The last three columns give the likelihood ratio test statistics, degrees of freedom and p-values for testing the full model (VI) against the other five

	logLik	AIC	BIC	LRT	df	p-value
jointFitBsp.pbc	−1840.58	3723.15	3801.76	10.84	3	0.013
jointFitBsp2.pbc	−1953.26	3948.52	4027.12	236.20	3	< 0.001
jointFitBsp3.pbc	−1837.83	3719.65	3802.00	5.34	2	0.069
jointFitBsp4.pbc	−1837.42	3718.85	3801.19	4.53	2	0.104
jointFitBsp5.pbc	−1953.03	3950.06	4032.40	235.74	2	< 0.001
jointFitBsp6.pbc	−1835.16	3718.32	3808.15			

since for the other models there is more evidence of poorer fit than in the full model (VI).

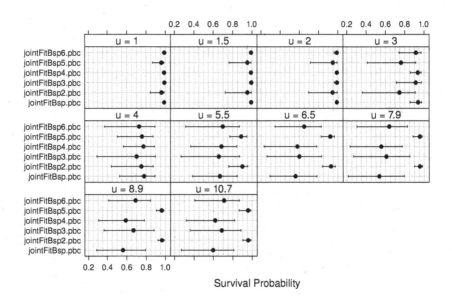

FIGURE 7.8: Dynamic predictions of survival probabilities for Patient 51 from the PBC dataset. Each panel depicts point estimates and the associated 95% confidence intervals of the probability of surviving one additional year after the last longitudinal response has been recorded, based on the six joint models.

7.4   Prospective Accuracy for Joint Models

The previous section demonstrated that different features of the marker process may be more strongly associated with the risk for an event than others. Information criteria, such as the AIC and BIC, can be useful when interest is in the overall predictive ability of the joint model encompassing both the longitudinal and survival parts. However, often the focus may primarily be in the survival outcome, and in particular in determining how good the longitudinal marker is in predicting this outcome. The answer to this question has received a lot of attention in the literature, where two main lines of research have emerged. The first one focuses on calibration measures and how well the model predicts the observed data (Graf et al., 1999; Schemper and Henderson, 2000; Henderson et al., 2002; Gerds and Schumacher, 2006), and the second one focusing on discrimination measures and how well the model can discriminate between patients who will experience the event in a short time frame, from patients who will experience it in a later time (Harrell et al., 1982; Heagerty et al., 2000; Heagerty and Zheng, 2005; Antolini et al., 2005; Pencina et al., 2008). In this section we focus on the latter family of measures, and we rely on a Receiver Operating Characteristic (ROC) approach to assess how well a longitudinal marker can discriminate between patients with low and high risk of having the event.

7.4.1 Discrimination Measures for Binary Outcomes

To introduce the basic concepts behind discrimination measures, we will first consider the simple binary response setting. In particular, let d_i denote the disease status indicator for subject i, that takes values 1 or 0 depending on whether or not the subject experienced the event of interest. Let also y_i denote a scalar marker measured at baseline that is believed to be strongly associated with the probability of disease. Our aim is to utilize the observed marker values to identify the subjects that have greater chance of being 'diseased'. To achieve this we construct an appropriate prediction rule that classifies subject i as diseased when her observed marker level exceeds a specific threshold, i.e., $y_i > c$. Based on this rule, we can now quantify the performance of the marker using the probabilities of correct classification conditional on the disease status. In particular, the probability that the marker correctly classifies a subject as diseased is called sensitivity (also known as the true positive rate):

$$\mathrm{TP}(c) = \Pr(y_i > c \mid d_i = 1),$$

whereas the probability that the marker correctly classifies a subject as non-diseased is called specificity:

$$1 - \mathrm{FP}(c) = \Pr(y_i \leq c \mid d_i = 0),$$

where $\mathrm{FP}(c) = \Pr(y_i > c \mid d_i = 0)$ denotes the false positive rate. Note that these probabilities measure the predictive accuracy of the specific rule $\{y_i > c\}$. To describe the overall discrimination capability of the marker we compute the sensitivity and specificity for all possible prediction rules $\{y_i > c, c \in \mathbb{R}_y\}$, where $\mathbb{R}_y \subseteq \mathbb{R}$ denotes the sample space of the marker, and $\mathbb{R}$ is the set of real numbers. This gives rise to the ROC curve, which is the plot of the true positive rate (sensitivity) against the false positive rate (1 − specificity) for varying c, and is formally defined as

$$\mathrm{ROC}(p) = \mathrm{TP}\{\mathrm{FP}^{-1}(p)\},$$

where p is in $[0, 1]$, and $\mathrm{FP}^{-1}(p) = \inf_c\{c : \mathrm{FP}(c) \leq p\}$. A generic example of an ROC curve is presented in Figure 7.9. The left panel displays boxplots of the marker levels in the diseased and nondiseased groups, and the right panel the corresponding ROC curve. The dashed line in the left panel corresponds to the rule $y_i > 35$, and the dashed lines in the right panel annotate the performance of this rule in terms of sensitivity and 1 − specificity. The higher the ROC curve is in the unit quadrant, the more accurate the predictions rules are.

A summary of the predictive accuracy index of the marker for all the

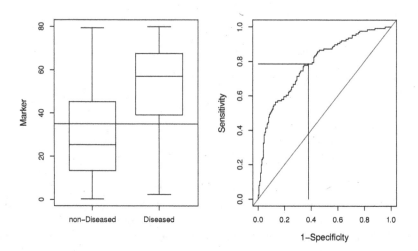

FIGURE 7.9: An example of an ROC curve. Left panel: boxplots of the marker levels in the diseased and nondiseased groups. Right panel: the ROC curve corresponding to this marker for all possible threshold values c. The dashed lines represent the prediction rule $y_i > 35$ that has sensitivity 0.79 and specificity 0.62.

possible threshold values c is given by the area under the ROC curve (AUC) defined as:

$$\text{AUC} = \int_0^1 \text{ROC}(p)\,dp.$$

A more intuitive interpretation of the AUC is provided by the equivalent formulation (Hanley and McNeil, 1982):

$$\text{AUC} = \Pr(y_i > y_j \mid d_i = 1, d_j = 0). \tag{7.13}$$

This postulates that for any random pair $\{i, j\}$ of 'comparable' subjects (i.e., subjects whose status can be ranked, such as the one being diseased and the other non-diseased), the AUC represents the probability that the ranking of the marker levels of the two subjects is concordant with the ranking of their disease status. An AUC equal to one indicates maximum discrimination, whereas AUC $= 0.5$ indicates random discrimination (i.e., the marker is no better in discriminating patients than flipping a coin). A key advantage of ROC methodology is that it can be used to compare different candidate markers. For example, for HIV-infected patients one might want to compare the CD4 cell count with the viral load, or whether the immediate change in CD4 that is observed around the time of infection provides better accuracy than the baseline level of the CD4. For more background information on ROC curves for continuous markers the reader is referred to Krzanowski and Hand (2009).

7.4.2 Discrimination Measures for Survival Outcomes

To extend the definitions of sensitivity and specificity from the binary setting presented in the previous section to survival data, we view an event time as a time-dependent binary outcome, taking the value 0 for all the time points prior to the event and the value 1 afterwards. In fact, this representation of survival times is equivalent to the counting process representation of time-to-event outcomes $N_i(t) = I(t \geq T_i^*)$, introduced in Section 3.5. The time-dependent nature of the binary outcome $N_i(t)$ allows for several potential definitions of sensitivity and specificity depending on the manner subjects are classified as either 'cases' or 'controls' at any particular time point t. A taxonomy of the different possibilities we have available in this context has been proposed by Heagerty and Zheng (2005). Focusing still on a scalar marker y_i that is used as a predictor for an event, the three main families of accuracy measures are

1. *Cumulative Sensitivity / Dynamic Specificity*:

$$\mathrm{TP}_t^{\mathbb{C}}(c): \qquad \mathrm{Pr}(y_i > c \mid T_i^* \leq t), \quad \text{and}$$
$$1 - \mathrm{FP}_t^{\mathbb{D}}(c): \qquad \mathrm{Pr}(y_i \leq c \mid T_i^* > t).$$

   Under these definitions at any fixed time t, the entire population is classified as either a case or a control on the basis of their event status at time t. In addition, each subject plays the role of a control for times $t < T_i^*$, but then contributes as a case for later times $t \geq T_i^*$.

2. *Incident Sensitivity / Static Specificity*:

$$\mathrm{TP}_t^{\mathbb{I}}(c): \qquad \mathrm{Pr}(y_i > c \mid T_i^* = t), \quad \text{and}$$
$$1 - \mathrm{FP}_{\tilde{t}}^{\mathbb{S}}(c): \qquad \mathrm{Pr}(y_i \leq c \mid T_i^* > \tilde{t}).$$

   These definitions have been adopted by Etzioni et al. (1999) and Slate and Turnbull (2000), and posit that each subject does not change status and is classified as either a case or a control. Cases are stratified according to the time the event occurs, and controls are defined as those subjects who are event free through a fixed follow-up period $(0, \tilde{t})$.

3. *Incident Sensitivity / Dynamic Specificity*:

$$\mathrm{TP}_t^{\mathbb{I}}(c): \qquad \mathrm{Pr}(y_i > c \mid T_i^* = t), \quad \text{and}$$
$$1 - \mathrm{FP}_t^{\mathbb{D}}(c): \qquad \mathrm{Pr}(y_i \leq c \mid T_i^* > t).$$

   Under this approach a subject can play the role of a control for all

$t < T_i^*$, but then plays the role of a case when $t = T_i^*$. Here, sensitivity measures the expected fraction of subjects with a marker level exceeding the threshold c among the subpopulation of individuals who have the event at t, while specificity measures the fraction of subjects with a marker level less or equal to c among those who survive beyond time t.

An important feature of all the above definitions is that they are time-dependent, meaning that the capability of the marker to discriminate between cases and controls changes as time progresses. After selecting definitions for the time-dependent sensitivity and specificity, ROC curves and the areas under these curves can be computed and interpreted in the same manner as in the binary context. These measures will also be time-varying and reflect how the accuracy of the marker evolves during follow-up.

7.4.3 Prediction Rules for Longitudinal Markers

Following Rizopoulos (2011) and Zheng and Heagerty (2007), we extend now the framework of the time-dependent accuracy measures of the previous section to the case of longitudinal markers. As it has been previously noted, an inherent characteristic of the studies that require a joint modeling approach to answer the scientific questions of interest is their dynamic nature. Namely, as longitudinal information is collected for a subject, we can continuously update the predictions of her survival probabilities. Taking this feature into account, it is often of medical relevance to distinguish patients that are about to experience the event within a time frame after their last measurement from patients that are going to surpass this time frame without an event. In this setting a useful property of the longitudinal marker would be to successfully discriminate between these patients. In particular, as before, we assume that we have collected a set of longitudinal measurements $\mathcal{Y}_i(t) = \{y_i(s); 0 \leq s < t\}$ up to time point t for subject i. We are interested in events occurring in the medically relevant time frame $(t, t + \Delta t]$ within which the physician can take an action (e.g., initiate or change treatment) to improve the survival chance of this patient. Using an appropriate function of the marker history $\mathcal{Y}_i(t)$, we can define a prediction rule to discriminate between patients of high and low risk for an event. For instance, for PBC patients we could consider values of the log serum bilirubin larger than a specific threshold as predictive for death. Since we are in a longitudinal context, we have the flexibility of determining which values of the longitudinal history $\mathcal{Y}_i(t)$ of the patient will contribute to the specification of the prediction rule. To allow for full generality we consider a vector of threshold values c, based on which we define

$$\mathcal{P}_i^s(t, k, c) = \{y_i(s) \geq c_s; k \leq s \leq t\}$$

as a 'success', i.e., the marker indicates that the event will occur, and

$$\mathcal{P}_i^f(t, k, c) = \mathbb{R}^{r(k,t)} \setminus \{y_i(s) \geq c_s; k \leq s \leq t\}$$

as a 'failure', where $\mathbb{R}^n$ denotes the n-dimensional Euclidean space, and $r(k,t)$ the number of longitudinal measurements taken in the interval $[k,t]$. The value of $k \geq 0$ specifies which past marker values of the longitudinal history contribute to the rule, and c_s denotes the threshold value at time point s. The convention in these prediction rules is that larger values for the marker are associated with higher risk for death. When the opposite is true, for instance in the case we are using the CD4 cell count as a marker for HIV-infected patients, these definitions should be adjusted accordingly.

To demonstrate the full generality of $\mathcal{P}_i^s(t,k,c)$ and the range of different possibilities we have available in defining prediction rules, we present three illustrative examples:

Ex1: The simplest and most frequently used prediction rule utilizes only the last available longitudinal measurement to drive decisions, that is,

$$\mathcal{P}_i^s(t,k,c) = \{y_i(t) \geq c\}.$$

This rule represents a time-dependent analogue of the prediction rules we have seen in Sections 7.4.1 and 7.4.2 for baseline markers. In particular, for any time point t we classify a patient in the high risk group for experiencing the event, if her observed marker level at the same time point exceeds a specific threshold c.

Ex2: Even though the previous rule is simple and easy to use in practice, its drawback is that it uses a single marker measurement, and therefore it discards useful information. A small extension is to use the marker values at two time points, for example:

$$\mathcal{P}_i^s(t,k,c) = \{y_i(t-1) \geq c\} \cap \{y_i(t) \geq c\}.$$

This rule classifies a patient at time t in the high risk group if her marker levels exceeded the same threshold value c at both time points t and $t-1$.

Ex3: A further enhancement over Example 2 is to allow the prediction rule to capture a worsening of the condition of the patient. This can be achieved by either an absolute increase prediction rule, such as,

$$\mathcal{P}_i^s(t,k,c) = \{y_i(t-1) \geq c\} \cap \{y_i(t) \geq c+\nu\}, \quad \nu > 0,$$

which formalizes the idea that there is a higher chance for a patient to experience the event if she shows an absolute increase in her marker levels of ν units, or a relative increase prediction rule, such as,

$$\mathcal{P}_i^s(t,k,c) = \{y_i(t-1) \geq c\} \cap \{y_i(t) \geq (1+\nu)c\}, \quad \nu > 0,$$

which analogously states that there is a higher chance for a patient to experience the event if she shows an increase in her marker levels of a magnitude of $(100 \times \nu)\%$.

We will call rules that are based on a single assessment of the marker, as in Example 1, *simple prediction rules*, and rules involving more than one marker evaluations, as in Examples 2 and 3, *composite prediction rules*. Since our interest here is in utilizing the observed marker levels $\mathcal{Y}_i(t)$ up to time t to predict events in the medically relevant interval $(t, t + \Delta t]$, the sensitivity and specificity are respectively defined as:

$$\text{TP}_t^{\Delta t}(c) = \Pr\{\mathcal{P}_i^s(t, k, c) \mid T_i^* > t, T_i^* \in (t, t + \Delta t]; \theta^*\}, \tag{7.14}$$

and

$$1 - \text{FP}_t^{\Delta t}(c) = \Pr\{\mathcal{P}_i^f(t, k, c) \mid T_i^* > t, T_i^* > t + \Delta t; \theta^*\}. \tag{7.15}$$

According to the categorization of Heagerty and Zheng (2005) presented in Section 7.4.2, the above specifications correspond to cumulative sensitivity and dynamic specificity, respectively. In addition, note that these accuracy measures are not only time-dependent but they also depend on the length of the medically relevant time interval Δt. This means that for the same t different models may exhibit different discrimination power for different Δt. As before, the overall discrimination capability of the longitudinal marker for all possible thresholds $c \in \mathbb{R}_y$ can be assessed using the corresponding ROC curve

$$\text{ROC}_t^{\Delta t}(p) = \text{TP}_t^{\Delta t}\{[\text{FP}_t^{\Delta t}]^{-1}(p)\},$$

where p is in $[0, 1]$ and $[\text{FP}_t^{\Delta t}]^{-1}(p) = \inf_c\{c : \text{FP}_t^{\Delta t}(c) \leq p\}$, and the area under the ROC curve:

$$\text{AUC}_t^{\Delta t} = \int_0^1 \text{ROC}_t^{\Delta t}(p) \, dp.$$

7.4.4   Discrimination Indices

An important feature of all the accuracy measures for survival data we have presented so far is that they describe how well a marker (baseline or time-dependent) can discriminate between patients at a specific follow-up time t. Therefore, at different time points the marker may exhibit different levels of discrimination, and thus a relevant question is how can we summarize the discriminative capability of the marker over the whole follow-up period. To evaluate the overall performance of baseline markers, Harrell et al. (1982) have proposed a concordance index based on a modification of the Kendall-Goodman-Kruskal-Somers type rank correlation coefficient (Goodman and Kruskal, 1979). This can be seen as an extension of the definition of the AUC (7.13) in the binary context with a time-dependent disease status. Namely, for a random pair of subjects $\{i, j\}$ whose true event times can be ordered such that subject i experienced the event before subject j, then we are interested in the probability that their marker levels are concordant with their event times, i.e.,

$$C_h = \Pr(y_i > y_j \mid T_i^* < T_j^*). \tag{7.16}$$

This global accuracy summary index is, in fact, related to the time-dependent ROC curves presented in Section 7.4.2. In particular, in this context Heagerty and Zheng (2005) have shown that the C_h index (7.16) can be equivalently derived as a weighted average of AUCs obtained from the incidence/dynamic definitions of sensitivity and specificity, respectively. More specifically, they showed that

$$C_h = \int_0^\infty \text{AUC}_t \, u(t) \, dt, \tag{7.17}$$

where $\text{AUC}_t = \Pr(y_i > y_j \mid T_i^* = t, T_j^* > t)$ and $u(t) = 2 \cdot p(t) \cdot \mathcal{S}(t)$. This equivalent definition of the C_h index opens the possibility for a family of global concordance summary measures, which are based on alternative specifications of the AUC and of the weight function $u(t)$. For example, concordance discrimination indices for time-dependent markers can be constructed using appropriate definitions of the AUC (Antolini et al., 2005). Following this approach, Rizopoulos (2011) has proposed a dynamic discrimination index based on the AUC derived by (7.14) and (7.15), namely:

$$C_{dyn}^{\Delta t} = \int_0^\infty \text{AUC}_t^{\Delta t} \, u(t) \, dt,$$

with

$$u(t) = \Pr(T_i^* > t) \Big/ \int \Pr(T_i^* > t) \, dt,$$

where $\Pr(T_i^* > t)$ is the marginal survival probability. The choice for this weight function was made on the grounds of accounting for the fact that not all time points contribute equally to the comparison because at later time points we expect less subjects to be still available. Other weight functions $u(t)$ may be utilized as well to define alternative versions of the dynamic discrimination index $C_{dyn}^{\Delta t}$, and the optimal choice in that regard remains an open question.

In practice we would typically restrict our attention to a fixed follow-up period $(0, \tau)$. In this case the $C_{dyn}^{\Delta t}$ index can be modified to account for finite follow-up:

$$[C_{dyn}^{\Delta t}]^\tau = \int_0^\tau \text{AUC}_t^{\Delta t} \, u^\tau(t) \, dt,$$

where $u^\tau(t) = u(t) / \int_0^\tau u(t) dt$. $[C_{dyn}^{\Delta t}]^\tau$ will still be connected to the probability that the predictions for a random pair of subjects are concordant with their outcomes, but given that the smaller event time occurs within the interval $(0, \tau)$.

7.4.5   Estimation under the Joint Modeling Framework

The estimation of sensitivity, specificity, and of the AUC in the binary setting described in Section 7.4.1 can be simply based on the calculation of the respective frequencies in the observed sample. For example, the sensitivity can be estimated as the proportion of subjects in the sample with $y_i > c$ from the subjects who were diseased. In the survival context, however, estimation of the prospective accuracy measures is complicated by censoring. In particular, note that these measures were defined with respect to the true event time variable T_i^*. However, when we are interested in estimating, say sensitivity at a specific time point t, and a subject was censored at $t' < t$, then we do not know her event status at t, and therefore she cannot be classified as neither case nor control. This means that we cannot simply count the number of cases and controls in the sample at hand for different prediction rules, as in the binary setting, but we rather need to estimate the bivariate distribution of the true event times and the longitudinal measurements $\{T_i^*, y_i\}$. In that respect, the joint modeling framework is greatly advantageous because it provides a complete specification for this distribution. That is, with joint models we can simultaneously account for both censoring and the endogenous nature of the longitudinal outcome, and, in addition, we can also easily adjust for other baseline covariates affecting the risk for an event by introducing them in design matrix W of the survival submodel.

For ease of exposition, we will only focus on the estimation of sensitivity, since the estimation of specificity proceeds in an analogous manner. We will follow a similar approach as in Sections 7.1 and 7.2, and derive an appropriate simulation scheme to produce a Monte Carlo estimate of sensitivity and its standard error. More specifically, we observe that (7.14) is written as (condition on covariates is assumed but omitted from the notation):

$$\Pr\{\mathcal{P}_i^s(t, k, c) \mid T_i^* > t, T_i^* \in (t, t + \Delta t]; \theta^*\}$$

$$= \frac{\Pr\{\mathcal{P}_i^s(t, k, c), T_i^* \in (t, t + \Delta t] \mid T_i^* > t; \theta^*\}}{1 - \Pr(T_i^* > t + \Delta t \mid T_i^* > t; \theta^*)}, \qquad (7.18)$$

where θ^*, as before, denotes the true parameter values. Under assumptions (4.7) and (4.8), and the joint model's definition, we can obtain further simplifications for the numerator and denominator. In particular, the numerator takes the form

$$\Pr\{\mathcal{P}_i^s(t, k, c), T_i^* \in (t, t + \Delta t] \mid T_i^* > t; \theta^*\}$$

$$= \int \Pr\{\mathcal{P}_i^s(t, k, c), T_i^* \in (t, t + \Delta t] \mid T_i^* > t, b_i; \theta^*\} p(b_i \mid T_i^* > t; \theta^*) \, db_i$$

$$= \int \Pr\{\mathcal{P}_i^s(t, k, c) \mid b_i; \theta^*\} \times \Pr\{T_i^* \in (t, t + \Delta t] \mid T_i^* > t, b_i; \theta^*\}$$

$$\times \, p(b_i \mid T_i^* > t; \theta^*) \, db_i, \qquad (7.19)$$

where

$$\Pr\{\mathcal{P}_i^s(t,k,c) \mid b_i; \theta^*\} = \prod_{s=k}^{t} \Phi\left\{\frac{c_s - m_i(s,b_i,\beta^*)}{\sigma^*}\right\},$$

with $\Phi(\cdot)$ denoting the standard normal cumulative distribution function, and

$$\Pr\{T_i^* \in (t, t+\Delta t] \mid T_i^* > t, b_i; \theta^*\} = 1 - \frac{\mathcal{S}_i\{t+\Delta t \mid \mathcal{M}_i(t+\Delta t, b_i); \theta^*\}}{\mathcal{S}_i\{t \mid \mathcal{M}_i(t, b_i); \theta^*\}}.$$

Similarly for the denominator, we obtain:

$$\Pr(T_i^* > t + \Delta t \mid T_i^* > t; \theta^*)$$

$$= \int \Pr(T_i^* > t + \Delta t \mid T_i^* > t, b_i; \theta^*)\, p(b_i \mid T_i^* > t; \theta^*)\, db_i$$

$$= \int \frac{\mathcal{S}_i\{t+\Delta t \mid \mathcal{M}_i(t+\Delta t, b_i); \theta^*\}}{\mathcal{S}_i\{t \mid \mathcal{M}_i(t, b_i); \theta^*\}}\, p(b_i \mid T_i^* > t; \theta^*)\, db_i. \quad (7.20)$$

Thus, we observe that sensitivity is rewritten as the ratio of the expected values of

$$\mathcal{E}_1(b_i, \theta) = \left[\prod_{s=k}^{t} \Phi\left\{\frac{c_s - m_i(s,b_i,\beta^*)}{\sigma^*}\right\}\right]\left[1 - \frac{\mathcal{S}_i\{t+\Delta t \mid \mathcal{M}_i(t+\Delta t, b_i); \theta^*\}}{\mathcal{S}_i\{t \mid \mathcal{M}_i(t, b_i, \theta); \theta^*\}}\right]$$

and

$$\mathcal{E}_2(b_i, \theta) = \mathcal{S}_i\{t+\Delta t \mid \mathcal{M}_i(t+\Delta t, b_i); \theta^*\}\Big/\mathcal{S}_i\{t \mid \mathcal{M}_i(t, b_i); \theta^*\}$$

with respect to the marginal posterior distribution $p(b_i \mid T_i^* > t; \theta^*)$. We should note that this posterior distribution is not the same as the one used in the derivation of the conditional survival probabilities (7.2) or in the predictions for the longitudinal outcome (7.9). In particular, in (7.2) and (7.9) the posterior of the random effects conditions on both $T_i^* > t$ and the observed longitudinal history $\mathcal{Y}_i(t)$, while in the above derivations for the time-dependent sensitivity it only conditions on $T_i^* > t$. This means that in order to apply a similar simulation scheme as in Section 7.1.2, we first need to express $p(b_i \mid T_i^* > t; \theta^*)$ in terms of $p(b_i \mid T_i^* > t, \mathcal{Y}_i(t); \theta^*)$. This is achieved by observing that the former distribution is proportional to:

$$p(b_i \mid T_i^* > t; \theta^*) \propto p(T_i^* > t \mid b_i; \theta^*)\, p(b_i; \theta^*)$$

$$= \int p(T_i^* > t, \mathcal{Y}_i(t) \mid b_i; \theta^*)\, p(b_i; \theta^*)\, d\mathcal{Y}_i(t)$$

$$= \int p(\mathcal{Y}_i(t) \mid b_i; \theta^*)\, \mathcal{S}_i\{t \mid \mathcal{M}_i(t, b_i); \theta^*\}\, p(b_i; \theta^*)\, d\mathcal{Y}_i(t). \quad (7.21)$$

Therefore, combining Equations (7.19), (7.20) and (7.21), and calculating their expectation with respect to the asymptotic posterior distribution of the parameters $\{\theta \mid \mathcal{D}_n\} \sim \mathcal{N}\{\hat{\theta}, \text{var}(\hat{\theta})\}$, we arrive at the following simulation scheme:

S1: Draw $\theta^{(l)} \sim \mathcal{N}\{\hat{\theta}, \text{var}(\hat{\theta})\}$.

S2: Draw $\mathcal{Y}_i^{(l)}(t) \sim \mathcal{N}\{X_i\beta^{(l)} + Z_i b_i^{(l-1)}, [\sigma^{(l)}]^2\}$.

S3: Draw $b_i^{(l)} \sim \{b_i \mid T_i^* > t, \mathcal{Y}_i^{(l)}(t), \theta^{(l)}\}$.

S4: Compute $\mathcal{E}_1(b_i^{(l)}, \theta^{(l)})$ and $\mathcal{E}_2(b_i^{(l)}, \theta^{(l)})$.

Steps 1–4 are repeated $l = 1, \ldots, L$ times, where L denotes the number of Monte Carlo samples. As before, Step 1 is used to account for the variability of the maximum likelihood estimates, in Step 2 we simulate plausible longitudinal histories under the joint model up to time t, and in Step 3 we simulate random effects realizations conditioning on the longitudinal history of $\mathcal{Y}_i^{(l)}(t)$ and $T_i^* > t$. The last step just entails the calculation of the realizations $\mathcal{E}_1(b_i^{(l)}, \theta^{(l)})$ and $\mathcal{E}_2(b_i^{(l)}, \theta^{(l)})$, the ratio of which gives the sensitivity. Again, similar to previous simulation schemes we have seen in this chapter, Step 3 is implemented using a Metropolis-Hastings algorithm with independent proposals from a multivariate t distribution centered at the empirical Bayes estimates $\hat{b}_i^{(t)}$, and with scale matrix the covariance matrix of these estimates $\text{var}(\hat{b}_i^{(l)})$. A small practical issue in the implementation of this simulation scheme has to do with the starting values for b_i. More specifically, in the simulation schemes presented in Sections 7.1.2 and 7.2, we take as an initial value for b_i the mode $\hat{b}_i^{(t)}$ of the target distribution from which we want to simulate, and therefore there is no need to use burn-in. However, taking the same initial value in the above scheme where our aim is to simulate from $\{b_i \mid T_i^* > t\}$, it will require some burn-in because this initial value may be away from the support of the target distribution.

The Monte Carlo estimate of sensitivity takes the form:

$$\widehat{\Pr}\{\mathcal{P}_i^s(t, k, c) \mid T_i^* > t, T_i^* \in (t, t + \Delta t]\} = \frac{\sum_l \mathcal{E}_1(b_i^{(l)}, \theta^{(l)})}{L - \sum_l \mathcal{E}_2(b_i^{(l)}, \theta^{(l)})},$$

with the corresponding standard error estimated using the Monte Carlo standard errors of $\mathcal{E}_1(b_i^{(l)}, \theta^{(l)})$ and $\mathcal{E}_2(b_i^{(l)}, \theta^{(l)})$, and the Delta method. In particular, we have

$$s.e.\left(\widehat{\Pr}\{\mathcal{P}_i^s(t,k,c) \mid T_i^* > t, T_i^* \in (t, t + \Delta t]\}\right) = \{gVg^\top\}^{1/2},$$

where

$$g = L\left[1/\{L - \sum_l \mathcal{E}_2(b_i^{(l)}, \theta^{(l)})\},\right.$$

$$\left.\sum_l \mathcal{E}_1(b_i^{(l)}, \theta^{(l)})/\{L - \sum_l \mathcal{E}_2(b_i^{(l)}, \theta^{(l)})\}^2\right],$$

and

$$\text{vech}(V) = L^{-1}\left[\text{var}\{\mathcal{E}_1(b_i^{(l)}, \theta^{(l)})\},\right.$$

$$\left.\text{cov}\{\mathcal{E}_1(b_i^{(l)}, \theta^{(l)}), \mathcal{E}_2(b_i^{(l)}, \theta^{(l)})\}, \text{ var}\{\mathcal{E}_2(b_i^{(l)}, \theta^{(l)})\}\right].$$

Having estimated both sensitivity and specificity, it is straightforward to construct the corresponding ROC curve and additionally calculate the AUC. Finally, for the estimation of the dynamic discrimination index $C_{dyn}^{\Delta t}$ we also require an estimate of the marginal survival function $\mathcal{S}(t) = \Pr(T_i^* > t)$. This can be obtained from either the fitted joint model using the approximate expression

$$\mathcal{S}(t) = \int \mathcal{S}_i(t \mid b_i; \hat{\theta}) \, p(b_i; \hat{\theta}) \, db_i \approx n^{-1} \sum_i \mathcal{S}_i(t \mid \hat{b}_i; \hat{\theta}),$$

as we have seen in Section 6.1 or using the Kaplan-Meier product limit estimator (3.2). In addition, the integral in the numerator of $C_{dyn}^{\Delta t}$, which does not have a closed-form solution, can be numerically approximated using either the trapezoidal rule, Simpson's rule or a Gaussian quadrature approach (Press et al., 2007).

7.4.6 *Implementation in* R

We illustrate the calculation of the time-dependent discrimination measures in the Liver Cirrhosis dataset. In particular, we are interested in investigating whether the prothrombin index is a potentially useful marker in discriminating between subjects who died within a short time interval after their last assessment and subjects who lived longer than that. We start by fitting a simple joint model to the data. For the longitudinal part, we assume linear evolutions in time for each subject, and we also allow for differences in the average evolutions between the two treatment groups. In addition, to capture sudden changes in the prothrombin index in the very early part of follow-up in each treatment group, we also include a separate indicator variable of the baseline measurement. The model takes the form:

$$y_i(t) \;=\; m_i(t) + \varepsilon_i(t)$$

$$=\; \beta_0 + \beta_1 \text{Predns}_i + \beta_2 t + \beta_3 \text{T0}_i + \beta_4 \{\text{Predns}_i \times t\}$$

$$+ \beta_5 \{\text{Predns}_i \times \text{T0}_i\} + b_{i0} + b_{i1} t + \varepsilon_i(t),$$

where `Predns` denotes the dummy variable for prednisone treatment group, and `T0` the dummy variable for the baseline measurement. The R code to fit the model is

```
> prothro$t0 <- as.numeric(prothro$time == 0)

> lmeFitBsp.pro <- lme(pro ~ treat * (time + t0), random = ~ time | id,
      data = prothro)
```

For the survival submodel we include as a time-independent covariate the treatment, and as time-dependent one the true underlying profile of the pro-thrombin index as estimated from the longitudinal model, i.e.,

$$h_i(t) \;=\; h_0(t) \exp\{\gamma \text{Predns}_i + \alpha m_i(t)\}.$$

which is fitted in R with the code:

```
> coxFit.pro <- coxph(Surv(Time, death) ~ treat, data = prothros,
      x = TRUE)
```

We fit the corresponding joint model assuming a piecewise-constant baseline risk function $h_0(t)$ with six knots placed at equally spaced percentiles of the observed event times:

```
> jointFitBsp.pro <- jointModel(lmeFitBsp.pro, coxFit.pro,
      timeVar = "time", method = "piecewise-PH-aGH")

> summary(jointFitBsp.pro)
```

. . .

```
Event Process
              Value Std.Err  z-value p-value
treatpredns  0.2211  0.1402   1.5772  0.1147
Assoct      -0.0406  0.0036 -11.2040 <0.0001
log(xi.1)    1.2221  0.2612   4.6793
log(xi.2)    1.1222  0.2650   4.2347
```

```
log(xi.3)      0.6148  0.2756    2.2306
log(xi.4)      0.6764  0.2710    2.4961
log(xi.5)      0.5626  0.2786    2.0196
log(xi.6)      1.2004  0.3202    3.7486
log(xi.7)      1.7162  0.3703    4.6346
. . .
```

We observe that the prothrombin index is strongly associated with the event outcome, with a unit decrease in the marker corresponding to a 1.04-fold increase in the risk for death (95% CI: 1.03; 1.05). The time-dependent sensitivity (7.14) and specificity (7.15), and the corresponding ROC curve and the AUC for this marker can be calculated in package **JM** using function rocJM(). This function has very similar syntax as the survfitJM() function we have used in Section 7.1.3, and accepts as main arguments a fitted joint model and a data frame that contains the baseline covariate information as well as the time points at which longitudinal measurements were supposed to be taken. To illustrate the use of this function, we focus on a representative subject from the placebo group who has provided five prothrombin index measurements at baseline, three months, one year, three years, and four years. We first build the data frame holding this information

```
> plcbData <- data.frame(
       id = 1,
       treat = factor("placebo", levels = levels(prothro$treat)),
       time = c(0, 0.25, 1, 3, 4)
  )
> plcbData$t0 <- as.numeric(plcbData$time == 0)
> plcbData
   id    treat time t0
1   1 placebo 0.00  1
2   1 placebo 0.25  0
3   1 placebo 1.00  0
4   1 placebo 3.00  0
5   1 placebo 4.00  0
```

The final required argument of function rocJM() is argument dt that specifies the length(s) Δt of the medically relevant time interval(s). With the following call we produce the estimates of the discrimination measures at the last available time point, i.e., $t = 4$, for Δt being equal to one, two, and four years, respectively:

```
> set.seed(123)

> ROCplcb <- rocJM(jointFitBsp.pro, dt = c(1, 2, 4), data = plcbData,
       M = 1000, burn.in = 500)
```

```
> ROCplcb
Areas under the time-dependent ROC curves

Estimation: Monte Carlo (500 samples)
Difference: absolute, lag = 1 (0)
Thresholds range: (-28, 306)

Case: 1
Recorded time(s): 0, 0.25, 1, 3, 4
  dt t + dt    AUC    Cut
  1        5 0.6799 80.216
  2        6 0.6944 81.552
  4        8 0.7321 85.560
```

By default rocJM() works under the simple prediction rule that is based on
the last available marker measurement to discriminate between cases and controls.[5] The output provides the time-dependent AUCs under the different options for dt. For this particular case we observe that at time $t = 4$, the option
$\Delta t = 4$ provides slightly better discrimination than the other two. Column
Cut contains the threshold values for the marker that maximize the product of
sensitivity and specificity under the different options for dt. Even though this
choice of the best threshold value is intuitively appealing and easy to calculate
we should note that it is not always optimal, and thus it is simply provided as
an indication. An alternative statistic that can be used to capture the performance of a specific prediction rule is the Youden's index, which is defined as
Sensitivity + Specificity − 1 (Youden, 1950; Kraemer, 2004). To report in the
output of rocJM() the best threshold according to Youden's formula, the user
should set the option optThr = "youden". Argument M specifies the number
of Monte Carlo samples in the simulation scheme described in Section 7.4.5,
and argument burn.in specifies the number of samples to be excluded from
the calculations. The corresponding ROC curves are produced by a simple call
to the plot() function, and are depicted in Figure 7.10.

```
> plot(ROCplcb, legend = TRUE)
```

As the AUCs also suggested, we observe that the ROC curve for $\Delta t = 4$
lies above the ROC curves for $\Delta t = 1$ and $\Delta t = 2$, indicating that at year
four the marker can discriminate a little bit better between patients who are
going to die before year eight from patients who are going to live longer than
eight years. To examine how the predictive performance of the marker evolves
during follow-up, we can produce the ROC curves at different time points t.
This can be achieved by suitably updating the data argument of rocJM()

---

[5]Note that in the case of the prothrombin index low values are indicative for an event,
and therefore the simple prediction is defined as $\mathcal{P}_i^s(t, k, c) = \{y_i(t) \leq c\}$.

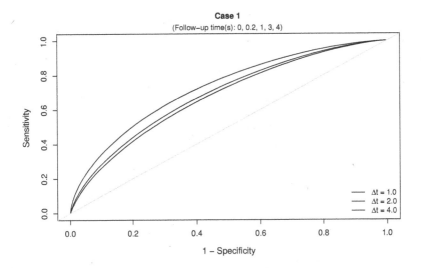

FIGURE 7.10: ROC curves at time $t = 4$ and three options for Δt under the simple prediction rule (based on the joint model fitted to the Liver Cirrhosis dataset).

using a `for`-loop. The following code illustrates this based on the `plcbData` data frame:

```
> ROCs <- vector("list", 5)

> for (i in seq_along(ROCs)) {
      set.seed(123)
      ROCs[[i]] <- rocJM(jointFitBsp.pro, dt = c(1, 2, 4),
          data = plcbData[seq_len(i), ], M = 1000, burn.in = 500)
  }
```

At each iteration, one extra row of `plcbData` is taken into account, and thus we obtain the estimates of sensitivity and specificity at $t = 0$, 0.25, 1, 3, and 4 years. The corresponding time-varying ROC curves starting from $t = 0.25$ years, and for the three different options of Δt, are graphically illustrated in Figure 7.11. The R code to produce this graph uses a similar `for`-loop:

```
> par(mfrow = c(2, 2), oma = c(0, 0, 2, 0))
> for (i in 2:5) {
      plot(ROCs[[i]], legend = TRUE)
  }
> mtext("Prediction rule: Simple", side = 3, line = -1, outer = TRUE)
```

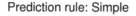

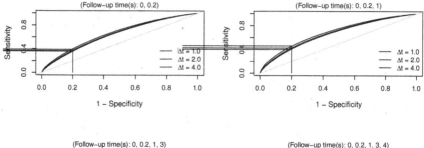

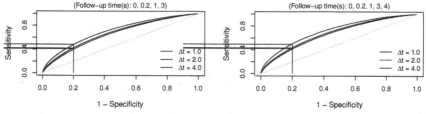

FIGURE 7.11: Time-dependent ROC curves for the liver cirrhosis dataset under the simple prediction rule. The horizontal solid lines denote the sensitivity levels corresponding false positive rate of 20%.

The horizontal solid lines represent the sensitivity levels under the three choices for Δt, when specificity is set to 80%. As time progresses, we see a clearer separation between the three Δt options, with $\Delta t = 4$ offering slightly better discrimination than $\Delta t = 1$ and 2. However, in general, under the simple prediction rule, the prothrombin index cannot very well separate patients who will die before $t + \Delta t$ from those who will not.

We continue our ROC analysis by investigating whether we can improve discrimination by considering a composite prediction rule. Following Example 3 given on p.199, we use the rule

$$\mathcal{P}_i^s(t, k, c) = \{y_i(t - k) \le c\} \cap \{y_i(t) \le 0.8c\},$$

which postulates that there is a higher chance for a patient to experience the event within the time interval $(t, t + \Delta t]$ when she shows a 20% decrease in her prothrombin levels between two subsequent visits, with $t - k$ denoting the time point of the next-to-last visit. To produce the ROCs and the AUCs under this prediction rule, we use arguments `diffType` and `rel.diff` of `rocJM()`. In the former we specify the option `"relative"` to denote that we are interested in a relative prediction rule, and in the latter we specify a numeric vector denoting the relation between the threshold values at the different time points. The corresponding syntax is

```
> set.seed(123)

> ROCplcb.Rel <- rocJM(jointFitBsp.pro, dt = c(1, 2, 4), data = plcbData,
      diffType = "relative", rel.diff = c(1, 0.8), M = 1000, burn.in = 500)



> ROCplcb.Rel
Areas under the time-dependent ROC curves

Estimation: Monte Carlo (500 samples)
Difference: relative, lag = 2 (1, 0.8)
Thresholds range: (-28, 306)

Case: 1
Recorded time(s): 0, 0.25, 1, 3, 4
 dt t + dt     AUC    Cut.1    Cut.2
  1      5 0.6725 102.928 82.3424
  2      6 0.6878 104.264 83.4112
  4      8 0.7290 108.272 86.6176
```

In the above call we have used again the full data frame **plcbData** meaning that the reported AUCs and the 'optimal' cut-points are for the last available time point $t = 4$. The ROC curves for the three options for Δt are presented in Figure 7.12, and are again obtained using a simple call to the **plot()** method:

```
> plot(ROCplcb.Rel, legend = TRUE)
```

Both the AUCs and the ROCs are very similar to the ones obtained from the simple prediction rule, and, in particular, we again observe that we achieve better discrimination for $\Delta t = 4$. We further investigate the performance of the composite prediction rule at different time points by producing the time-varying accuracy measures. These are produced with a similar **for**-loop as the one used for the simple rule, with the resulting time-varying ROCs depicted in Figure 7.13.

```
> ROCs.r <- vector("list", 5)
> for (i in seq_along(ROCs)) {
      set.seed(123)
      ROCs.r[[i]] <- rocJM(jointFitBsp.pro, dt = c(1, 2, 4),
          data = plcbData[seq_len(i), ], diffType = "relative",
          rel.diff = c(1, 0.8), M = 1000, burn.in = 500)
  }
```

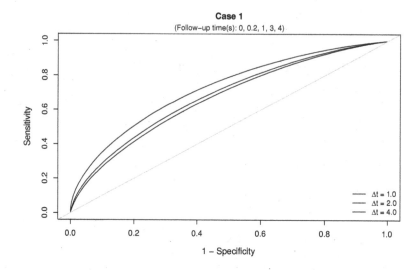

FIGURE 7.12: ROC curves at time $t = 4$ and three options for Δt under the composite prediction rule assuming 20% decrease in prothrombin levels between visits (based on the joint model fitted to the Liver Cirrhosis dataset).

```
> par(mfrow = c(2, 2), oma = c(0, 0, 2, 0))
> for (i in 2:5) {
    plot(ROCs.r[[i]], legend = TRUE, main = "Prediction rule: Simple")
  }
> mtext("Prediction rule: Composite", side = 3, line = -1, outer = TRUE)
```

A comparison between Figure 7.11 and Figure 7.13 shows that the time-varying ROCs curves under the two rules are almost identical suggesting that in this particular example we do not gain much by considering the composite prediction rule.

As a final step of our ROC analysis, and motivated by the observations made in Section 7.3 regarding the influence of the chosen parameterization on the predictions for the survival outcome, we explore how discrimination is affected by the posited association structure between the longitudinal and event time outcomes. In particular, assuming the same linear mixed model to describe the underlying longitudinal evolutions of the prothrombin index in time, we will consider three joint models, with corresponding survival sub-models:

$$\text{(I)} \quad h_i(t) = h_0(t) \exp\{\gamma \mathbf{Predns}_i + \alpha_1 m_i(t)\}$$
$$\text{(II)} \quad h_i(t) = h_0(t) \exp\{\gamma \mathbf{Predns}_i + \alpha_2 m_i'(t)\}$$
$$\text{(III)} \quad h_i(t) = h_0(t) \exp\{\gamma \mathbf{Predns}_i + \alpha_1 m_i(t) + \alpha_2 m_i'(t)\}$$

Prediction rule: Composite

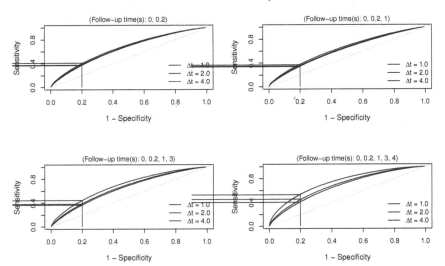

FIGURE 7.13: Time-dependent ROC curves for the liver cirrhosis dataset under the composite prediction rule.

Model (I) is the model we have used so far in our analysis and assumes that the risk for death at time t is related to the true value of the prothrombin index at the same time point. Model (II) postulates that the risk at t is associated with the slope of the true longitudinal trajectory at this time point, and Model (III) assumes that the risk depends on both the current value of the marker and the current slope of the marker's trajectory. As before, in order to fit Models (II) and (III) we need first to define the list that contains the R formulas defining the fixed- and random-effects parts of $m_i'(t)$. In our particular example, we have that

$$m_i(t) = \beta_0 + \beta_1 \texttt{Predns}_i + \beta_2 t + \beta_3 \texttt{TO}_i + \beta_4\{\texttt{Predns}_i \times t\}$$

$$+ \beta_5\{\texttt{Predns}_i \times \texttt{TO}_i\} + b_{i0} + b_{i1}t,$$

and therefore,

$$m_i'(t) = \beta_2 + \beta_4 \texttt{Predns}_i + b_{i1}.$$

We translate $m_i'(t)$ in a pair of R formulas for the fixed and random parts in the following list:

```
> dform2 <- list(fixed = ~ treat, indFixed = c(3, 5),
    random = ~ 1, indRandom = 2)
```

The components `indFixed` and `indRandom` in the above list give the position indexes of the fixed- and random-effects coefficients vectors β and b_i, respectively, of the original $m_i(t)$ that are used in the specification of $m_i'(t)$. That is, from the fixed-effects coefficients vector β of $m_i(t)$ we require the third and fifth element for the fixed-effects part in the specification of $m_i'(t)$, and analogously the second element of the random-effects coefficients vector b_i. The corresponding joint models are fitted with the syntax

```
> jointFitBsp2.pro <- update(jointFitBsp.pro,
    parameterization = "slope", derivForm = dform2)

> jointFitBsp3.pro <- update(jointFitBsp.pro,
    parameterization = "both", derivForm = dform2)
```

Using similar calls to `rocJM()` as before, we estimate the ROCs and AUCs under these two joint models for a placebo patient at time $t = 4$, for $\Delta t = 1$, 2 and 4, and using the composite prediction rule that classifies patients as 'cases' when they show a relative decrease of 20% in their prothrombin levels between the two last visits. Namely, for Model (II) the call is

```
> set.seed(123)

> ROCplcb.Rel2 <- rocJM(jointFitBsp2.pro, dt = c(1, 2, 4),
    data = plcbData, directionSmaller = TRUE, diffType = "relative",
    rel.diff = c(1, 0.8), M = 1000, burn.in = 500)


> ROCplcb.Rel2
Areas under the time-dependent ROC curves

Estimation: Monte Carlo (500 samples)
Difference: relative, lag = 2 (1, 0.8)
Thresholds range: (-28, 306)

Case: 1
Recorded time(s): 0, 0.25, 1, 3, 4
 dt t + dt    AUC    Cut.1    Cut.2
  1       5 0.6543 105.600 84.4800
  2       6 0.6599 105.600 84.4800
  4       8 0.6766 109.608 87.6864
```

and for Model (III) the respective call is

```
> set.seed(123)

> ROCplcb.Rel3 <- rocJM(jointFitBsp3.pro, dt = c(1, 2, 4),
      data = plcbData, diffType = "relative", rel.diff = c(1, 0.8),
      M = 1000, burn.in = 500)



> ROCplcb.Rel3
Areas under the time-dependent ROC curves

Estimation: Monte Carlo (500 samples)
Difference: relative, lag = 2 (1, 0.8)
Thresholds range: (-28, 306)

Case: 1
Recorded time(s): 0, 0.25, 1, 3, 4
 dt t + dt     AUC    Cut.1    Cut.2
  1       5 0.7105  90.904  72.7232
  2       6 0.7244  93.576  74.8608
  4       8 0.7566 100.256  80.2048
```

The additional argument `directionSmaller` included in the call for Model
(II) is used to define the direction of the inequality in the prediction rule,
here that lower values for the prothrombin index are indicative for an event.
This was not required to be set before, and also is not required in Model (III)
because `rocJM()` determines it by the sign of the association coefficient for the
current value term $m_i(t)$. Comparing the AUCs for the different Δt options
under the three models (the AUCs for Model (I) are presented on p.211), we
observe that the parameterization that combines both the current value term
$m_i(t)$ and the slope term $m_i'(t)$ seems to offer a bit better discrimination to
some extend than the parameterizations that have each one of these terms
separately. The same conclusion is also reached by the corresponding ROC
curves for the three models, presented in Figure 7.14, from which it can be
seen that for a specificity of 80%, Model (III) offers higher sensitivity rates
than the other two models, especially for $\Delta t = 4$. Nevertheless, even with
this improvement the prothrombin index does not prove to be a marker that
can successfully discriminate 'cases' from 'controls'. To investigate whether
Model (III) offers better discrimination than the other two models over the
main period of interest of ten years, and not only at $t = 4$, we calculate the
dynamic discrimination index, presented in Section 7.4.4, i.e.,

$$[C_{dyn}^{\Delta t}]^{\tau} = \frac{\int_0^{\tau} \text{AUC}_t^{\Delta t} \, S(t) \, dt}{\int_0^{\tau} S(t) \, dt},$$

for $\tau = 10$. As an illustration we calculate $[C_{dyn}^{\Delta t}]^{10}$ for a placebo patient and
for $\Delta t = 4$. The first step to achieve this is to calculate the time-dependent

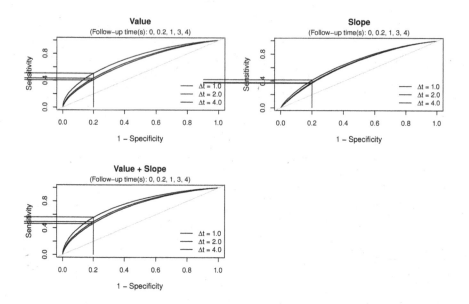

FIGURE 7.14: Time-dependent ROC curves for the liver cirrhosis dataset under the composite prediction rule and three different parameterizations for the joint model. The horizontal lines denote the sensitivity levels for a specificity of 80%.

AUCs at different time points over the ten year period. We have chosen the baseline, three months, half year, one year, and yearly thereafter until year ten; the required information is included in the following data frame:

```
> plcbData2 <- data.frame(
      id = 1,
      treat = factor("placebo", levels = levels(prothro$treat)),
      time = c(0, 0.25, 0.5, 1:10)
 )
> plcbData2$t0 <- as.numeric(plcbData2$time == 0)
```

As done previously, the time-dependent AUCs are calculated in R using a `for`-loop which at each iteration considers one additional row of the data frame `plcbData2`:

```
> ROCs.MI <- ROCs.MII <- ROCs.MIII <- vector("list", nrow(plcbData2))
```

```
> for (i in seq_along(ROCs.MI)) {
    set.seed(123)
    ROCs.MI[[i]] <- rocJM(jointFitBsp.pro, dt = 4,
        data = plcbData2[seq_len(i), ], diffType = "relative",
        rel.diff = c(1, 0.8), M = 1000, burn.in = 500)

    ROCs.MII[[i]] <- rocJM(jointFitBsp2.pro, dt = 4,
        data = plcbData2[seq_len(i), ], directionSmaller = TRUE,
        diffType = "relative", rel.diff = c(1, 0.8),
        M = 1000, burn.in = 500)

    ROCs.MIII[[i]] <- rocJM(jointFitBsp3.pro, dt = 4,
        data = plcbData2[seq_len(i), ], diffType = "relative",
        rel.diff = c(1, 0.8), M = 1000, burn.in = 500)
}
```

The results of each iteration for the three models are saved in the lists
`ROCs.MI`, `ROCs.MII`, and `ROCs.MIII`, respectively. In the following step we
extract $\text{AUC}_t^{\Delta t}$ from these lists and calculate the marginal function $\mathcal{S}(t)$:

```
> AUCs.MI <- sapply(ROCs.MI, "[[", "AUCs")
> AUCs.MII <- sapply(ROCs.MII, "[[", "AUCs")
> AUCs.MIII <- sapply(ROCs.MIII, "[[", "AUCs")
> sf <- survfit(Surv(Time, death) ~ treat, data = prothros,
        subset = treat == "placebo")
> Surv.Plcb <- summary(sf, times = c(0, 0.25, 0.5, 1:10))$surv
```

In particular, the `sapply()` statements extract the `AUCs` component across all
the elements for each of the three lists, and function `survfit()` from package
survival computes the Kaplan-Meier estimate for the Liver Cirrhosis dataset.
In `survfit()` we use the `subset` argument in order to estimate $\mathcal{S}(t)$ only
for the placebo patients, and then we use the `summary()` method to return
$\hat{S}_{KM}(t)$ at the specific time points of interest. We approximate the integrals in
the numerator and denominator of $[\text{C}_{dyn}^{\Delta t}]^{10}$ using the trapezoidal rule, which
is, in general, defined as:

$$\int_a^b f(x)dx \approx (b-a)\frac{f(a) + f(b)}{2}.$$

To achieve better precision, we approximate the integrals for each one of the
twelve sub-intervals defined by the 13 time points in `plcbData2`, that is, we
rewrite $[\text{C}_{dyn}^{\Delta t}]^{10}$ as

$$[\text{C}_{dyn}^{\Delta t}]^{10} = \frac{\int_0^{0.25} \text{AUC}_t^{\Delta t}\mathcal{S}(t)dt + \int_{0.25}^{0.5} \text{AUC}_t^{\Delta t}\mathcal{S}(t)dt + \ldots + \int_9^{10} \text{AUC}_t^{\Delta t}\mathcal{S}(t)dt}{\int_0^{0.25} \mathcal{S}(t)dt + \int_{0.25}^{0.5} \mathcal{S}(t)\, dt + \ldots + \int_9^{10} \mathcal{S}(t)dt},$$

and then we approximate with the trapezoidal rule each one of the above
integrals. We can flexibly define the limits a and b for each of the integrals in
R using the `head()` and `tail()` functions, i.e.,

```
> times <- c(0, 0.25, 0.5, 1:10)
> a <- head(times, -1)
> b <- tail(times, -1)
> rbind(a, b)
   [,1] [,2] [,3] [,4] [,5] [,6] [,7] [,8] [,9] [,10] [,11] [,12]
a 0.00 0.25  0.5    1    2    3    4    5    6     7     8     9
b 0.25 0.50  1.0    2    3    4    5    6    7     8     9    10
```

In a similar manner and using the definition of the trapezoidal rule, the sum of the twelve integrals in the denominator of $[C_{dyn}^{\Delta t}]^{10}$ is derived as

```
> Denom <- sum((b - a) * (head(Surv.Plcb, -1) + tail(Surv.Plcb, -1)) / 2)
```

Analogously, we also derive the sum of the twelve integrals in the numerator of $[C_{dyn}^{\Delta t}]^{10}$ based on the time-varying AUCs of each of the three joint models:

```
> Numer.MI <- sum((b - a) * (head(AUCs.MI * Surv.Plcb, -1) +
    tail(AUCs.MI * Surv.Plcb, -1)) / 2)

> Numer.MII <- sum((b - a) * (head(AUCs.MII * Surv.Plcb, -1) +
    tail(AUCs.MII * Surv.Plcb, -1)) / 2)

> Numer.MIII <- sum((b - a) * (head(AUCs.MIII * Surv.Plcb, -1) +
    tail(AUCs.MIII * Surv.Plcb, -1)) / 2)
```

Finally, the dynamic discrimination indices are simply obtained by calculating the corresponding ratios:

```
> Numer.MI / Denom # Cdyn Model (I)
[1] 0.7209312
> Numer.MII / Denom # Cdyn Model (II)
[1] 0.6824211
> Numer.MIII / Denom # Cdyn Model (III)
[1] 0.7293451
```

Comparing the values of the three indices that summarize the discrimination capability over the whole ten year follow-up period, we observe that the increased accuracy Model (III) showed at $t = 4$ over the other two models is diminished. In particular, Models (I) and (III) offer practically the same level of discrimination, which is a bit better than the one offered by Model (II). This implies that, for the patients under study, the current value of the prothrombin index $m_i(t)$ seems to play a more prominent role with respect to discrimination than the slope of the true trajectory $m_i'(t)$.

Appendix A

A Brief Introduction to R

This appendix provides a brief introduction to specific aspects of R that will provide users the minimal background knowledge required to fit joint models in their own data. It should be stressed that no attempt is made to provide a thorough introduction to R; interested readers are referred instead to the Introduction to R manual that ships together with every installation of R, and the fine texts of Venables and Ripley (2002), and Dalgaard (2008). Additional material can be found online at: `http://cran.r-project.org/other-docs.html`.

A.1 Obtaining and Installing R and R Packages

The R software and documentation is freely distributed under the GNU general public licence and can be obtained from the Comprehensive R Archive Network (CRAN) accessible via the website: `http://cran.r-project.org/`. R may be build from source but there are also binary versions for Windows, Mac OS X, and the main flavors of Linux. Installation of the binary distributions is typically straightforward for users familiar with the relevant platform's standard installation tools.

Add-on freely available packages are also available via CRAN. For example, package **JM** that is primarily used in this book can be installed with the command

```
> install.packages("JM")
```

It is also generally advisable to use the most recent version of the installed packages, which can be obtained by running the command

```
> update.packages()
```

A.2   Simple Manipulations

A.2.1   Basic R Objects

The basic data objects in R are vectors, with the two main types being numeric vectors holding quantitative information and character vectors holding qualitative information. Vectors can be defined by means of the `c()` function; for example, the following syntax defines a numeric vector of six elements

```
> x <- c(1, 3, 5, 7, 2, NA)
> x
[1]  1  3  5  7  2 NA
```

The last entry `NA` stands for 'not available' and is the missing data identifier in R. The symbol `"<-"` is called the assignment operator and is used to store the result of function `c()` in the object `x`. A character vector can be similarly defined using the `c()` function, but the entries need to be input within quotes (either single or double):

```
> y <- c("male", "male", "female")
> y
[1] "male"    "male"    "female"
```

An additional type of objects used to specify a discrete grouping of the components of other vectors of the same length are the factors. These are defined using the `factor()` function, e.g.,

```
> f <- factor(c(1,2,2,1,1,2), levels = c(1,2,3),
    labels = c("apple", "orange", "banana"))
> f
[1] apple  orange orange apple  apple  orange
Levels: apple orange banana
```

In this example we define a categorical grouping of the input numeric vector `c(1,2,2,1,1,2)` identified by the value of the `levels` argument, with labels specified by the `labels` argument. Note that even though there is no occurrence of value 3 corresponding to the level 'banana', the factor object `f` is explicitly set to include this possibility.

Vectors can also be organized to a rectangular format and defining in that way matrices of appropriate dimensions. The basic functions to create matrices in R are the `matrix()`, and `rbind()` and `cbind()` functions. The first one takes as input a vector and transforms to a matrix by giving it a dimension attribute, whereas the latter two bind together in row-wise or column-wise order, respectively, vectors of the same length. The following syntax illustrates the use of these functions by constructing a matrix with elements the integers from one to nine (to automatically create this sequence of integers we use the `":"` function):

```
> matrix(1:9, nrow = 3, ncol = 3)
     [,1] [,2] [,3]
[1,]   1    4    7
[2,]   2    5    8
[3,]   3    6    9
> cbind(1:3, 4:6, 7:9)
     [,1] [,2] [,3]
[1,]   1    4    7
[2,]   2    5    8
[3,]   3    6    9
```

Both functions produce exactly the same output, but in the first case we have a vector of nine elements, which is organized in a 3×3 matrix, whereas in the second case we bind together in column-wise order three vectors with three elements each. We observe that by default `matrix()` organizes the elements of the input vector in a column-wise order. This can be overwritten using the `by.row` argument of that function.

A defining characteristic of the previously defined vectors and matrices is that all of their elements need to be of the same type, that is, we cannot have a vector where its first element is numeric and the second one is a character. A more flexible type of R objects that overcomes this constraint are `lists`, which are defined using the `list()` function. For instance, the following syntax defines a list with four elements, two of type numeric, at positions one and three, and two of type character at positions two and four:

```
> L <- list(1, "a", 2, "b")
> L
[[1]]
[1] 1

[[2]]
[1] "a"

[[3]]
[1] 2

[[4]]
[1] "b"
```

A special type of lists are the data frames, which constitute the fundamental data structure used by most of R's modeling software. Similar to lists, data frames can hold different types of objects, but the restriction is that these should be vectors of the same length, such that they can be organized in a rectangular format (as in a matrix):

```
> DF <- data.frame(id = 1:5,
    sex = c("male", "male", "male", "female", "female"),
    age = c(28, 32, 35, 29, 24))
> DF
  id    sex age
1  1   male  28
2  2   male  32
3  3   male  35
4  4 female  29
5  5 female  24
```

Lists can be considered as the most powerful objects in R because each element of a list can be any valid R object. For example, the following syntax constructs a list in which the first element is a numeric vector, the second one a numeric matrix, the third one a data frame with two variables, one numeric and one factor, and the last element is an other list with two elements, a numeric vector and a character vector (output not shown):

```
> list(
    x = 1:10,
    mat = matrix(1:16, nrow = 4, ncol = 4),
    dat = data.frame(x = 1:3, f = factor(c("m", "f", "m"))),
    lis = list(y = 2:5, ch = c("a", "ab", "abc"))
)
```

A.2.2   Indexing

Data manipulations for all the above defined objects are primarily performed using indexing operations. There are three basic types of indexing, namely, position indexing, logical indexing, and name indexing. Each of these types of indexing is performed using the square brackets operator [...]. More specifically, with position indexing we extract elements of an object at specific positions; for instance, from the x vector defined above, we can extract its first and third element (i.e., the elements at position one and three) using the syntax

```
> x[c(1,3)]
[1] 1 5
```

Similarly to vectors, for matrices and data frames, we can extract rows or columns by specifying their position (i.e., number). To distinguish between rows and columns we use a comma inside the square brackets syntax. For example, the first two rows of the numeric matrix defined earlier are extracted with

```
> mat <- matrix(1:9, nrow = 3, ncol = 3)

> mat[1:2, ]
     [,1] [,2] [,3]
[1,]    1    4    7
[2,]    2    5    8
```

whereas, the last two columns of the data frame DF are extracted with

```
> DF[, 2:3]
     sex age
1   male  28
2   male  32
3   male  35
4 female  29
5 female  24
```

Logical indexing is used to extract components of R objects based on logical expressions. For instance, to extract the elements of the x vector which are greater or equal to three, we use the syntax:

```
> x >= 3
[1] FALSE  TRUE  TRUE  TRUE FALSE    NA
```

```
> x[x >= 3]
[1]  3  5  7 NA
```

The first line is a logical vector of the same length as x, with elements TRUE and FALSE according to whether the corresponding element of x satisfied the logical condition. Using this logical vector inside the square brackets the indexing operator will extract the elements of x corresponding to the TRUE entries of the logical vector.

Name indexing is used on named R objects. In particular, any object in R can have names for its elements; for example, the following syntax constructs a named numeric vector with three elements

```
> z <- c("a" = 1, "b" = 2, "c" = 3)

> z
a b c
1 2 3
```

In comparison to the vector x we have defined before, the elements of vector z have names. Name indexing proceeds by specifying within the square brackets indexing operator a character vector with the names of the elements we wish to extract, e.g.,

```
> z[c("b", "d")]
   b <NA>
   2  NA
```

Thus, the above syntax extracts from z the elements with names "b" and "d". However, because no element in z has the name "d", we obtain as a result a missing value.

A.3   Import and Manipulate Data Frames

The basic function to read data ASCII files in R is read.table(). This function has several arguments that control how the data will be imported into R. These can be viewed in the online help file of the function, which is accessible using the code help("read.table"). Additional functions to import datasets from other statistical software packages are provided by recommended package **foreign**, and other add-on packages from CRAN.

After importing a dataset and before starting with the analysis, it is typically required to perform several data manipulation steps. Some examples of basic data manipulations in R are illustrated below using the data frame aids.id from package **JM**. This data frame can be loaded using the code data(aids.id, package = "JM").

* The first step before starting working with a dataset, is to have a look at the variables this contains, and decide whether some data manipulations will be required. To print the whole dataset we can just type its name in the R console. However, in the majority of the cases, this will not be that useful because the dataset will probably contain many rows and columns. To have a better look of the type of information included in the data frame, it will suffice to just print some of its rows. This easily achieved with function head() that prints the first six rows of a data frame, e.g.,

```
> head(aids.id)
```

	patient	Time	death	CD4	obstime	drug	gender	prevOI
1	1	16.97	0	10.677078	0	ddC	male	AIDS
2	2	19.00	0	6.324555	0	ddI	male	noAIDS
3	3	18.53	1	3.464102	0	ddI	female	AIDS
4	4	12.70	0	3.872983	0	ddC	male	AIDS
5	5	15.13	0	7.280110	0	ddI	male	AIDS
6	6	1.90	1	4.582576	0	ddC	female	AIDS

	AZT	start	stop	event
1	intolerance	0	6.0	0
2	intolerance	0	6.0	0
3	intolerance	0	2.0	0
4	failure	0	2.0	0
5	failure	0	2.0	0
6	failure	0	1.9	1

Another useful function that explicitly outputs information regarding the type of variables in a data frame is function str(). For aids.id it gives

```
> str(aids.id)
```

```
data.frame:        467 obs. of  12 variables:
 $ patient: Factor w/ 467 levels "1","2","3","4",..: 1 2 3 4..
 $ Time   : num  17 19 18.5 12.7 15.1 ...
 $ death  : int  0 0 1 0 0 1 0 1 1 0 ...
 $ CD4    : num  10.68 6.32 3.46 3.87 7.28 ...
 $ obstime: int  0 0 0 0 0 0 0 0 0 0 ...
 $ drug   : Factor w/ 2 levels "ddC","ddI": 1 2 2 1 2 1 1 2 ..
 $ gender : Factor w/ 2 levels "female","male": 2 2 1 2 2 1 ..
 $ prevOI : Factor w/ 2 levels "noAIDS","AIDS": 2 1 2 2 2 2 ..
 $ AZT    : Factor w/ 2 levels "intolerance",..: 1 1 1 2 2 2..
 $ start  : int  0 0 0 0 0 0 0 0 0 0 ...
 $ stop   : num  6 6 2 2 2 1.9 2 2 2 2 ...
 $ event  : num  0 0 0 0 0 1 0 0 0 0 ...
```

For instance, we can see that Time is a continuous variable of type numeric, whereas variable gender is a factor.

* To extract a variable from the data frame, we use the symbol $, which is a shorthand for the name indexing operator we have seen in the previous section. For instance, the following code extracts variable sex from aids.id:

```
> aids.id$sex
```

* With a similar code we can also transform a variable. For instance, the following code defines a new variable, with name `logTime`, in the data frame which is the natural logarithm of the `Time` variable:

```
> aids.id$logTime <- log(aids.id$Time)
```

* To convert a **numeric** variable into a `factor` we use the `factor()` function. For example, the following code transforms variable `death` into a `factor`:

```
> aids.id$death <- factor(aids.id$death, levels = 0:1,
      labels = c("alive", "dead"))
```

* Subsets of the original data frame are usually constructed using indexing and logical expressions. For instance,

– `aidsNew1` contains only variables `Time`, `death` and `drug` from the original `aids.id`:

```
> aidsNew1 <- aids.id[c("Time", "death", "drug")]
```

– `aidsNew2` contains only the patients with observed event times greater than three months:

```
> aidsNew2 <- aids.id[aids.id$Time > 3, ]
```

– `aidsNew3` contains only the male patients:

```
> aidsNew3 <- aids.id[aids.id$gender == "male", ]
```

– `aidsNew4` contains only the female patients with baseline square root CD4 cell count greater than five:

```
> aidsNew4 <- aids.id[aids.id$gender == "female" &
      aids.id$CD4 > 5, ]
```

A.4   The Formula Interface

Statistical models in R are defined using the formula interface. In general, an R formula has the form

```
>      response ~ terms
```

where **response** denotes the response variable(s) of interest, and **terms** represents the additive components of a general linear model. These could also include transformations of the response variable and the predictors. Table A.1 shows several examples of the R formula syntax. For example, the following code:

```
> lm(log(blood.pressure) ~ ns(age, 3) + sex * hdl, data = BPdata)
```

fits a linear regression model (using function `lm()`), with response variable the natural logarithm of **blood.pressure** and predictors **age** expanded in a natural cubic spline basis with two internal knots (using function `ns()` from package **splines**), **sex**, **hdl** cholesterol, and the interaction term between **sex** and **hdl**.

TABLE A.1: Correspondence between the formula interface of R and the mathematical formulation of the linear predictor of a model (y denotes the response variable)

Model Terms	R formula syntax
$y = \beta_0 + \beta_1 \text{age} + \beta_2 \text{female}$	`y ~ age + sex`
$y = \beta_1 \text{age} + \beta_2 \text{female} + \beta_2 \text{male}$	`y ~ age + sex - 1`
$y = \beta_0 + \beta_1 \text{age} + \beta_2 \text{female}$ $+ \beta_3 \text{age} \times \text{female}$	`y ~ age + sex + age:sex` or `y ~ age * sex`
$y = \beta_0 + \beta_1 \text{age} + \beta_2 \text{caucasian}$ $+ \beta_3 \text{female} + \beta_4 \text{age} \times \text{female}$ $+ \beta_5 \text{caucasian} \times \text{female}$	`y ~ (age + race) * sex`
$y = \beta_0 + \beta_1 \text{age} + \beta_2 \text{caucasian}$ $+ \beta_3 \text{female} + \beta_4 \text{age} \times \text{female}$ $+ \beta_5 \text{caucasian} \times \text{female}$ $+ \beta_6 \text{age} \times \text{caucasian}$	`y ~ (age + race + sex)^2`
$y = \beta_0 + \beta_1 \text{age} + \beta_2 \text{age}^2 + \beta_3 \text{age}^3$	`y ~ age + I(age^2) + I(age^3)` or `y ~ poly(age, 3)`

Appendix B

The EM Algorithm for Joint Models

In this appendix we provide the technical details behind the EM algorithm that is used to maximize the log-likelihood of joint models. For the remainder of this appendix it is assumed that the reader is familiar with the contents of Section 4.3.2.

B.1 A Short Description of the EM Algorithm

The Expectation-Maximization (EM) algorithm is a very general iterative algorithm for maximum likelihood estimation in incomplete-data problems. The range of problems that can be attacked by the EM is remarkably broad, and includes problems that are not usually considered to involve missing data. The intuitive idea behind the EM algorithm is that the log-likelihood corresponding to the complete data is typically much simpler to maximize, often in close form. To take advantage of this feature, the algorithm has two steps: the Expectation (E) step and the Maximization (M) step. In the E step we fill in the missing data and we replace, in fact, the log-likelihood of the observed data with a surrogate function. This surrogate function is then maximized in the M-step. However, the price we pay for this simplification is that the EM algorithm is iterative because the reconstruction of the missing data in the E-step is bound to be slightly wrong if the parameters do not already equal to their maximum likelihood estimates.

In a nutshell each EM algorithm proceeds as follows: Let Y denote the

229

complete data vector, which is decomposed in an observed part Y^o and a missing part Y^m. Our aim is to estimate the parameters θ of the complete data model, but using only the observed information. In the E-step we compute the expected value of the complete data log-likelihood:

$$Q(\theta \mid \theta^{(it)}) = E\{\log p(y; \theta) \mid y^o; \theta^{(it)}\}$$

$$= \int \log p(y^m, y^o; \theta) \, p(y^m \mid y^o; \theta^{(it)}) \, dy^m,$$

and in the M-step we obtain the updated parameters by

$$\theta^{(it+1)} = \arg\max_{\theta} Q(\theta \mid \theta^{(it)}).$$

One of the great advantages of the EM algorithm is its numerical stability. In particular, as it has been shown by Dempster et al. (1977), at each iteration the EM algorithm leads to an increase of the observed data log-likelihood, i.e., $\log p(y^o; \theta^{(it+1)}) \geq \log p(y^o; \theta^{(it)})$, and avoids wildly overshooting or undershooting the maximum of the likelihood along its current direction of search. However, an important drawback of the EM is its slow rate of convergence in a neighborhood of the maximum point. This rate directly reflects the amount of missing data in a problem. For a brief historic review of the genesis of this algorithm, the reader is referred to Little and Rubin (2002, Section 8.2), whereas a more detailed presentation along with the more general family of Minorization-Maximization algorithms is given in Lange (2004, Chapters 6 and 7).

B.2   The E-step for Joint Models

We will illustrate the use of the EM algorithm to derive the maximum likelihood estimates of the standard joint model presented in Chapter 4, since the adaption of the E- and M-steps for all the extensions we have seen in Chapter 5 is rather straightforward. In particular, we consider the model:

$$\begin{cases} h_i(t) &= h_0(t) \exp\left[\gamma^\top w_i + \alpha\{x_i^\top(t)\beta + z_i^\top(t)b_i\}\right], \\[2mm] y_i(t) &= x_i^\top(t)\beta + z_i^\top(t)b_i + \varepsilon_i(t) \\[2mm] b_i &\sim \mathcal{N}(0, D), \quad \varepsilon_i(t) \sim \mathcal{N}(0, \sigma^2), \end{cases}$$

$\theta = (\theta_t^\top, \theta_y^\top, \theta_b^\top)^\top$, with $\theta_y = (\beta^\top, \sigma^2)^\top$, $\theta_t = (\gamma^\top, \alpha, \theta_{h_0}^\top)^\top$, with θ_{h_0} denoting the parameters in the baseline risk function $h_0(\cdot)$, and $\theta_b = \text{vech}(D)$.

   To apply the EM recipe in joint models we treat the random effects as 'missing data'. In particular, our aim is to find the parameter values $\hat{\theta}$ that maximize the observed data log-likelihood $\ell(\theta) = \sum_i \log p(T_i, \delta_i, y_i; \theta)$, but by maximizing instead the expected value of the complete data log-likelihood, i.e.,

$$
\begin{aligned}
Q(\theta \mid \theta^{(it)}) &= \sum_i \int \log p(T_i, \delta_i, y_i, b_i; \theta) \, p(b_i \mid T_i, \delta_i, y_i; \theta^{(it)}) \, db_i \\
&= \sum_i \int \Big\{ \log p(T_i, \delta_i \mid b_i; \theta_t, \beta) + \log p(y_i \mid b_i; \theta_y) \\
&\qquad + \log p(b_i; \theta_b) \Big\} p(b_i \mid T_i, \delta_i, y_i; \theta^{(it)}) \, db_i.
\end{aligned}
$$

As explained in Section 4.3.5, the integral with respect to the random effects as well as the integral with respect to time in the definition of the survival function involved in term $p(T_i, \delta_i \mid b_i; \theta_t, \beta)$ do not have closed-form solutions. Therefore, for the evaluation of $Q(\theta \mid \theta^{(it)})$ numerical integration procedures must be employed, such as Gaussian quadrature rules or Monte Carlo sampling.

B.3 The M-step for Joint Models

Due to the fact that the complete data log-likelihood is split into three parts, i.e.,

$$
\log p(T_i, \delta_i, y_i, b_i; \theta) = \log p(T_i, \delta_i \mid b_i; \theta_t, \beta) + \log p(y_i \mid b_i; \theta_y) + \log p(b_i; \theta_b),
$$

maximization of $Q(\theta \mid \theta^{(it)})$ with respect to θ involves only the piece(s) in which the respective parameter appears. The following expressions required in the specification of the M-step are presented using the integrals with respect to time and the random effects. For the actual calculation of these expressions, these integrals need to be approximated with the methods mentioned in Section 4.3.5. More specifically, for the measurement error variance in the longitudinal measurement model and the covariance matrix of the random effects are updated in the M-step according to the closed-form expressions

$$
\begin{aligned}
\hat{\sigma}^2 &= N^{-1} \sum_i \int (y_i - X_i\beta - Z_i b_i)^\top (y_i - X_i\beta - Z_i b_i) p(b_i \mid T_i, \delta_i, y_i; \theta) \, db_i \\
&= N^{-1} \sum_i (y_i - X_i\beta)^\top (y_i - X_i\beta - 2Z_i \tilde{b}_i) + \mathrm{tr}(Z_i^\top Z_i \widetilde{vb}_i) + \tilde{b}_i^\top Z_i^\top Z_i \tilde{b}_i,
\end{aligned}
$$

$$
\hat{D} = n^{-1} \sum_i \widetilde{vb}_i + \tilde{b}_i \tilde{b}_i^\top,
$$

where $N = \sum_i n_i$, $\tilde{b}_i = E(b_i \mid T_i, \delta_i, y_i; \theta^{(it)}) = \int b_i p(b_i \mid T_i, \delta_i, y_i; \theta^{(it)}) db_i$, and $\widetilde{vb}_i = \mathrm{var}(b_i \mid T_i, \delta_i, y_i; \theta^{(it)}) = \int (b_i - \tilde{b}_i)^2 p(b_i \mid T_i, \delta_i, y_i; \theta^{(it)}) db_i$. Under the above formulation of the joint model, we cannot obtain closed-form solutions of the score equations for the fixed effects β and the parameters of the survival submodel θ_t. Thus, for these parameters the M-step is implemented via a one-step Newton-Raphson update, i.e.,

$$\hat{\beta}^{(it+1)} = \hat{\beta}^{(it)} - \{\partial S(\hat{\beta}^{(it)})/\partial\beta\}^{-1} S(\hat{\beta}^{(it)}),$$

$$\hat{\theta}_t^{(it+1)} = \hat{\theta}_t^{(it)} - \{\partial S(\hat{\theta}_t^{(it)})/\partial\theta_t\}^{-1} S(\hat{\theta}_t^{(it)}),$$

where $\hat{\beta}^{(it)}$ and $\hat{\theta}_t^{(it)}$ denote the values of β and θ_t at the current iteration, respectively, and $\partial S(\hat{\beta}^{(it)})/\partial\beta$ and $\partial S(\hat{\theta}_t^{(it)})/\partial\theta_t$ denote the corresponding blocks of the Hessian matrix, evaluated at $\hat{\beta}^{(it)}$ and $\hat{\theta}_t^{(it)}$, respectively. The components of the score vector corresponding to β and θ_t have the form

$$S(\beta) = \sum_i X_i^\top \{y_i - X_i\beta - Z_i\tilde{b}_i\}/\sigma^2 + \alpha\delta_i x_i(T_i)$$

$$- \exp(\gamma^\top w_i) \int \int_0^{T_i} h_0(s)\alpha x_i(s) \exp\left[\alpha\{x_i^\top(s)\beta + z_i^\top(s)b_i\}\right]$$

$$\times p(b_i \mid T_i, \delta_i, y_i; \theta) \, ds \, db_i,$$

$$S(\gamma) = \sum_i w_i \left[\delta_i - \exp(\gamma^\top w_i) \int \int_0^{T_i} h_0(s) \exp\left[\alpha\{x_i^\top(s)\beta + z_i^\top(s)b_i\}\right]\right.$$

$$\left. \times p(b_i \mid T_i, \delta_i, y_i; \theta) \, ds \, db_i\right],$$

$$S(\alpha) = \sum_i \delta_i \{x_i^\top(T_i)\beta + z_i^\top(T_i)\tilde{b}_i\}$$

$$- \exp(\gamma^\top w_i) \int \int_0^{T_i} h_0(s)\{x_i^\top(s)\beta + z_i^\top(s)b_i\} \exp\left[\alpha\{x_i^\top(s)\beta + z_i^\top(s)b\right.$$

$$\times p(b_i \mid T_i, \delta_i, y_i; \theta) \, ds \, db_i,$$

$$S(\theta_{h0}) = \sum_i \delta_i \frac{\partial \log h_0(T_i; \theta_{h0})}{\partial\theta_{h0}^\top}$$

$$- \exp(\gamma^\top w_i) \int \int_0^{T_i} \frac{\partial h_0(s; \theta_{h0})}{\partial\theta_{h0}^\top} \exp\left[\alpha\{x_i^\top(s)\beta + z_i^\top(s)b_i\}\right]$$

$$\times p(b_i \mid T_i, \delta_i, y_i; \theta) \, ds \, db_i.$$

The corresponding blocks of the Hessian matrix $\partial S(\beta)/\partial \beta$ and $\partial S(\theta_t)/\partial \theta_t$, respectively, can be computed using a central difference approximation (Press et al., 2007, Section 5.7).

Appendix C

Structure of the JM Package

In this appendix we give an overview of the main functions in package **JM**. Even though we describe the main usage of these functions, we purposely do not provide all of their respective arguments because on future versions of the package some of these may change and/or additional arguments may be introduced. The definite reference for their syntax and output is the online manual of the package.

C.1 Methods for Standard Generic Functions

The main fitting function of package **JM** is function `jointModel()` that fits a wide variety of joint models for longitudinal and event time data. The two main arguments of this function are an object of class `"lme"` representing a linear mixed-effects model fitted using function `lme()` from package **nlme**, and an object of class `"coxph"` representing a Cox proportional hazards model fitted using function `coxph()` from package **survival**. In the call to `coxph()` it is required to set the option `x = TRUE` in order the design matrix of the Cox model to be included in the model object, but it is also advisable to set the option `model = TRUE` such that the entire model frame (and not only the design matrix) is returned. In addition, the user needs to specify the `timeVar` argument, which is the name of the time variable in the linear mixed model. The `method` argument controls the type of survival submodel and the numerical integration method. For a more detailed presentation of the different options for the `method` argument, the reader is referred to Section 4.2.

Function `jointModel()` returns an R list of class `"jointModel"`, for which there are S3 methods defined for several of the standard generic functions in R. These are enlisted below:

Functions `print()` and `summary()` return the results of a fitted joint model. The former function only prints the estimated parameters for the longitudinal and survival submodels, whereas the latter provides a more detailed output, including summary statistics for the dataset used to fit the model and Wald tests for the regression coefficients of the two submodels.

Functions `coef()`, `fixef()` extract the estimated coefficients for the two submodels from a fitted joint model. For the survival process both provide the same output, but for the longitudinal model, the former returns the subject-specific regression coefficients (i.e., the fixed effects plus their corresponding random effects estimates), whereas the latter only returns the estimated fixed effects.

Function `ranef()` computes the empirical Bayes estimates for the random effects for each subject. These may be the mean or the mode of the posterior distribution of the random effects given the observed data. The function also computes estimates for the dispersion of the posterior of the random effects, with available options the posterior variance and the inverse Hessian matrix (calculated as the second order derivative of the log posterior with respect to the random effects). Examples using this function can be found in Section 4.5.

Function `vcov()` extracts the estimated variance-covariance matrix of the maximum likelihood estimates. An example using this function can be found in Section 4.4.1.

Functions `fitted()` and `residuals()` compute several kind of fitted values and residuals, respectively, for the two outcomes. For the longitudinal submodel, subject-specific and marginal fitted values and residuals are available. In addition, for the longitudinal submodel, function `residuals()` can be used to compute the multiply-imputed residuals that account for nonrandom dropout (see Section 6.3 for more details). For the relative risk submodel, function `fitted()` can be used to return the marginal or subject-specific estimates of the survival, cumulative hazard, and log cumulative hazard functions, whereas function `residuals()` computes the martingale and Cox-Snell residuals. Examples using this function can be found in Sections 6.1.1, 6.1.2, and 6.2.

Function `anova()` computes Wald and likelihood ratio tests (LRT) based on fitted joint models. When a single joint model object is supplied, marginal Wald tests for all regression coefficients are performed, whereas when two fitted joint models are supplied, the function performs the corresponding LRT. In the latter case, the user is primarily responsible to provide nested joint models in order for the LRT to be valid (i.e., the code does minimal checking to validate this). Examples using this function can be found in Sections 4.4.1 and 5.1.

Function `plot()` produces diagnostic plots for the longitudinal and survival process. These include, among others, the scatterplot of subject-specific residuals versus the subject-specific fitted values, and the QQ-plot of the subject-specific residuals for the longitudinal outcome, and the fitted marginal survival function for the time-to-event. Examples using this function can be found in Sections 6.1.1 and 5.3.

Function `predict()` produces subject-specific and marginal predictions for the longitudinal outcome, along with associate confidence or prediction confidence intervals. The subject-specific predictions are produced conditionally on the fact that the subject was still alive up to a specific time point. Examples using this function can be found in Sections 4.4.2, 7.2, and 7.3.

Function `logLik()` extracts the log-likelihood value of the fitted model, including as an attribute the number of parameters, and function `AIC()` can be used to compute the Akaike's and Bayesian information criteria.

C.2   Additional Functions

Function `survfitJM()` produces subject-specific predictions (along with associated confidence intervals) of conditional survival probabilities. The estimated probabilities and confidence intervals can be depicted using the corresponding `plot()` method. Examples using this function can be found in Sections 7.1.3 and 7.3.

Function `rocJM()` produces estimates, based on a joint model, of time-dependent sensitivity and specificity, and the corresponding areas under the ROC for investigating the discriminative capability of the longitudinal outcome in distinguishing between patients who will or will not fail within a prespecified time interval. The corresponding `plot()` method produce the plots of the ROC curves. Examples using this function can be found in Section 7.4.6.

Function `wald.strata()` performs a Wald test for stratified joint models testing the null hypothesis of no differences between the baseline hazard functions in different strata. An example using this function can be found in Section 5.3.

Function `xtable()` returns the LaTeX code to produce the table of estimated coefficients, standard errors, and p-values from a fitted joint model. This is based on the generic function `xtable()` from package **xtable** (Dahl, 2012).

Function `weibull.frailty()` fits a Weibull model for multivariate survival data using a Gamma distributed frailty term to account for the associations. An example using this function can be found in Section 6.3.2.

Function `piecewiseExp.ph()` takes a fitted Cox model and fits the corresponding relative risk model with a piecewise-constant baseline hazard (4.3) using the Poisson regression equivalence. An example using this function can be found in Section 4.4.1.

Bibliography

Aalen, O. (1976). Nonparametric inference in connection with multiple decrement models. *Scandinavian Journal of Statistics* **3**, 15–27.

Aalen, O., Borgan, O., and Gjessing, H. (2008). *Survival and Event History Analysis: A Process View Point.* Springer-Verlag, New York.

Abrams, D., Goldman, A., Launer, C., Korvick, J., Neaton, J., Crane, L., Grodesky, M., Wakefield, S., Muth, K., Kornegay, S., Cohn, D., Harris, A., Luskin-Hawk, R., Markowitz, N., Sampson, J., Thompson, M., and Deyton, L. (1994). A comparative trial of didanosine and zalcitabine in patients with human immunodeficiency virus infection who are intolerant of or have failed zidovudine therapy. *New England Journal of Medicine* **330**, 657–662.

Agresti, A., Caffo, B., and Ohman-Strickland, P. (2004). Examples in which misspecification of a random effects distribution reduces efficiency, and possible remedies. *Computational Statistics & Data Analysis* **47**, 639–653.

Akaike, H. (1974). A new look at the statistical model identification. *IEEE Transactions on Automatic Control* **19**, 716–723.

Albert, P. and Follmann, D. (2000). Modeling repeated count data subject to informative dropout. *Biometrics* **56**, 667–677.

Albert, P., Follmann, D., Wang, S., and Suh, E. (2002). A latent autoregressive model for longitudinal binary data subject to informative missingness. *Biometrics* **58**, 631–642.

Allignol, A. and Latouche, A. (2012). *CRAN Task View: Survival Analysis.* Version 2011-03-27. http://cran.r-project.org/view=Survival.

Altschuler, B. (1970). Theory for the measurement of competing risks in animal experiments. *Mathematical Biosciences* **6**, 1–11.

Andersen, P., Borgan, O., Gill, R., and Keiding, N. (1993). *Statistical Models Based on Counting Processes.* Springer-Verlag, New York.

Andersen, P. and Gill, R. (1982). Cox's regression model for counting processes: A large sample study. *Annals of Statistics* **10**, 1100–1120.

Antolini, L., Boracchi, P., and Biganzoli, E. (2005). A time-dependent discrimination index for survival data. *Statistics in Medicine* **24**, 3927–3944.

239

Barlow, W. and Prentice, R. (1988). Residuals for relative risk regression. *Biometrika* **75**, 65–74.

Bates, D., Maechler, M., and Bolker, B. (2011). *lme4: Linear mixed-effects models using S4 classes.* R package version 0.999375-42. http://cran.r-project.org/package=lme4.

Booth, J. and Hobert, J. (1999). Maximizing generalized linear mixed model likelihoods with an automated Monte Carlo EM algorithm. *Journal of the Royal Statistical Society, Series B* **61**, 265–285.

Breslow, N. (1972). Discussion of paper 'Regression models and life-tables' by D. Cox. *Journal of the Royal Statistical Society, Series B* **34**, 216–217.

Breslow, N. and Clayton, D. (1993). Approximate inference in generalized linear mixed models. *Journal of the American Statistical Association* **88**, 9–25.

Breslow, N., Lubin, J., Marek, P., and Langholz, B. (1983). Multiplicative models and cohort analysis. *Journal of the American Statistical Association* **78**, 1–12.

Brown, E. and Ibrahim, J. (2003). A Bayesian semiparametric joint hierarchical model for longitudinal and survival data. *Biometrics* **59**, 221–228.

Brown, E., Ibrahim, J., and DeGruttola, V. (2005). A flexible B-spline model for multiple longitudinal biomarkers and survival. *Biometrics* **61**, 64–73.

Cavender, J., Rogers, W., Fisher, L., Gersh, B., Coggin, J., and Myers, W. (1992). Effects of smoking on survival and morbidity in patients randomized to medical or surgical therapy in the Coronary Artery Surgery Study (CASS): 10-year follow-up. *Journal of the American College of Cardiology* **20**, 145–157.

Chi, Y.-Y. and Ibrahim, J. (2006). Joint models for multivariate longitudinal and multivariate survival data. *Biometrics* **62**, 432–445.

Copas, J. and Li, H. (1997). Inference for non-random samples (with discussion). *Journal of the Royal Statistical Society, Series B* **59**, 55–95.

Cox, D. (1972). Regression models and life-tables (with discussion). *Journal of the Royal Statistical Society, Series B* **34**, 187–220.

Cox, D. and Hinkley, D. (1974). *Theoretical Statistics.* Chapman & Hall, London.

Cox, D. and Oakes, D. (1984). *Analysis of Survival Data.* Chapman & Hall, London.

Cox, D. and Snell, E. (1968). A general definition of residuals. *Journal of the Royal Statistical Society, Series B* **30**, 248–275. .

Creemers, A., Hens, N., Aerts, M., Molenberghs, G., Verbeke, G., and Kenward, M. (2010). A sensitivity analysis for shared-parameter models for incomplete longitudinal data. *Biometrical Journal* **52**, 111–125.

Dafni, U. and Tsiatis, A. (1998). Evaluating surrogate markers of clinical outcome measured with error. *Biometrics* **54**, 1445–1462.

Dahl, D. (2012). ***xtable**: Export tables to LaTeX or HTML*. R package version 1.7-0. http://cran.r-project.org/package=xtable.

Dalgaard, P. (2008). *Introductory Statistics with R*, 2nd edition. Springer-Verlag, New York.

DeGruttola, V. and Tu, X. (1994). Modeling progression of CD-4 lymphocyte count and its relationship to survival time. *Biometrics* **50**, 1003–1014.

Demidenko, E. (2004). *Mixed Models: Theory and Applications*. Wiley, Hoboken.

Dempster, A., Laird, N., and Rubin, D. (1977). Maximum likelihood from incomplete data via the EM algorithm. *Journal of the Royal Statistical Society, Series B* **39**, 1–38.

Dempster, A., Rubin, D., and Tsutakawa, R. (1981). Estimation in covariance components models. *Journal of the American Statistical Association* **76**, 341–353.

Dierckx, P. (1993). *Curve and Surface Fitting with Splines*. Oxford University Press, New York.

Diggle, P., Farewell, D., and Henderson, R. (2007). Analysis of longitudinal data with drop-out: objectives, assumptions and a proposal (with discussion). *Journal of the Royal Statistical Society, Series C* **56**, 499–550.

Diggle, P., Heagerty, P., Liang, K.-Y., and Zeger, S. (2002). *Analysis of Longitudinal Data*, 2nd edition. Oxford University Press, New York.

Diggle, P. and Kenward, M. (1994). Informative dropout in longitudinal data analysis (with discussion). *Journal of the Royal Statistical Society, Series C* **43**, 49–93.

Ding, J. and Wang, J.-L. (2008). Modeling longitudinal data with nonparametric multiplicative random effects jointly with survival data. *Biometrics* **64**, 546–556.

Dobson, A. and Henderson, R. (2003). Diagnostics for joint longitudinal and dropout time modeling. *Biometrics* **59**, 741–751.

Duchateau, L. and Janssen, P. (2008). *The Frailty Model*. Springer-Verlag, New York.

Efron, B. and Tibshirani, R. (1994). *An Introduction to the Bootstrap.* Chapman & Hall/CRC Press, Boca Raton.

Elashoff, R., Li, G., and Li, N. (2008). A joint model for longitudinal measurements and survival data in the presence of multiple failure types. *Biometrics* **64,** 762–771.

Etzioni, R., Pepe, M., Longton, G., Hu, C., and Goodman, G. (1999). Incorporating the time dimension in receiver operating operating characteristic curve. *Medical Decision Making* **19,** 242–251.

Faucett, C., Schenker, N., and Elashoff, R. (1998). Analysis of censored survival data with intermittently observed time-dependent binary covariates. *Journal of the American Statistical Association* **93,** 427–437.

Faucett, C. and Thomas, D. (1996). Simultaneously modelling censored survival data and repeatedly measured covariates: A Gibbs sampling approach. *Statistics in Medicine* **15,** 1663–1685.

Fieuws, S., Verbeke, G., Maes, B., and Vanrenterghem, Y. (2008). Predicting renal graft failure using multivariate longitudinal profiles. *Biostatistics* **9,** 419–431.

Fisher, L. and Lin, D. (1999). Time-dependent covariates in the Cox proportional-hazards regression model. *Annual Review of Public Health* **20,** 145–157.

Fitzmaurice, G., Laird, N., and Ware, J. (2004). *Applied Longitudinal Analysis.* Wiley, Hoboken.

Fleming, T. and Harrington, D. (1984). Nonparametric estimation of the survival distribution. *Communications in Statistics: Theory and Methods* **13,** 2469–2486.

Fleming, T. and Harrington, D. (1991). *Counting Processes and Survival Analysis.* Wiley, New York.

Follmann, D. and Wu, M. (1995). An approximate generalized linear model with random effects for informative missing data. *Biometrics* **51,** 151–168.

Gallant, A. and Nychka, D. (1987). Seminonparametric maximum likelihood estimation. *Econometrica* **55,** 363–390.

Garre, F., Zwinderman, A., Geskus, R., and Sijpkens, Y. (2008). A joint latent class changepoint model to improve the prediction of time to graft failure. *Journal of the Royal Statistical Society, Series A* **171,** 299–308.

Gay, D. (1990). *Usage summary for selected optimization routines.* AT&T Bell Laboratories, Murray Hill, NJ. Computing Science Technical Report No. 153.

Gelman, A. and Hill, J. (2007). *Data Analysis Using Regression and Multilevel/Hierarchical Models.* Cambridge University Press, New York.

Gelman, A., Van Mechelen, I., Verbeke, G., Heitjan, D., and Meulders, M. (2005). Multiple imputation for model checking: Completed-data plots with missing and latent data. *Biometrics* **61**, 74–85.

Gerds, T. and Schumacher, M. (2006). Consistent estimation of the expected Brier score in general survival models with right-censored event times. *Biometrical Journal* **48**, 1029–1040.

Goodman, L. and Kruskal, W. (1979). *Measures of Association for Cross Classification.* Springer-Verlag, New York.

Graf, E., Schmoor, C., Sauerbrei, W., and Schumacher, M. (1999). Assessment and comparison of prognostic classification schemes for survival data. *Statistics in Medicine* **18**, 2529–2545.

Greenwood, M. (1926). The natural duration of cancer. *Reports on Public Health and Medical Subjects* **33**, 1–26.

Greven, S., Crainiceanu, C., Küchenhoff, H., and Peters, A. (2008). Restricted likelihood ratio testing for zero variance components in linear mixed models. *Journal of Computational and Graphical Statistics* **17**, 870–891.

Hand, D. and Crowder, M. (1996). *Practical Longitudinal Data Analysis.* Chapman & Hall/CRC Press, Boca Raton.

Hanley, J. and McNeil, B. (1982). The meaning and the use of the area under a receiver operating characteristic (ROC) curve. *Radiology* **143**, 29–36.

Hanson, T., Branscum, A., and Johnson, W. (2011). Predictive comparison of joint longitudinal-survival modeling: A case study illustrating competing approaches (with discussion). *Lifetime Data Analysis* **17**, 3–28.

Harrell, F. (2001). *Regression Modeling Strategies: With Applications to Linear Models, Logistic Regression, and Survival Analysis.* Springer-Verlag, New York.

Harrell, F., Callif, R., Pryor, D., Lee, K., and Rosati, R. (1982). Evaluating the yield of medical tests. *Journal of the American Medical Association* **247**, 2543–2546.

Harville, D. (1974). Bayesian inference for variance components using only error contrasts. *Biometrika* **61**, 383–385.

Harville, D. (1977). Maximum likelihood approaches to variance component estimation and to related problems. *Journal of the American Statistical Association* **72**, 320–340.

Hauptmann, M., Wellmann, J., Lubin, J., Rosenberg, P., and Kreienbrock, L. (2000). Analysis of exposure-time-response relationships using a spline weight function. *Biometrics* **56**, 1105–1108.

Heagerty, P. and Kurland, B. (2001). Misspecified maximum likelihood estimates and generalized linear mixed models. *Biometrika* **88**, 973–985.

Heagerty, P., Lumley, T., and Pepe, M. (2000). Time-dependent ROC curves for censored survival data and a diagnostic marker. *Biometrics* **56**, 337–344.

Heagerty, P. and Zheng, Y. (2005). Survival model predictive accuracy and ROC curves. *Biometrics* **61**, 92–105.

Heckman, J. (1976). The common structure of statistical models of truncation, sample selection, and limited dependent variables and a simple estimator for such models. *Annals of Economic and Social Measurement* **5**, 475–492.

Hedeker, D. and Gibbons, R. (2006). *Longitudinal Data Analysis*. Wiley, Hoboken.

Henderson, R., Diggle, P., and Dobson, A. (2000). Joint modelling of longitudinal measurements and event time data. *Biostatistics* **1**, 465–480.

Henderson, R., Diggle, P., and Dobson, A. (2002). Identification and efficacy of longitudinal markers for survival. *Biostatistics* **3**, 33–50.

Herndon, J. and Harrell, F. (1996). The restricted cubic spline hazard model. *Communications in Statistics – Theory and Methods* **19**, 639–663.

Hogan, J. and Laird, N. (1997). Mixture models for the joint distribution of repeated measures and event times. *Statistics in Medicine* **16**, 239–258.

Hogan, J. and Laird, N. (1998). Increasing efficiency from censored survival data by using random effects to model longitudinal covariates. *Statistical Methods in Medical Research* **7**, 28–48.

Hougaard, P. (2000). *Analysis of Multivariate Survival Data*. Springer-Verlag, New York.

Hsieh, F., Tseng, Y.-K., and Wang, J.-L. (2006). Joint modeling of survival and longitudinal data: likelihood approach revisited. *Biometrics* **62**, 1037–1043.

Hu, W., Li, G., and Li, N. (2009). A Bayesian approach to joint analysis of longitudinal measurements and competing risks failure time data. *Statistics in Medicine* **28**, 1601–1619.

Huang, X., Li, G., Elashoff, R., and Pan, J. (2011). A general joint model for longitudinal measurements and competing risks survival data with heterogeneous random effects. *Lifetime Data Analysis* **17**, 80–100.

Huang, X., Stefanski, L., and Davidian, M. (2009). Latent-model robustness in joint models for a primary endpoint and a longitudinal process. *Biometrics* **64**, 719–727.

Ibrahim, J., Chen, M., and Sinha, D. (2001). *Bayesian Survival Analysis.* Springer-Verlag, New York.

Ibrahim, J. and Molenberghs, G. (2009). Missing data methods in longitudinal studies: A review. *Test* **18**, 1–43.

Jansen, I., Hens, N., Molenberghs, G., Aerts, M., Verbeke, G., and Kenward, M. (2006). The nature of sensitivity in monotone missing not at random models. *Computational Statistics & Data Analysis* **50**, 830–858.

Jansen, I. and Molenberghs, G. (2008). A flexible marginal modelling strategy for non-monotone missing data. *Journal of the Royal Statistical Society, Series A* **171**, 347–373.

Jiang, J. (2010). *Linear and Generalized Linear Mixed Models and Their Applications.* Springer-Verlag, New York.

Kalbfleisch, J. and Prentice, R. (2002). *The Statistical Analysis of Failure Time Data,* 2nd edition. Wiley, New York.

Kaplan, E. and Meier, P. (1958). Nonparametric estimation for incomplete observations. *Journal of the American Statistical Association* **93**, 457–481.

Kenward, M. (1998). Selection models for repeated measurements with non-random dropout: An illustration of sensitivity. *Statistics in Medicine* **17**, 2723–2732.

Kenward, M. and Molenberghs, G. (1998). Likelihood based frequentist inference when data are missing at random. *Statistical Science* **13**, 236–247.

Klein, J. and Moeschberger, M. (2003). *Survival Analysis - Techniques for Censored and Truncated Data.* Springer-Verlag, New York.

Kraemer, H. (2004). Reconsidering the odds ratio as a measure of 2×2 association in a population. *Statistics in Medicine* **23**, 257–270.

Krzanowski, W. and Hand, D. (2009). *ROC Curves for Continuous Data.* Chapman & Hall/CRC Press, Boca Raton.

Kurland, B. and Heagerty, P. (2005). Directly parameterized regression conditioning on being alive: Analysis of longitudinal data truncated by deaths. *Biostatistics* **6**, 241–258.

Kurland, B., Johnson, L., Egleston, B., and Diehr, P. (2009). Longitudinal data with follow-up truncated by death: Match the analysis method to research aims. *Statistical Science* **24**, 211–222.

Laird, N. and Ware, J. (1982). Random-effects models for longitudinal data. *Biometrics* **38**, 963–974.

Lange, K. (2004). *Optimization.* Springer-Verlag, New York.

Lawless, J. (2002). *Statistical Models and Methods for Lifetime Data*, 2nd edition. Wiley, New York.

Lesaffre, E. and Spiessens, B. (2001). On the effect of the number of quadrature points in a logistic random-effects model: An example. *Journal of the Royal Statistical Society, Series C* **50**, 325–335.

Li, N., Elashoff, R., Li, G., and Saver, J. (2010). Joint modeling of longitudinal ordinal data and competing risks survival times and analysis of the NINDS rt-PA stroke trial. *Statistics in Medicine* **29**, 546–557.

Liang, K.-Y. and Zeger, S. (1986). Longitudinal data analysis using generalized linear models. *Biometrika* **73**, 13–22.

Lin, H., McCulloch, C., and Mayne, S. (2002). Maximum likelihood estimation in the joint analysis of time-to-event and multiple longitudinal variables. *Statistics in Medicine* **21**, 2369–2382.

Lin, H., McCulloch, C., and Rosenheck, R. (2004). Latent pattern mixture models for informative intermittent missing data in longitudinal studies. *Biometrics* **60**, 295–305.

Lin, H., Turnbull, B., McCulloch, C., and Slate, E. (2002). Latent class models for joint analysis of longitudinal biomarker and event process: Application to longitudinal prostate-specific antigen readings and prostate cancer. *Journal of the American Statistical Association* **97**, 53–65.

Lindstrom, M. and Bates, D. (1988). Newton-Raphson and EM algorithms for linear mixed-effects models for repeated measures data. *Journal of the American Statistical Association* **83**, 1014–1022.

Lipsitz, S., Fitzmaurice, G., Ibrahim, J., Gelber, R., and Lipshultz, S. (2002). Parameter estimation in longitudinal studies with outcome-dependent follow-up. *Biometrics* **58**, 621–630.

Litière, S., Alonso, A., and Molenberghs, G. (2007). Type I and type II error under random-effects misspecification in generalized linear mixed models. *Biometrics* **63**, 1038–1044.

Litière, S., Alonso, A., and Molenberghs, G. (2008). The impact of a misspecified random-effects distribution on the estimation and the performance of inferential procedures in generalized linear mixed models. *Statistics in Medicine* **27**, 3125–3144.

Little, R. (1993). Pattern-mixture models for multivariate incomplete data. *Journal of the American Statistical Association* **88**, 125 – 134.

Little, R. (1994). A class of pattern-mixture models for normal incomplete data. *Biometrika* **81**, 471 – 483.

Little, R. (1995). Modeling the drop-out mechanism in repeated-measures studies. *Journal of the American Statistical Association* **90**, 1112 – 1121.

Little, R. and Rubin, D. (2002). *Statistical Analysis with Missing Data*, 2nd edition. Wiley, New York.

Liu, L. and Huang, X. (2009). Joint analysis of correlated repeated measures and recurrent events processes in the presence of death, with application to a study on acquired immune deficiency syndrome. *Journal of the Royal Statistical Society, Series C* **58**, 65 – 81.

Liu, L., Huang, X., and O'Quigley, J. (2008). Analysis of longitudinal data in the presence of informative observational times and a dependent terminal event, with application to medical cost data. *Biometrics* **64**, 950 – 958.

Ma, G., Troxel, A., and Heitjan, F. (2004). An index of local sensitivity to non ignorable drop-out in longitudinal modelling. *Statistics in Medicine* **24**, 2129 – 2150.

McCullagh, P. and Nelder, J. (1989). *Generalized Linear Models*, 2nd edition. Chapman & Hall, London.

McCulloch, C. (1997). Maximum likelihood algorithms for generalized linear mixed models. *Journal of the American Statistical Association* **92**, 162 – 170.

McCulloch, C., Searle, S., and Neuhaus, J. (2008). *Generalized, Linear, and Mixed Models*, 2nd edition. Wiley, New Jersey.

Molenberghs, G., Beunckens, C., Sotto, C., and Kenward, M. (2008). Every missingness not at random model has a missingness at random counterpart with equal fit. *Journal of the Royal Statistical Society, Series B* **70**, 371 – 388.

Molenberghs, G. and Kenward, M. (2007). *Missing Data in Clinical Studies*. Wiley, New York.

Molenberghs, G. and Verbeke, G. (2005). *Models for Discrete Longitudinal Data*. Springer-Verlag, New York.

Molenberghs, G. and Verbeke, G. (2007). Likelihood ratio, score, and Wald tests in a constrained parameter space. *The American Statistician* **61**, 22 – 27.

Murtaugh, P., Dickson, E., Van Dam, G., Malincho, M., Grambsch, P., Langworthy, A., and Gips, C. (1994). Primary biliary cirrhosis: prediction of short-term survival based on repeated patient visits. *Hepatology* **20**, 126–134.

Nash, J. (1990). *Compact Numerical Methods for Computers. Linear Algebra and Function Minimisation*. Adam Hilger, New York.

Nelson, W. (1972). Theory and applications of hazard plotting for censored failure data. *Technometrics* **14**, 945–965.

Neuhaus, J., Hauck, W., and Kalbfleisch, J. (1992). The effects of mixture distribution misspecification when fitting mixed-effects logistic models. *Biometrika* **79**, 755–762.

Neuhaus, J., Kalbfleisch, J., and Hauck, W. (1994). Conditions for consistent estimation in mixed-effects models for binary matched-pairs data. *Canadian Journal of Statistics* **22**, 139–148.

Neuhaus, J., McCulloch, C., and Boylan, R. (2011). A note on type II error under random effects misspecification in generalized linear mixed models. *Biometrics* **67**, 654–656.

Nobre, J. and Singer, J. (2007). Residuals analysis for linear mixed models. *Biometrical Journal* **6**, 863–875.

Pencina, M., D'Agostino, Sr, R., D'Agostino, Jr, R., and Vasan, R. (2008). Evaluating the added predictive ability of a new marker: from area under the ROC curve to reclassification and beyond. *Statistics in Medicine* **27**, 157–172.

Pinheiro, J. and Bates, D. (1995). Approximations to the log-likelihood function in the nonlinear mixed-effects model. *Journal of Computational and Graphical Statistics* **4**, 12–35.

Pinheiro, J. and Bates, D. (2000). *Mixed-Effects Models in S and S-PLUS*. Springer-Verlag, New York.

Pinheiro, J., Bates, D., DebRoy, S., Sarkar, D., and R Development Core Team (2012). *nlme: Linear and nonlinear mixed-effects models*. R package version 3.1-103. http://cran.r-project.org/package=nlme.

Pinheiro, J. and Chao, E. (2006). Efficient laplacian and adaptive gaussian quadrature algorithms for multilevel generalized linear mixed models. *Journal of Computational and Graphical Statistics* **15**, 58–81.

Prentice, R. (1982). Covariate measurement errors and parameter estimates in a failure time regression model. *Biometrika* **69**, 331–342.

Prentice, R. (1989). Surrogate endpoints in clinical trials: Definition and operation criteria. *Statistics in Medicine* **8**, 431–440.

Press, W., Teukolsky, S., Vetterling, W., and Flannery, B. (2007). *Numerical Recipes: The Art of Scientific Computing*, 3rd edition. Cambridge University Press, New York.

Proust-Lima, C., Diakite, A., and Liquet, B. (2011). *lcmm: Estimation of various latent class mixed models and joint latent class mixed models*. R package version 1.4-3. http://cran.r-project.org/package=lcmm.

Proust-Lima, C., Joly, P., Dartigues, J., and Jacqmin-Gadda, H. (2009). Joint modelling of multivariate longitudinal outcomes and a time-to-event: A nonlinear latent class approach. *Computational Statistics & Data Analysis* **53**, 1142–1154.

Proust-Lima, C. and Taylor, J. (2009). Development and validation of a dynamic prognostic tool for prostate cancer recurrence using repeated measures of posttreatment PSA: A joint modeling approach. *Biostatistics* **10**, 535–549.

Pulkstenis, E., Ten Have, T., and Landis, R. (1998). Model for the analysis of binary longitudinal pain data subject to informative dropout through remediation. *Journal of the American Statistical Association* **93**, 438–450.

Putter, H., Fiocco, M., and Geskus, R. (2007). Tutorial in biostatistics: Competing risks and multi-state models. *Statistics in Medicine* **26**, 2389–2430.

Rao, P. (1997). *Variance Components: Mixed Models, Methodologies and Applications*. Chapman & Hall/CRC Press, Boca Raton.

Raudenbush, S., Yang, M., and Yosef, M. (2000). Maximum likelihood for generalized linear models with nested random effects via high-order, multivariate Laplace approximations. *Journal of Computational and Graphical Statistics* **9**, 141–157.

R Development Core Team (2012). *R: A Language and Environment for Statistical Computing*. R Foundation for Statistical Computing, Vienna, Austria. ISBN 3-900051-07-0. http://www.r-project.org/.

Rizopoulos, D. (2010). **JM**: An R package for the joint modelling of longitudinal and time-to-event data. *Journal of Statistical Software* **35 (9)**, 1–33.

Rizopoulos, D. (2011). Dynamic predictions and prospective accuracy in joint models for longitudinal and time-to-event data. *Biometrics* **67**, 819–829.

Rizopoulos, D. (2012a). Fast fitting of joint models for longitudinal and event time data using a pseudo-adaptive Gaussian quadrature rule. *Computational Statistics & Data Analysis* **56**, 491–501.

Rizopoulos, D. (2012b). *JM: Shared parameter models for the joint modelling of longitudinal and time-to-event data.* R package version 1.0-0. http://cran.r-project.org/package=JM.

Rizopoulos, D. and Ghosh, P. (2011). A Bayesian semiparametric multivariate joint model for multiple longitudinal outcomes and a time-to-event. *Statistics in Medicine* **30**, 1366–1380.

Rizopoulos, D. and Lesaffre, E. (2012). Introduction to the special issue on joint modelling techniques. *Statistical Methods in Medical Research* **00**, 00–00, doi: 10.1177/0962280212445800.

Rizopoulos, D., Verbeke, G., and Lesaffre, E. (2009). Fully exponential Laplace approximations for the joint modelling of survival and longitudinal data. *Journal of the Royal Statistical Society, Series B* **71**, 637–654.

Rizopoulos, D., Verbeke, G., Lesaffre, E., and Vanrenterghem, Y. (2008). A two-part joint model for the analysis of survival and longitudinal binary data with excess zeros. *Biometrics* **64**, 611–619.

Rizopoulos, D., Verbeke, G., and Molenberghs, G. (2008). Shared parameter models under random effects misspecification. *Biometrika* **95**, 63–74.

Rizopoulos, D., Verbeke, G., and Molenberghs, G. (2010). Multiple-imputation-based residuals and diagnostic plots for joint models of longitudinal and survival outcomes. *Biometrics* **66**, 20–29.

Robins, J., Hernan, M., and Brumback, B. (2000). Marginal structural models and causal inference in epidemiology. *Epidemiology* **11**, 550–560.

Robins, J., Scharfstein, D., and Rotnitzky, A. (1999). Sensitivity analysis for selection bias and unmeasured confounding in missing data and causal inference models. In Halloran, M. and Berry, D., editors, *Statistical Models in Epidemiology: The Environment and Clinical Trials.* Springer-Verlag, New York.

Rosenberg, P. (1995). Hazard function estimation using B-splines. *Biometrics* **51**, 874–887.

Rubin, D. (1976). Inference and missing data. *Biometrika* **63**, 581–592.

Ruppert, D., Wand, M., and Carroll, R. (2003). *Semiparametric Regression.* Cambridge University Press, Cambridge.

Sahu, S., Dey, D., Aslanidou, H., and Sinha, D. (1997). A Weibull regression model with gamma frailties for multivariate survival data. *Lifetime Data Analysis* **3**, 123–137.

Sarkar, D. (2008). *Lattice: Multivariate Data Visualization with R.* Springer, New York.

Schemper, M. and Henderson, R. (2000). Predictive accuracy and explained variation in Cox regression. *Biometrics* **56**, 249–255.

Schwarz, G. (1978). Estimating the dimension of a model. *Annals of Statistics* **6**, 461–464.

Searle, S., Casella, G., and McCulloch, C. (1992). *Variance Components.* Wiley, New York.

Self, S. and Liang, K.-Y. (1987). Asymptotic properties of maximum likelihood estimators and likelihood ratio tests under nonstandard conditions. *Journal of the American Statistical Association* **82**, 605–610.

Self, S. and Pawitan, Y. (1992). Modeling a marker of disease progression and onset of disease. In Jewell, N., Dietz, K., and Farewell, V., editors, *AIDS Epidemiology: Methodological Issues*. Birkhaüser, Boston.

Skrondal, A. and Rabe-Hesketh, S. (2004). *Generalized Latent Variable Modeling: Multilevel, Longitudinal, and Structural Equation Models.* Chapman & Hall/CRC Press, Boca Raton.

Slate, E. and Turnbull, B. (2000). Statistical models for longitudinal biomarkers of disease onset. *Statistics in Medicine* **19**, 617–637.

Snijders, T. and Bosker, R. (1999). *Multilevel Analysis: An Introduction to Basic and Advanced Multilevel Modeling.* Sage Publications, London.

Song, X., Davidian, M., and Tsiatis, A. (2002). A semiparametric likelihood approach to joint modeling of longitudinal and time-to-event data. *Biometrics* **58**, 742–753.

Stram, D. and Lee, J.-W. (1994). Variance components testing in the longitudinal mixed-effects models. *Biometrics* **50**, 1171–1177.

Sun, J. (2006). *The Statistical Analysis of Interval-censored Failure Time Data.* Springer-Verlag, New York.

Sweeting, M. and Thompson, S. (2011). Joint modelling of longitudinal and time-to-event data with application to predicting abdominal aortic aneurysm growth and rupture. *Biometrical Journal* **53**, 750–763.

Sylvestre, M.-P. and Abrahamowicz, M. (2009). Flexible modeling of the cumulative effects of time-dependent exposures on the hazard. *Statistics in Medicine* **28**, 3437–3453.

Tableman, M. and Kim, J. (2003). *Survival Analysis Using S: Analysis of Time-to-Event Data.* Chapman & Hall/CRC Press, Boca Raton.

Takkenberg, J., van Herwerden, L., Eijkemans, M., Bekkers, J., and Bogers, A. (2002). Evolution of allograft aortic valve replacement over 13 years: Results of 275 procedures. *European Journal of Cardio-Thoracic Surgery* **21**, 683–691.

Takkenberg, J., van Herwerden, L., Galema, T., Bekkers, J., Kleyburg-Linkers, V., Eijkemans, M., and Bogers, A. (2006). Serial echocardiographic assessment of neoaortic regurgitation and root dimensions after the modified Ross procedure. *Journal of Heart Valve Disease* **15**, 100–106.

Therneau, T. and Grambsch, P. (2000). *Modeling Survival Data: Extending the Cox Model.* Springer-Verlag, New York.

Therneau, T., Grambsch, P., and Fleming, T. (1990). Martingale based residuals for survival models. *Biometrika* **77**, 147–160.

Therneau, T. and Lumley, T. (2012). ***survival:*** *Survival analysis including penalised likelihood.* R package version 2.36-12. http://cran.r-project.org/package=survival.

Thomas, D. (1988). Models for exposure-time-response relationships with applications to cancer epidemiology. *Annual Reviews of Public Health* **9**, 451–482.

Tierney, L. and Kadane, J. (1986). Accurate approximations for posterior moments and marginal densities. *Journal of the American Statistical Association* **81**, 82–86.

Troxel, A., Harrington, D., and Lipsitz, S. (1998). Analysis of longitudinal data with non-ignorable non-monotone missing values. *Journal of the Royal Statistical Society, Series C* **74**, 425–438.

Troxel, A., Lipsitz, S., and Harrington, D. (1998). Marginal models for the analysis of longitudinal measurements with nonignorable non-monotone missing data. *Biometrika* **85**, 661–672.

Troxel, A., Ma, G., and Heitjan, F. (2004). An index of local sensitivity to nonignorability. *Statistica Sinica* **14**, 1221–1237.

Tseng, Y.-K., Hsieh, F., and Wang, J.-L. (2005). Joint modelling of accelerated failure time and longitudinal data. *Biometrika* **92**, 587–603.

Tsiatis, A. and Davidian, M. (2001). A semiparametric estimator for the proportional hazards model with longitudinal covariates measured with error. *Biometrika* **88**, 447–458.

Tsiatis, A. and Davidian, M. (2004). Joint modeling of longitudinal and time-to-event data: An overview. *Statistica Sinica* **14**, 809–834.

Tsiatis, A., DeGruttola, V., and Wulfsohn, M. (1995). Modeling the relationship of survival to longitudinal data measured with error: Applications to survival and CD4 counts in patients with AIDS. *Journal of the American Statistical Association* **90**, 27–37.

Tsonaka, R., Rizopoulos, D., Verbeke, G., and Lesaffre, E. (2010). Non-ignorable models for intermittently missing categorical longitudinal responses. *Biometrics* **66**, 834–844.

Tsonaka, R., Verbeke, G., and Lesaffre, E. (2009). A semi-parametric shared parameter model to handle non-monotone non-ignorable missingness. *Biometrics* **65**, 81–87.

Vacek, P. (1997). Assessing the effect of intensity when exposure varies over time. *Statistics in Medicine* **16**, 505–513.

van der Vaart, A. (1998). *Asymptotic Statistics*. Cambridge University Press, New York.

Venables, W. and Ripley, B. (2002). *Modern Applied Statistics with S*, 4th edition. Springer-Verlag, New York.

Verbeke, G. and Lesaffre, E. (1997). The effect of misspecifying the random effects distribution in linear mixed models for longitudinal data. *Computational Statistics & Data Analysis* **23**, 541–556.

Verbeke, G. and Molenberghs, G. (2000). *Linear Mixed Models for Longitudinal Data*. Springer-Verlag, New York.

Verbeke, G. and Molenberghs, G. (2003). The use of score tests for inference on variance components. *Biometrics* **59**, 254–262.

Verbeke, G., Molenberghs, G., and Beunckens, C. (2008). Formal and informal model selection with incomplete data. *Statistical Science* **23**, 201–218.

Viviani, S., Rizopoulos, D., and Alfò, M. (2012). Local sensitivity to nonignorability in shared parameter models, Submitted.

Vonesh, E., Greene, T., and Schluchter, M. (2006). Shared parameter models for the joint analysis of longitudinal data and event times. *Statistics in Medicine* **25**, 143–163.

Wang, Y. and Taylor, J. (2001). Jointly modeling longitudinal and event time data with application to acquired immunodeficiency syndrome. *Journal of the American Statistical Association* **96**, 895–905.

White, H. (1982). Maximum likelihood estimation of misspecified models. *Econometrica* **50**, 1–26.

Whittemore, A. and Killer, J. (1986). Survival estimation using splines. *Biometrics* **42**, 495–506.

Wickham, H. (2007). Reshaping data with the **reshape** package. *Journal of Statistical Software* **21 (12)**, 1–20.

Wienke, A. (2011). *Frailty Models in Survival Analysis.* Chapman & Hall/CRC Press, Boca Raton.

Williamson, P., Kolamunnage-Dona, R., Philipson, P., and Marson, A. (2008). Joint modelling of longitudinal and competing risks data. *Statistics in Medicine* **27**, 6426–6438.

Wolkewitz, M., Allignol, A., Schumacher, M., and Beyersmann, J. (2010). Two pitfalls in survival analyses of time-dependent exposure: A case study in a cohort of Oscar nominees. *The American Statistician* **64**, 205–211.

Wu, M. and Bailey, K. (1988). Analysing changes in the presence of informative right censoring caused by death and withdrawal. *Statistics in Medicine* **7**, 337–346.

Wu, M. and Bailey, K. (1989). Estimation and comparison of changes in the presence of informative right censoring: conditional linear model. *Biometrics* **45**, 939–955.

Wu, M. and Carroll, R. (1988). Estimation and comparison of changes in the presence of informative right censoring by modeling the censoring process. *Biometrics* **44**, 175–188.

Wulfsohn, M. and Tsiatis, A. (1997). A joint model for survival and longitudinal data measured with error. *Biometrics* **53**, 330–339.

Xu, J. and Zeger, S. (2001). Joint analysis of longitudinal data comprising repeated measures and times to events. *Applied Statistics* **50**, 375–387.

Yao, F. (2008). Functional approach of flexibly modelling generalized longitudinal data and survival time. *Journal of Statistical Planning and Inference* **138**, 995–1009.

Ye, W., Lin, X., and Taylor, J. (2008a). A penalized likelihood approach to joint modeling of longitudinal measurements and time-to-event data. *Statistics and Its Interface* **1**, 33–45.

Ye, W., Lin, X., and Taylor, J. (2008b). Semiparametric modeling of longitudinal measurements and time-to-event data–a two stage regression calibration approach. *Biometrics* **64**, 1238–1246.

Youden, W. (1950). Index for rating diagnostic tests. *Cancer* **3**, 32–35.

Yu, M., Taylor, J., and Sandler, H. (2008). Individualized prediction in prostate cancer studies using a joint longitudinal-survival-cure model. *Journal of the American Statistical Association* **103**, 178–187.

Zeng, D. and Cai, J. (2005). Asymptotic results for maximum likelihood estimators in joint analysis of repeated measurements and survival time. *The Annals of Statistics* **33**, 2132 – 2163.

Zheng, Y. and Heagerty, P. (2007). Prospective accuracy for longitudinal markers. *Biometrics* **63**, 332 – 341.

Index